Electronic Health Records

A Practical Guide for Professionals and Organizations

Fourth Edition

D0565426

Margret K. Amatayakul,
MBA, RHIA, CHPS, CPHIT, CPEHR, FHIMSS

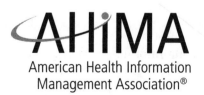

American Health Information
Management Association®

ISBN 978-1-58426-219-0
AHIMA Product No. AB102608

AHIMA Staff:
Claire Blondeau, MBA, Senior Editor
Katie Greenock, Editorial and Production Coordinator
Pamela Woolf, Project Editor
Lou Ann Wiedemann, MS, RHIA, CPEHR, Director of Professional Practice Resources, Reviewer
Ken Zielske, Director of Publications

AHIMA strives to recognize the value of people from every racial and ethnic background as well as all genders, age groups, and sexual orientations by building its membership and leadership resources to reflect the rich diversity of the American population. AHIMA encourages the celebration and promotion of human diversity through education, mentoring, recognition, leadership, and other programs.

American Health Information Management Association
233 North Michigan Avenue, Suite 2150
Chicago, IL 60601-5800

ahima.org

Contents

About the Author

Margret K. Amatayakul, MBA, RHIA, CHPS, CPHIT, CPEHR, FHIMSS has more than 40 years of experience in national and international healthcare information management. She is a leading authority on electronic health record (EHR) strategies for healthcare organizations and has extensive experience in EHR selection and project management.

After having served as director of medical record services at the Illinois Eye and Ear Infirmary, associate professor at the University of Illinois at the Medical Center, associate executive director of the American Health Information Management Association, and executive director of the Computer-based Patient Record Institute, Amatayakul formed her own consulting firm, Margret\A Consulting, LLC, in 1999. She provides information systems consulting services, freelance writing, and educational programming to the healthcare industry.

Amatayakul earned her bachelor's degree from the University of Illinois at the Medical Center and her master's degree in business administration, with concentrations in marketing and finance, from the University of Illinois at Chicago. She is a much-sought-after speaker, has published extensively, and has an impressive list of professional service awards to her credit. She is active in national policy setting and standards initiatives, served on the board of directors of the Healthcare Information and Management Systems Society (HIMSS), is on the faculty and board of examiners of Health IT Certification, and continues to serve the health informatics community as adjunct faculty of the College of St. Scholastica.

The author can be contacted at margret@margret-a.com.

Foreword

The electronic health record (EHR) is the "bridge to everywhere." Not only does it bridge disparate information systems it also bridges the processes of healthcare from departmental islands to the view of an institution or multiple institutions. In so doing, it bridges the diverse roles of many of medical specialties and allied healthcare occupations. To begin to meet its potential value, the EHR must also bridge the gap between the complexity of medical data and decision-making and the limitations of unaided human cognition. To fully realize its potential, the EHR must be a key enabler in bridging the chasm between growing medical knowledge and daily practice in institutions, clinics and offices around the country.

In world transportation systems, we don't build bridges with guesses and opportunistic projects. We engineer them by relying on science created through the accumulated experience of all the bridge builders that have gone before. We construct them with an evolving set of techniques created by a full knowledge of the techniques that have been used before. And we operate and maintain them using standard procedures and guidelines that have proven effective around the world. This is as it should be when so many people rely on safe, long-lived bridges for their economic and personal well-being.

So it is in designing, building, implementing and operating the bridges that are our EHRs. While there is plenty of room for innovation, it would be folly to undertake any of these tasks without thoroughly understanding the body of experience that has gone before.

In her fourth edition of *Electronic Health Records: A Practical Guide for Professionals and Organizations,* Margret "A." expands and revises one of the industry's most substantial repositories of knowledge about all phases of building and using an EHR.

In early chapters, she establishes a foundation of terminology and quickly moves to identify current realities and future possibilities and separates these from simple hype. She further provides a grounding in the broader field of information systems life cycles and then elaborates the special needs and characteristics that differentiate EHR systems from most other information systems.

She next takes on the important basis upon which successful EHR implementations must rely—project management approaches, strategic planning, migration from the current state and the special approaches that must be used to identify how the EHR will fit into and enable improvements in care delivery processes.

After addressing this fundamental basis, she goes on to selecting, negotiating for, implementing and operating the EHR system. Finally, after parsing the differences in projects for enterprise-wide and ambulatory EHR systems, she closes by establishing the broader context of EHRs within health information exchanges, the Nationwide Health Information Network, and cooperating with personal health records (PHRs).

Margret Amatayakul is a health information management professional who very early recognized the potential importance of EHRs. Throughout the evolution of these systems she has focused her work on establishing and contributing to a communal understanding of their importance and challenges. Having been at the center of this field as it evolved from vision to reality, she is an ideal person to contribute this important compendium of information on the science and practice of building, implementing and operating EHR systems. This fourth edition will be of value to students and healthcare and IT professionals as they are drawn into the challenges and healthcare improvements enabled by EHRs. "Old pros" who already experienced the challenge of using EHR systems to bridge the many people and processes of healthcare will also enjoy finding this information organized and reiterated to improve their understanding.

Wes Rishel
Vice-President and Distinguished Analyst
Gartner Group, Inc.

Preface

It is clear that electronic health records (EHRs) are no longer a novelty for organizations on the "bleeding edge" of change. Instead, most healthcare executives are recognizing that EHRs are becoming essential for doing business today.

With the federal government establishing a goal of an EHR for all Americans by 2014, several states following up with similar mandates, legislation to provide incentives for using e-prescribing in the ambulatory environment and ultimately sanctions for not using it, there certainly has been a tremendous surge of EHR activity. There is both risk and reward in that. Key lessons we've learned in even just the past 2 years include:

- Convergence on vision and greater appreciation that an EHR is more a program in support of clinical transformation than a specific project that has a defined beginning and end

- Expansion of the EHR concept beyond that of only the record of episodic care to knowledge generation and use

- Greater acceptance of health information sharing across the continuum of care, including for consumer empowerment

- Recognition that it is virtually impossible to keep up with data collection requirements of various programs without clinical information systems that capture accurate and complete data in a form capable of being processed by a computer

- The need to attend to all aspects of EHR utilization, including not only clinical but evidentiary

Although the era of EHR is upon us, there are still many healthcare professionals and organizations seeking guidance on EHR definition, migration path, planning, selection, and implementation. The changes that accompany the computerization of health information are huge. Many healthcare professionals still find it a challenge to fully adapt to computers that store information securely out of sight and require structured data entry and controlled vocabularies to dictate what information is collected, who collects it, and how it is recorded. Clinical guidelines and protocols embedded in EHR systems provide clinical decision support for patient safety and quality outcomes.

More than ever before, EHR system creation and use encompasses the need for all stakeholders to work together. Although its basis is clinical information, the EHR is used not only by clinicians, but also by virtually every other health professional who manages healthcare payment, risk, quality, research, education, and operations. Patients, too, are increasingly gaining access to their health information and making important contributions to their personal healthcare by doing so. Indeed, the preface to the first edition of this book spoke extensively about the power of information and the fear that giving up paper records somehow would result in a power shift in the healthcare community. If any power shift has occurred, it has resulted in patient and provider empowerment. The right EHR focuses on providing the right data, in the right presentation, with the right worflow, for the right decision making, to achieve the right outcomes. In addition, EHRs serve as the foundation for population health and, ultimately, the potential for a nationwide health information network.

Objectives of This Practical Guide

Electronic Health Records: A Practical Guide for Professionals and Organizations, Fourth Edition is intended to be a guide for individuals who are interested or involved in the EHR planning and implementation process, whether in a healthcare organization, working for a vendor, or in a policy-making position. This book covers the elements of the EHR process in chronological fashion, from developing a migration path to implementation and ongoing management of systems. It also addresses the essential elements in achieving value at whatever point the organization is in planning for, adopting what has already been implemented, or moving along the migration path to new and enhanced components. Along the way, it provides a solid background about EHR history, trends, and common pitfalls. Where the third edition added chapters on specific application strategies and case studies for different care settings, this edition increases emphasis on the importance of planning, devotes an entire chapter to health information exchange (HIE), and adds a new chapter on personal health records (PHRs).

Although not intended for use exclusively as a textbook, *Electronic Health Records: A Practical Guide for Professionals and Organizations*, Fourth Edition can help translate complex discussions about EHRs into everyday, understandable language. This book is designed to facilitate board or executive management appreciation for the EHR, clinician understanding of the level of change to expect from an EHR, operational managers accepting making change happen, information technologists new to the healthcare environment understanding its unique characteristics, and politicians and government officials gaining insight into the scope and complexity of EHRs.

Chapter 1 defines the EHR, identifies early attempts at development, and relates current status. Chapter 2 provides a grounding in information systems theory and systems development life cycle to reinforce the notion that an EHR project is not the acquisition of a single application but, rather, a system of components that must work together.

Chapter 3 discusses challenges to adoption, with the intent of overcoming myths and capitalizing on lessons learned.

Chapter 4 describes the importance of EHR project management and identifies the roles of the various stakeholders in EHR planning and implementation. (Those familiar with the third edition will find that this chapter combines former chapter 4 and chapter 13.) Chapter 5 encourages the process of setting goals to achieve not only a financial return on investment, but also an impact on quality of care that is the cornerstone of clinical transformation brought about by an EHR. Chapter 6 then offers a unique structure for strategically planning the EHR as a migration path. It emphasizes the importance of coordinating EHR planning with the organization's strategic initiatives and the fact that an EHR project is not just about implementing hardware and software, but addressing the people, policy, and process issues to achieve EHR goals.

Chapters 7 through 10 cover the various forms of assessments that serve as the baseline for EHR planning. Chapter 7 has been considerably expanded to focus not only on the importance of but the "how to's" of healthcare processes and workflow analysis. Chapter 8 provides information on conducting a functional needs assessment. Chapter 9 describes the data, information, and file structures necessary for an EHR. Chapter 10 provides a primer on computer concepts, communications technologies, Internet services, data storage and retrieval, and data security necessary to support the EHR.

Chapters 11 through 13 address EHR costs, benefits, selection strategies, and implementation tactics. Chapter 11 includes cost and benefits worksheets and specific methodologies for describing an EHR's benefits portfolio, including determining return on investment and impact on quality. Chapter 12 provides detailed advice on how to select an EHR vendor and tips on contract negotiation. Chapter 13 provides a summary of the implementation requirements and ongoing activities associated with continuing to build a comprehensive EHR.

Chapters 14 through 16 focus on specific EHR applications. Chapter 14 highlights bridge strategies to achieve early wins from automation and complement more comprehensive initiatives. Chapter 15 describes acute care applications, such as computerized provider order entry, barcode medication administration, point-of-care charting, and clinical decision support. Chapter 16 describes EHR in the ambulatory care environment, including clinical messaging, EHR and practice management system integration, and e-prescribing.

Finally, chapters 17 and 18 address two important, new initiatives in healthcare computing. Chapter 17 summarizes the federal government and private-sector initiatives being implemented to support HIE and describes the technology needed to support HIE organizations and how those may ultimately serve as the foundation for a nationwide health information network. Chapter 18 is new and provides a comprehensive view of personal health records (PHRs).

Although the book covers the steps in EHR planning and implementation in a logical sequence from the beginning of a project to the end, each reader may want to focus on certain chapters. Each reader brings a different background to the EHR project. Some will be knowledgeable about computers and simply want to know more about the healthcare context and unique features of EHR systems; others may need a refresher on the latest information technology.

Any Web sites listed in this book were current and valid as of the date of publication. However, Web page addresses and the information on them may change or disappear at any time and for any number of reasons. The reader is encouraged to perform general Web searches to locate any site addresses listed here that are no longer valid.

Note to educators: Instructor materials for this book include lesson plans, chapter slides, test banks, and other useful resources. The instructor materials are available in online format from the individual book pages in AHIMA's bookstore and through the Assembly on Education (AOE) Community of Practice (CoP). Instructors who are AHIMA members can sign up for this private community by clicking the Help icon within the CoP home page and requesting additional information on becoming an AOE CoP member. An instructor who is not an AHIMA member or an AHIMA member who is not an instructor may contact the publisher at publications@ahima.org. The instructor materials are not available to students enrolled in college or university programs.

Acknowledgments

The first edition of this book acknowledged the contribution of Rita Finnegan, past president and former executive director of AHIMA. It was Rita who brought me into the field of health information management (HIM) and achieved AHIMA support for the Institute of Medicine's first patient record study that led to my involvement in the formation of the Computer-based Patient Record Institute (CPRI) and to extend my network of associates and influence well beyond traditional boundaries.

As noted in both the second and third editions of this book, that network has only continued to grow and be enriched through many colleagues, clients, and students who teach me so much. These opportunities help me to achieve my professional goal of seeing EHRs become the basic supporting infrastructure for healthcare, wherever it may occur.

This fourth edition not only recognizes the pace at which the world of e-health is evolving, but marks four decades of my passion for what we now call EHRs. Likewise, it marks four decades of support from my husband, Paul, who still is always two steps ahead of me in new technology adoption. How could I not keep going?

Chapter 1
Introduction to Electronic Health Records

The last few years have seen a tremendous surge in adoption of electronic health records (EHRs). Although it is still difficult to determine precisely how many hospitals and physicians use an EHR because of variations in definition and standards for measuring actual use vs. implementation, it is clear that health information technology (HIT) in general and EHRs in particular are making a difference in health outcomes. EHRs today have "much enhanced utility in patient care, in management of the healthcare system, and in extension of knowledge" (IOM 1991, 3). EHRs represent a **clinical transformation**— not just changing documentation practices but in using health information in new ways to support care delivery. Despite great strides, however, the road to achieving EHRs for all or even most Americans by 2014, as the Federal Government outlined, is still a long journey. The EHR is not a simple computer application; rather, it represents a carefully constructed set of systems that are highly integrated and require a significant investment of time, money, process change, and human factor reengineering. Furthermore, the EHR is less a project than a program. Because the EHR is a clinical information system and clinical knowledge is constantly changing, the EHR requires continual maintenance. This chapter:

- Provides a framework and conceptual model to describe the EHR

- Identifies benefits envisioned for, and being realized by, EHR implementation

- Reviews the origins of various efforts to achieve the envisioned benefits of an EHR

- Discusses the current status of EHR development and how barriers to acquisition, implementation, and adoption are being addressed

- Describes the need for an organization to plan a migration path of information applications, technology, and operations needed to achieve the EHR

- Overviews the stages of EHR implementation

Key Terms

Adoption
Aggregated data
Ancillary
Bar code
Bedside terminals
Clinical data repository
Clinical data warehouse
Clinical decision
    support system
Clinical documentation
    systems
Clinical information
    systems (CIS)
Clinical messaging
Clinical transformation
Computer-based
    patient record
Computers on wheels
    (COWs)
Context sensitive
Continuity of care
    documents (CCD)
Continuity of care
    records (CCR)

Data mining
Data reuse
Data warehouse
Departmental systems
Discrete data
E-visits
Electronic medical
    record
Electronic medication
    administration
    record
Electronic prescribing
Enterprise-wide MPI
Health information
    exchange (HIE)
Human–computer
    interfaces
Implementation
Infrastructure
Integrated delivery
    network
Intranet
Knowledge sources
Longitudinal

Natural language
    processing
Personal health records
Point-of-care (POC)
    charting systems
Portals
Predictive modeling
Presentation layer
Radio frequency
    identification
Report wizards
Report writers
Rules engine
Smart peripherals
Source systems
Specialized source
    systems
Storage systems
Structured data
Supporting
    infrastructure
System
Unstructured data

Electronic Health Record Definition

Defining the EHR has not been simple. Despite forward progress in implementing EHRs, there continues to be disagreement about terminology used (for example, electronic medical record vs. electronic health record vs. clinical information system) and what each term may mean. However, most agree that the EHR is more of an information system framework that can be implemented in a variety of ways, providing many different functions and achieving a multiplicity of purposes rather than a single application.

Criteria for an EHR

Early efforts to define the EHR by the Institute of Medicine (IOM) suggest that an EHR:

- Integrates data from multiple sources
- Captures data at the point of care
- Supports clinical decision making

When these criteria are embodied in components that work in harmony, the result may be considered the EHR, as illustrated in figure 1.1.

Fundamental to this set of criteria is the notion that an EHR is a system. In general systems theory, a **system** is a set of interrelated elements that work together to achieve a goal. The human body is an example of a system. Each component of the body serves a distinct purpose, such as the integumentary system affording internal organ protection or the musculoskeletal system providing structure and mobility. What is different between the human body's system components and the set of information systems that should support an EHR is that many of the information systems have been developed independently and often are not interrelated. Part of the challenge in creating an EHR is to achieve interoperability among these disparate systems; that is, data from one application must be able to be shared with another application in a meaningful way for the applications to work together.

Components of the EHR

In contemplating what an EHR is, it is necessary to understand what information system (IS) components comprise an EHR. Figure 1.2 displays a conceptual model that depicts the

Figure 1.1.   EHR criteria

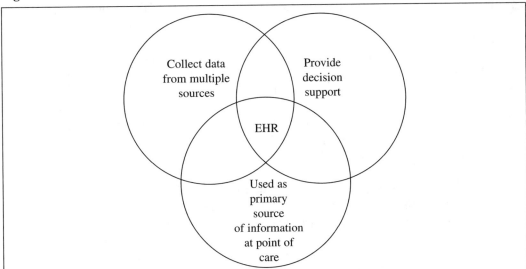

Figure 1.2.   Conceptual model of EHR

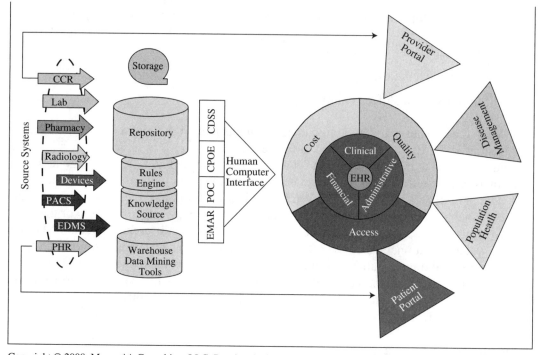

components that capture and integrate data and support caregiver decision making. However, because the EHR is as much a set of functions that provide value as it is technical system components, the conceptual model shows the relationship of the technical components to the value of the EHR. The value of integrating clinical, financial, and administrative data contributes significantly to improvements in quality, cost, and access to healthcare. Furthermore, the EHR is not limited to a single location but, rather, should include remote access for providers and consumers. It should be capable of integrating data across providers for continuity of care and from **personal health records** (PHRs) to form a **longitudinal** view of an individual's health status and healthcare. Information from episodes of care (for example, a clinic visit, a hospitalization, a long-term care stay) should support population health and feedback information that provides new knowledge.

From a technical perspective, the components of the EHR include:

- **Source systems** that *capture data* to support the EHR **infrastructure**. These source systems include all administrative, financial, and departmental systems that relate in any way to the health record. Examples of basic source systems include laboratory information systems (LIS), pharmacy information systems (PIS), radiology information systems (RIS), nutrition and food service information systems, and many other **ancillary**, or **departmental systems**. Some distinguish **specialized source systems** by clinical specialty, such as for cardiology or labor and delivery, or by type of services, such as intensive care unit (ICU) or emergency services.

Source systems may also include **smart peripherals**, such as smart infusion pumps or robotics.

- **Clinical information systems (CIS)** are another category of systems that *capture and process data* to support specific clinical functionality. In hospitals, clinical systems may be separate modules for different types of functions, such as computerized provider order entry (CPOE), electronic medication administration record (EMAR) (or bar code medication administration record [BC-MAR] for full, closed-loop medication administration management), results management, **point-of-care (POC) charting systems** (for example, nurse assessment, history and physical examination), and **clinical decision support system** (CDSS) for integrating data with clinical decision support rules for supplying reminders, alerts, context-sensitive order sets and templates, and other clinical guidance. In clinics or other ambulatory environments, complementary functions include POC charting, e-prescribing (e-Rx), order entry (O/E), and care planning—often all rolled into one application.

- A **supporting infrastructure** *integrates data*. Although each of the CIS described above can stand on their own, most organizations want to be able to integrate data from all source systems. A relational database, called a **clinical data repository** (CDR), serves this function. It is a relational database optimized to manage data transactions, such as the entry of an order or the retrieval of a laboratory result or the viewing of consultant's note. A **rules engine** supplies the CDR with programming logic for clinical decision support to be applied to the various data within the repository. **Knowledge sources** make information available from various external sources to work with data collected through the EHR, such as a drug knowledge database that describes the active ingredients of drugs and how they impact or may be impacted by various physiological states. Another integrating structure is a **data warehouse**, in which specific data can be mined (that is, aggregated and analyzed) to provide new knowledge. Components that integrate data also generate reports, often aided by special **report writers**, or **report wizards**, that enable the compilation of data into various reports. Finally, **storage systems** must archive data.

- **Presentation layer** software and **human–computer interfaces** help capture data at the POC and, by virtue of access to data, rules, knowledge, and mined data, support clinical decision making. The presentation layer of an application is that part that provides for data entry and retrieval functions. This software enables templates, icons, and various other data display characteristics. The human–computer interface is the input device by which users enter and retrieve data, such as a computer workstation, personal computers (PC), notebook/laptop computers, tablet computers, personal digital assistants (PDAs), voice recognition, handwriting recognition, and so on.

- Connectivity supports the capture and integration of data. A growing use of the EHR across the continuum of care, for quality measurement and reporting, and for population health is necessitating hardware and software that enables transmission of data across local and wide area networks in a secure and privacy-protected manner. The result has been the creation of various forms of **health information exchange (HIE)** among disparate organizations; new technology for connectivity, such as **portals** that provide remote access to the health record for physicians or patients, **continuity of care records (CCR)** or **continuity of care documents (CCD)** exchanged among referring providers, and PHRs to which providers and individuals contribute data and which assist individuals in managing consent for disclosure of information. HIE may also include the ability for health plans to contribute comprehensive problem lists and medication lists to providers or individuals' PHRs and for providers to contribute data to public health departments for population health.

The end result of implementing the technical components of the EHR is that quality, cost, and access to healthcare are enhanced through clinical, financial, and administrative data support. The American Health Information Management Association's (AHIMA's) A Vision from the e-HIM Future: A Report from the AHIMA e-HIM Task Force (see Appendix A) states that "health information will be used concurrently for multiple and diverse purposes, including healthcare delivery and treatment, outcomes measurement, finance, and support of health services and policy research, clinical trials, and disease prevention and surveillance at the individual, community, national, and international levels" (AHIMA 2003). As the HIM profession approaches 2010, the healthcare industry has transitioned even further to a focus on patient-centric and evidence-based healthcare with rapid momentum to improvements in adoption of EHRs and health information exchanges (HIEs). Furthermore, as observed in AHIMA's *Vision 2016: A Blueprint for Quality Education in HIM*, the widespread use of digital data systems and the distribution of technology to the patient and family are giving rise to the proliferation of PHRs as a point of information aggregation and consumer-directed patient care services. In such an environment, health information processes of providing health data sources, ensuring access, addressing privacy and security concerns, managing quality, and defining health information content, ownership, and other legal issues are becoming increasingly more sophisticated, scientific, complex, and even global.

Origins of the EHR

The concept of the EHR has existed since the early use of computers in healthcare and has undergone a significant transformation over time. Figure 1.3 illustrates the major milestones in the history of EHR implementation.

Figure 1.3.   History of EHR implementation

1970s	1980s	1990s	2000s
Academic Experiments	Feeder Systems	EHR Hype and Components	Integration and Connectivity

Copyright © 2008, Margret\A Consulting, LLC. Reprinted with permission.

Pioneers of the EHR

The first major efforts to automate clinical information occurred in the late 1960s and early 1970s. Several forward-thinking universities and companies recognized the value of emerging information technology (IT) for healthcare.

Some of the early attempts at automating the health record were highly successful and are precursors of current products. For example, efforts by Wiederhold at Stanford University and El Camino Hospital conducted with scientists at the Lockheed Company are often cited among the forerunners of the first commercial products. This early CIS effort was subsequently taken over and further developed by the Technicon Corporation (subsequently TDS Healthcare Systems Corporation, which is now part of the suite of products available from Eclipsys, Inc.).

Another pioneering provider–vendor partnership took place at Latter Day Saints (LDS) Hospital, now Intermountain Healthcare, with the HELP system on which 3M has based products. Other organizations that have contributed significantly to research in the design of CIS include Massachusetts General Hospital in Boston, Kaiser Permanente in Oakland, California, and Regenstrief Institute in Indianapolis (Shortliffe and Perreault 2001).

The National Library of Medicine (NLM) also contributed greatly to early efforts and continues to play an extremely active role in data and vocabulary development. Its Integrated Advanced Information Management Systems (IAIMS) grants have helped—and continue to help—fund many EHR-related projects. (For a comprehensive history of medical informatics, see M.F. Collen's *A History of Medical Informatics in the U.S. 1950–1990*.)

Early Limiting Factors

For the most part, applicability of the early EHR projects was limited to the environments in which they were created. Products often could not be "commercialized" or made readily able to be implemented in other settings because they were so closely linked to processes at one organization.

Furthermore, in the early days of computer use, most healthcare organizations lacked the source systems—the laboratory, radiology, pharmacy, and other ancillary services—to supply an EHR with the data needed to provide users with much value. Thus, the automation that ensued in the 1980s focused on the relatively simpler, but critical, source systems and those that produced more immediate payback. Initially, these were administrative and financial systems such as registration–admission/discharge/transfer (R–ADT), master person index (MPI), and accounts receivable (A/R). Later, departmental systems for laboratory, radiology, pharmacy, dietary, materials management, and others were developed and implemented. In general, new interest in automating the health record itself waned as other systems were being implemented.

Landmark Effort

In the mid 1980s, frustrated by the inadequacies of the paper health record and slow progress toward automating clinical data, the IOM initiated a study on "improving the patient record in light of new technology." In 1991, the IOM released a report of its study titled "The Computer-based Patient Record: An Essential Technology for Health Care." The IOM coined the term *computer-based patient record* (CPR), more commonly referred to now as the EHR. At the time, the CPR represented a huge leap from the concept of documentation that primarily supported the provider to documentation that focused on the person receiving care. The IOM's landmark work laid the conceptual foundation for a vision of a system that would:

> provide a longitudinal (that is, lifelong) record of events that may have influenced a person's health (IOM 1991, 137) and reside[s] in a system specifically designed to support users by providing accessibility to complete and accurate data, alerts, reminders, clinical decision support systems, links to medical knowledge, and other aids (IOM 1991, 11)

Interestingly, the IOM decided to follow up its 1991 report with another report in 1997. This revised edition includes several important observations:

> Despite this milieu of rapid change, the vision outlined in this report by the Committee on Improving the Patient Record remains remarkably on target, and the case for CPRs is stronger today than it was 6 years ago.
>
> Today there are several examples of quite robust hospital-based CPR systems developed by individual institutions, and commercial systems have moved toward achieving the 12 attributes of CPRs outlined in the original report. Plenty of room remains, however, to combine the depth of systems developed by institutions with easily modified, modular architecture, readily available technology, and the use of national standards. Even as CPR systems become increasingly robust, there is not, nor is there likely to be, a single CPR product that meets all the needs of a provider organization. Thus, organizations seeking CPRs face significant challenges in integrating various systems to achieve the full functionality they need. Moreover, CPR diffusion goes far beyond technology within an organization and relies at least as much on a change in culture that requires motivated, educated leadership within institutions.
>
> . . . varying degrees of progress can be observed on the seven recommendations originally made . . . [Despite some progress, a] coordinated national program for CPR advancement in the United States could be based on the seven recommendations presented in the original report (IOM 1997, vi–ix).

Wake-up Call

Despite ever greater demands on information capabilities called for in the IOM patient record reports, it was not until 1999 when the IOM published another landmark work, *To Err Is Human*, that the scope of patient safety and quality of care issues stunned the nation into true action. This report highlighted one study that estimated that medical errors kill some 44,000 people in U.S. hospitals each year and another study that put the estimate at closer to 98,000 deaths per year. Headlines in the national papers observed that even considering the lower estimate of deaths from medical mistakes, they exceeded those from highway accidents, breast cancer, or AIDS. Deaths from medication errors alone, estimated at 7,000 annually, were noted to exceed workplace injuries. The report emphasized that there were no "magic bullets," but that building a culture of safety—without attaching blame to individuals—was critical. The report recommended that well-understood safety principles should be adopted, such as designing jobs and working conditions for safety; standardizing and simplifying equipment, supplies, and processes; and avoiding reliance on memory through automated information and decision support systems (IOM 1999, 22, 34).

EHR Vision

Following this wake-up call, the Department of Health and Human Services (HHS) sought further guidance from the IOM on the key care delivery–related capabilities of an EHR system that could be contributed to a standard functional model. This work was subsequently contributed to the Health Level Seven (HL7) standards organization for development of a standard functional model for an EHR system, released as a draft standard for trial use in 2004, and finalized as an ANSI standard in 2007. The HL7 EHR System Functional Model (Appendix B) is also heavily referenced by the Certification Commission for Health Information Technology (CCHIT), which began certifying EHR products in 2006.

The IOM's 2003 Key Capabilities of an EHR system describes the EHR as including:

- Longitudinal collection of electronic health information for and about persons, where health information is defined as information pertaining to the health of an individual or healthcare provided to an individual

- Immediate electronic access to person- and population-level information by authorized, and only authorized, users

- Provision of knowledge and decision-support that enhance the quality, safety, and efficiency of patient care

- Support of efficient processes for healthcare delivery (IOM 2003)

The IOM's contributions to the vision of the EHR are significant not only because they have addressed a specific need for standards development and certification support, but also because they have defined the scope of the transition to the EHR. This transition is characterized by the following key quotes from the original IOM report:

- "Merely automating the form, content, and procedures of current patient records will perpetuate their deficiencies and will be insufficient to meet emerging user needs" (IOM 1991, 2)

- The [EHR] "encompasses a broader view of the patient record than is current today, moving from the notion of a location or device for keeping track of patient care events to a resource with much enhanced utility in patient care (including the ability to provide an accurate longitudinal account of care), in management of the healthcare system, and in extension of knowledge" (IOM 1991, 3)

- The [EHR] is "the core of healthcare information systems. Such systems must be able to transmit data to other types of clinical and administrative information systems within healthcare institutions; they must also be able to transmit data to and accept data from other healthcare institutions or secondary databases" (IOM 1991, 51)

EHR Terminology

A number of terms have come to be associated with the means to accomplish the IOM's goals. Some of these terms are generic; others are vendor specific.

As noted earlier, the IOM coined the term **computer-based patient record** (CPR), which it defined as "an electronic patient record that resides in a system specifically designed to support users by providing accessibility to complete and accurate data, alerts, reminders, clinical decision support systems, links to medical knowledge, and other aids" (IOM 1997).

Another popular term is **electronic medical record** (EMR). This term continues to be widely used; however, even here there are discrepancies. In hospitals, EMR is sometimes used to describe systems based on document imaging or electronic document management systems in hospitals and to distinguish those from systems called EHR that are template-based for structured data entry. Alternatively, physician offices frequently use the term EMR to describe even the most sophisticated of systems for use in the ambulatory environment.

A new distinction made between EMR and EHR is the degree of interoperability that exists. The National Alliance for Health Information Technology (The Alliance) offers the following definitions:

- *Electronic medical record*: An electronic record of health-related information on an individual that can be created, gathered, managed, and consulted by authorized clinicians and staff within one healthcare organization.

- *Electronic health record*: An electronic record of health-related information on an individual that conforms to nationally recognized interoperability standards and that can be created, managed, and consulted by authorized clinicians and staff across more than one healthcare organization.

EHR is the term used in this book, and is the term chosen in the IOM "Key Capabilities of an Electronic Health Record System" (2003), the term used by HL7 in its EHR System Functional Model, and the term used by CCHIT in its product certification. Given the widespread use of the term EHR in these leadership organizations, the term EHR and the goals of structured and standardized data collection that benefit patients wherever they may be treated seems an appropriate goal for all healthcare delivery organizations.

EHR Migration Path

Although the variety of terms initially may have come about to distinguish a migration path from components that largely achieve a paperless state to that which provides much enhanced utility, the terms actually do not do justice to the need for a migration path.

Because the EHR is a system of many source systems, supporting infrastructure, and connectivity capabilities, there is not necessarily a single approach or standard timeline to compiling the components of an EHR system. Every organization needs to create its own migration path. The path to achieving an EHR system must recognize the existing infrastructure in any given organization, the culture and resources of the organization, and the goals the organization expects to achieve from an EHR. Migration paths also will vary significantly depending on whether the organization is a hospital, a clinic, an **integrated delivery network** (IDN), or some other type of provider facility, and the extent to which it participates in HIE. Finally, a hospital may want to consider the CCHIT certification process that is also following something of a migration path as it starts to certify inpatient

Figure 1.4.   CCHIT EHR construct

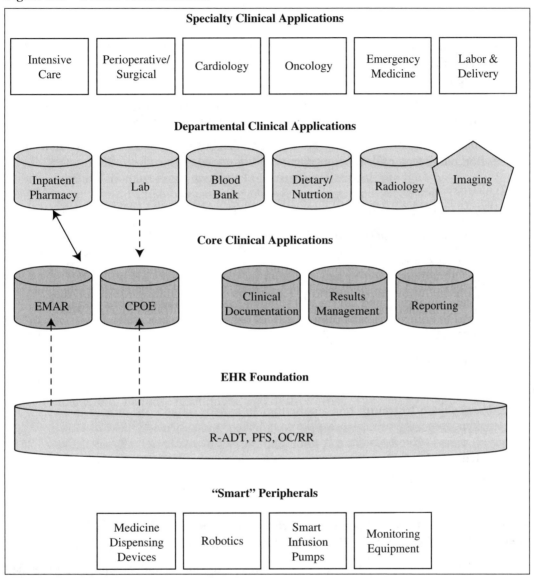

EHRs. Figure 1.4 identifies the components CCHIT envisions for an EHR and what it started certifying as EHR in its first year (2007) of inpatient product certification.

The following types of components are reflected in CCHIT's EHR construct and often are adopted in a migration path similar to the sequence suggested, with special variations between acute care and ambulatory care environments:

- Registration-admission, discharge, transfer (R-ADT), or its ambulatory equivalent, practice management system (PMS)

- Patient financial services (PFS), or its ambulatory equivalent billing systems
- Order communication/results retrieval (OC/RR)
- Departmental clinical applications (for example, lab, blood bank, inpatient pharmacy, dietary/nutrition, radiology/imaging [picture archiving and communication systems–PACS])
- Specialty clinical applications (for example, intensive care, perioperative/surgical, cardiology, oncology, emergency medicine, labor and delivery)
- Smart peripherals (for example, medicine dispensing devices, robotics, smart infusion pumps, monitoring equipment)
- EDMS
- Clinical messaging/provider-patient portals
- Clinical documentation (or, POC charting)
- CPOE and e-Rx
- EMAR/BC-MAR
- Results management
- Reporting
- Clinical data repository
- Clinical decision support
- Clinical warehousing
- PHRs
- HIE
- Population health

Registration-Admission, Discharge, Transfer (R-ADT), or its Ambulatory Equivalent, Practice Management System (PMS)

R-ADT, and for a clinic or physician office, PMS, is the most fundamental system needed to register patients, record their demographic and insurance information, and track their admission status or schedule visits. These functions also include a MPI, which may serve multiple entities within an integrated delivery network and is then referred to as an **enterprise-wide MPI** (EMPI).

Patient Financial Services (PFS), or its Ambulatory Equivalent Billing Systems

Another foundational system, of course, is one that receives charges and generates claims. These systems may also support eligibility checking to validate insurance coverage, determine co-payment requirements, and potentially deductible amounts. The systems also can check claims status with an insurance company, receive electronic remittance advice, manage any required prior authorizations, and—in experimental stages right now but expected in the future—process electronic claims attachments. In the ambulatory environment, the PMS often integrates patient registration, scheduling, MPI, and billing.

Order Communication/Results Retrieval Systems (OC/RR)

OC/RR systems provide the capability of transmitting orders to various ancillary departments and viewing results of laboratory and other diagnostic studies or the status of orders. OC/RR systems go a long way toward integrating the various source systems for operational purposes. However, they are essentially paper based because they rely on handwritten orders transcribed into a computer by clerical or nursing staff and diagnostic studies results typically generated in a paper or print file format.

OC/RR systems afford the functionality of automatically transmitting orders instead of telephoning, using a courier, faxing internally, or sending via a pneumatic tube, and provide access to results from multiple locations. These systems are often among the first information systems acquired in a hospital after the R-ADT and PFS, and their existence is essential for an EHR. If these systems are from different vendors, as they may well be, they often have separate interface programs written to be able to share patient demographic data.

Departmental Clinical Applications

Obviously, OC/RR systems are designed to communicate with systems that will receive and process the orders and generate results. There may be a myriad of such systems, also called ancillary, or source systems. The three major systems in a hospital include laboratory information system (LIS), (inpatient/clinical) pharmacy information system (PIS), and radiology information system (RIS). Other systems that frequently follow these include blood bank, dietary/nutrition and food services, and imaging (to capture radiology and other clinical images), which are called picture archiving and communication systems (PACS).

Departmental clinical applications serve two primary functions: The first function is to manage the department. So, for example, the LIS receives an order for a lab test and then provides considerable support for generating specimen collection lists, labels for specimen vials, connectivity with autoanalyzers, calibration of devices, quality checks, and even staff scheduling. A clinical pharmacy information system would do similar and equivalent functions, including maintaining the inventory of drugs, tracking drug expiration dates, and so on. The second function these clinical applications serve is to generate the clinical results they have processed (and associated charges). Hence, although the ultimate purpose of an LIS is to generate lab results, it does so with support for many other functions to get to the point it can generate the results, or dispense the medication if it is a clinical pharmacy information system, or supply a tray of nutritionally correct food for a patient on a soft diet.

Specialty Clinical Applications

Although there may be a fine line between what might be considered a departmental clinical application and a specialty clinical application, the distinction has been made by CCHIT as they set about to certify EHR products in hospitals and ambulatory environments. Where departmental clinical applications serve any patient, specialty clinical applications serve patients with specific disease states or level of nursing care required. Applications such as intensive care, perioperative/surgical, and emergency medicine obviously serve patients with many diseases or injuries, but have special staffing needs and services. Cardiology, oncology, labor and delivery, and psychiatry are examples where vendors have created niche products because their functions are highly focused. Hospitals and ambulatory settings may acquire these products over a considerable period of time, depending on their patient populations.

Smart Peripherals

Many medical devices are now able to be directly connected to an information system to enable capture of their information into the EHR. Monitoring equipment—both for use in a hospital or other care delivery organization as well as in a home—may supply information from fetal monitoring to blood pressure or blood sugar levels. Robotics in labs and pharmacies, in particular, are able to automate and hence reduce errors in human handling of specimen and drug dispensing. Robotics used as couriers can be programmed to find nursing units or even patient rooms. Again, these are not necessarily systems that are acquired early in a migration path, because their acquisition timing may be heavily dependent on the organization's mission and goals.

Electronic Document Management Systems (EDMS)

Electronic document management systems (EDMS) represent a wide range of functionality. Some merely capture images of the forms in the paper record for storage in a computer system for later retrieval. These are captured via a document scanning system. Others enable electronic feed (formerly referred to as COLD [computer output to laser disk] feed) to compile any digital documents (for example, typed documents from a transcription system, voice files from a dictation system, electronically generated documents from a speech recognition system, print files such as from a lab system or wave form files from a monitoring system, e-fax, and e-mail into an automated archive.

Most systems currently enable indexing of the forms, or even the data content on the forms to aid retrieval of information. An EDMS enables sophisticated indexing and direction of forms to a given patient's electronic file folder.

EDMS can be integrated with workflow technology as well. Workflow technology helps direct work on documents. For example, it can determine when a record is ready for coding and put it into the appropriate coder's work queue. Simultaneously, the patient financial services department may access the documents for reference or to generate a claims attachment. However sophisticated the ability to select blocks of text to view or how easily work may be distributed for processing, it must be kept in mind that EDMS primarily affords access to what was originally paper record content from multiple locations. It is often used as an interim technology or bridge strategy along a migration path to the EHR or as a supplemental technology to achieve a totally paperless environment.

Clinical Messaging Systems/Provider-Patient Portals

Clinical messaging systems add to OC/RR and EDMS systems the dimension of real-time access to information through Web-based technology. The Web-based technology may be applied within the organization's own internal network, or **intranet**, or may entail the exchange of information through a secure Web portal from the Internet.

Clinical messaging systems are often used to provide connectivity between a hospital and the offices of its medical staff members, although there is growing interest in using clinical messaging for communications with patients. These include a patient portal for secure email exchange and other applications such as **e-visits**, where providers may be reimbursed for certain types of patients to substitute an e-visit with a visit to the office.

Core Clinical Applications

Acquisition of core clinical applications generally initiates what most (and certainly the CCHIT) consider to be the components essential for an EHR. However, the sequence in which these components are acquired vary tremendously.

Clinical Documentation

Clinical documentation systems, also called **point-of-care (POC) charting systems** are those in which clinicians enter data as they are taking care of patients. These include nurse assessments, history and physical exams, progress notes, vital signs, and so on. POC charting systems in hospitals are now focused primarily on nursing staff documentation. For ambulatory EHRs, however, they are used by all clinicians, especially physicians and nurses. Data entered into POC systems may be structured or unstructured.

- **Structured data**, also called **discrete data**, refer to data that have been predefined in a table or checklist (figure 1.5) for recording the patient's problem from a drop-down menu or components of the history of present illness (HPI) using a checklist. Structured data enable standard values to be supplied for specific variables, so that the data

Figure 1.5.   Structured data entry in an EHR

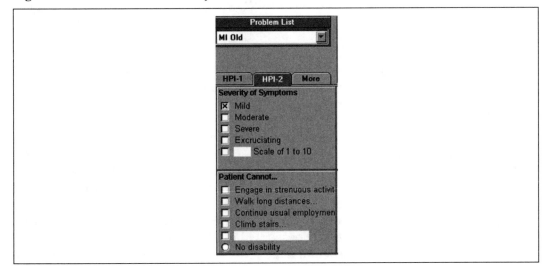

Figure 1.6.   Illustration of "type-ahead" function

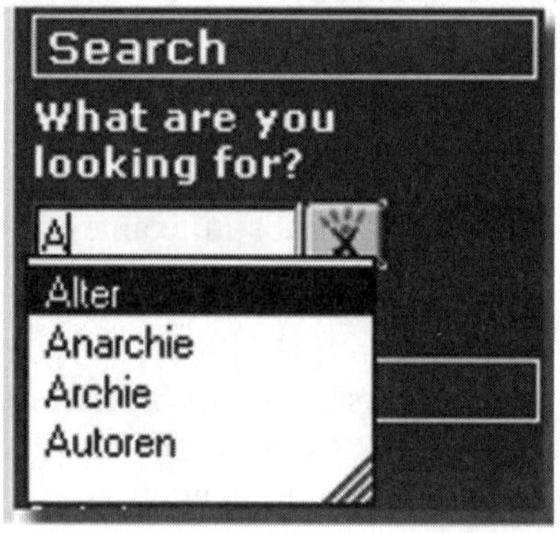

can be used in clinical decision support systems and provide standard meaning for reporting purposes. A user selects the data values desired for each variable using a mouse, arrows on the keyboard, touch screen, voice command, or other human–computer interface. In other cases, the user may be asked to enter a number or numeric score. For example, to record the severity of symptoms, a nurse may select a numeric score from 1 to 10 from a standard pain scale. It is important to note that the purpose of structured data entry is to help ensure standardization. It is interesting that in healthcare, there are actually two pain scales. One consists of scores from 1 to 10 and is used by nurses; the other consists of scores from 1 to 4 and is used by physical therapists. When setting up structured data entry, it is important to ensure that the appropriate scale, scoring system, or code set is specified in some way.

- **Unstructured data** essentially refers to narrative data, such as illustrated by the empty box in the section under "Patient Cannot..." in figure 1.5. Here, an area is reserved for caregivers to key in or dictate anything they want to record. Such unstructured data is more difficult to use in searches and generally is not converted into tabular or graphical form.

Early in their introduction, POC charting systems required significant changes in workflow. They were often time-consuming and difficult to use. Attempts were made to use so-called **bedside terminals** because returning to a small number of terminals at a nursing station was inadequate.

Today, POC charting systems have become much more sophisticated. Data entry may be performed using handheld devices, many of which are wireless, or notebook computers secured to carts (commonly referred to as **computers on wheels**, or **COWs**; or wireless on wheels, or WOWs). Data also may be captured by using smart text (or what would be called macros in word processing), where only a code is entered to represent an entire word or phrase, or by a "type-ahead" function, where typing the first few letters in a desired word presents a list of words from which to choose, as illustrated in figure 1.6. The most sophisticated systems would apply **natural language processing**, which permits narrative text to be converted to structured data for processing by the computer. This last form of data entry is still very much in the developmental stage.

Computerized Provider Order Entry (CPOE) Systems and E-Prescribing (e-Rx)

CPOE systems are intended for use by physicians and other providers (for example, physician assistants, nurse practitioners, and nurse midwives, according to their licensure) to enter orders directly into the computer system and be given prompts, reminders, or alerts about the order entered. These systems enhance legibility to avoid errors, and their decision support capability enhances patient safety and healthcare efficiencies. Decision support might include calculating the appropriate dose of a medication, especially for pediatrics, or indicating that a medication is contraindicated under certain circumstances, such as when the patient is known to be allergic to it, is taking another medication, is being prepped for a certain diagnostic study, or has liver or kidney disease. The CPOE system might identify that a specific drug is not covered by the patient's insurance and might offer equivalents. CPOE has been promoted very heavily for patient safety purposes to avoid medication errors, but it also can be helpful in identifying duplicate orders for services, providing cost comparisons of diagnostic studies, and alerting providers to needed preventive care services.

In a clinic or other ambulatory care setting, CPOE systems may include the ability to initiate diagnostic studies, order referrals, schedule next appointments, and task staff within the setting for other functions, such as surgical assistance. In addition, **electronic prescribing** (e-Rx) systems provide the ability to write a prescription and have it transmitted (or electronically faxed) directly to a retail pharmacy system.

Electronic/Bar Code Medication Administration Record (EMAR/BC-MAR)

Electronic medication administration record (EMAR) is the automation of many of the processes associated with medication administration in a hospital. In its most basic form, it is a printout generated by the pharmacy system that nurses can use to identify what medications should be administered to a patient and to document the administration. More sophisticated forms of EMAR use **bar code** or **radio frequency identification** (RFID) technology to add the dimension of positive identification of the patient, the medication being administered, and the nurse administering the drug. (When such technology is used it is referred to as BC-MAR.) In addition to identification and documentation, such BC-MAR systems provide alerts for medication timing, information about the medication itself should a nurse feel the need to better understand potential patient reactions, and aids workflow in scheduling medication administration. These systems are important for improving patient safety through the "medication five rights:" ensuring the right patient, right drug, right time, right dose, and right route.

Results Management

Although OC/RR systems enable viewing and printing of lab results, and so on, more sophisticated processing of such results when they are produced as structured data is feasible. For example, if lab results are generated as structured data, they may be graphed or structured into a table. If medication administration and vital signs data are saved as structured data (from BC-MAR and POC charting systems), they can be combined with lab results in structured form to evaluate the impact of the medication on the patient's condition. Such systems are obviously more sophisticated than results reporting systems, and therefore they are considered separate clinical systems by the CCHIT.

Reporting

Another clinical component that a care delivery organization may acquire is special report-writing software. If there is one fault in current EHR applications, it is that they are almost exclusively focused on direct care delivery functionality, with little attention to generating a printout of the legal health record and limited ability to develop useful reports for a variety of patient care, quality, or other functions. For example, if a provider wanted to generate an ad hoc report to compare treatment modalities for a specific disease state, most EHRs would require use of special report-writing software that requires a fair amount of programming skill to use effectively. A few vendors have recognized this and are now creating wizards to enable an organization to develop more reports on an ad hoc basis. Still, more sophisticated analytics generally require a clinical data warehouse in addition to the clinical data repository used to collect data from multiple locations for care delivery transactions.

Clinical Data Repository (CDR)

A **clinical data repository** (CDR) is a relational database that has been optimized for processing many transactions. Such transactions may be as simple as viewing a lab results or as complicated as analyzing data in a HPI against knowledge sources and generating a differential diagnosis. But the key is that a CDR is intended to support direct care delivery functions. In an ambulatory EHR, because all data are collected into a relational database optimized for processing transactions, by definition the system is using a clinical data repository. However, in an inpatient environment with the many different source systems, each having its own database, acquiring a CDR is often not done until such time as many of the core clinical applications are in place. It is at that time that the need for integrating data from all the different sources systems becomes crucial—both for ease of access as well as to support clinical decision support software.

Clinical Decision Support (CDS)

Clinical decision support (CDS) refers to any software that processes information to provide assistance with making a clinical decision. So for example, a physician may be able to access lab results while thinking about what drug to order, but it is not until software is integrated into the ordering function to remind the physician that a lab test should be performed to evaluate the efficacy of a certain drug in light of the patient's physiology that the system can be said to have CDS. CDS may be included in various core clinical applications. However, it is not until all data are compiled into a CDR that CDS affords the most help. Carrying the drug ordering example further, a CDS system that operates on a CDR would evaluate the drug against the patient's actual lab results and only remind the physician if there are no current labs or if the lab results are out of range for the given drug. In this case, a CDS system would work with all data in the CDR.

There are different forms of CDS. Some support may be in the form of active decision support, such as alerts or reminders to which the user must respond. Other CDS is considered passive because the user chooses to use it or not. CDS is generated by preprogrammed logic, or rules. For example, if a patient presents to an emergency department with chest pain, a CDS system may remind the physician to check all applicable body systems for the cause of the patient's pain (for example, heart, gastrointestinal, lungs). Alerts about allergies, contraindications, or a drug being off-formulary are common forms of CDS found in CPOE and e-Rx systems. Another example might be support for coding in a physician office EHR system, where the complexity of the patient encounter must be reflected in the evaluation and management (E/M) CPT code and ultimately contributes to the level of reimbursement for the visit.

The help provided through a CDS system also may be in the form of a clinical practice guideline, protocol, or care pathway. The CDS system not only offers the ability to chart against these guidelines or pathways but also makes them **context sensitive** so that only the parts of the guidelines that are applicable to the given patient are offered for charting. For example, female anatomy would not be presented as part of a physical exam for a male patient. Moreover, the CDS system may tap external knowledge sources to provide more comprehensive information. For example, if a physician is unfamiliar with a new drug offered as an alternative suggestion, he or she may be able to click a link to a reference that provides more complete information. A physician faced with an unusual set of symptoms and signs may look for reference material on the Web to develop a differential diagnosis, or there may be a special form of CDS that provides specific support for differential diagnosis. A pharmacist may need to make suggestions for alternative medications when a patient has an allergy or research the efficacy of various drugs when there is an unusual diagnosis. The CDS system may produce tailored instructions for the patient.

CDS should be contrasted with executive decision support, which is typically a stand-alone system that analyzes a large volume of **aggregated data** and provides trending information. Executive decision support is typically retrospective, providing quality improvement, productivity, staffing, and marketing information for executives. CDS is concurrent (provided at the time data are entered) or even prospective (when presenting "best practices" in anticipation of care). Clinical data, however, also may be aggregated for quality improvement studies, predictive modeling, or clinical research.

Clinical Data Warehouse (CDW)

Another advanced component of EHR systems may include a **clinical data warehouse** (CDW). This is a relational database, but one that has been optimized for performing sophisticated analysis on data. A CDW may be used to conduct **data mining**, for example, to look for new patterns in information that may be useful for clinical research. **Predictive modeling** has been widely performed by health plans to analyze information that may suggest the likelihood of needing health services. Although most hospitals and providers contribute data to external CDWs—via claims—some hospitals and large clinics may acquire a CDW, especially if they want to perform analytics for quality improvement or conduct clinical or health services research.

Personal Health Records (PHRs)

Personal health records (PHRs) are systems designed to support patient-entered data. If they are associated with a provider, they may serve as a means for patients to access their own health records (or summaries of their records) or to provide information to their providers about their health status, via a Web portal. Stand-alone PHR systems are not associated with a provider. These may be anything from a fax-back system to one that supports structured data entry by a patient on an independent Web site.

Health Information Exchange (HIE)

Health information exchange (HIE) refers to seamless exchange of health information across disparate organizations, often where the organizations have signed agreements to participate in a HIE organization, such as a local health information organization (LHIO) or regional health information organization (RHIO), which provides HIE services. These include patient identification functionality, record locator services, identity management and security services, and data exchange management. Some of the HIEs are managing the release of information functionality via patient consent afforded through the service or even via their PHRs.

Population Health

Population health also is facilitated through accurate, complete, and timely capture and reporting of public health data, including data relating to homeland security. Population health data collection may be initiated in the provider setting and linked automatically to a state data collection system. Population health may be served by decision support provided to caregivers through alerts from public health departments, such as to notify them of a new strain of virus or to remind them to seek certain information from patients who present with certain symptoms. A precursor to population health may be disease management, wherein providers and health plans share data about patients/health plan members who would benefit from certain educational programs or special monitoring.

EHR Adoption Status

EHRs have gone through a number of stages throughout the course of their history. Initial interest later led to disappointment but eventually a better sense of reality, and now a distinction between a system having been implemented and one that is fully adopted. Still, it is difficult to accurately describe the current state of EHR adoption because of the nature of organizations' various migration paths to EHR. For example, a hospital may have clinical documentation performed by all nurses all the time and CPOE implemented but only used by half of the physicians—how does one describe this hospital's current EHR status?

Media Hype

The release of the first IOM patient record study report in 1991 initially led to much media hype. Vendors flooded trade shows and publications with promotions for EHR products.

Information systems leadership surveys identified EHR projects as top priority for healthcare institutions, yet few went full speed ahead.

It was often assumed that an EHR product could be purchased and implemented in much the same way as departmental systems for keeping track of patient accounts, reporting laboratory results, and abstracting health records. Although many of these source systems now have become quite complex, they typically are more confined to a single department or a single set of functions.

Disappointment

As EHR project teams started evaluating institutional readiness for the EHR and assessing vendors' products, they found that the project was not as simple as installing departmental systems. They came to understand that the EHR is a highly complex concept. Virtually every system in the organization would touch, and be touched by, the EHR. Many organizations simply had not integrated all the necessary source systems to support the EHR. Furthermore, for an EHR to provide benefit, all clinicians had to use it in place of the paper health record and use information in new and different ways. Clinicians had never before been touched by any system in the way they would be affected by an EHR.

Finally, vendor offerings were typically found to be less complete than anticipated. Early in the evolution of the EHR, many vendors developed only an EHR concept and were looking for organizations to be development partners. Some vendors had one component of the EHR but could not integrate it with other applications into an organization's total operations. Unfortunately, many vendors failed to recognize the complexity of the EHR system. Few vendors took the time to study the nature of clinical information or the flow of clinical data through the healthcare delivery system. Still fewer attempted to introduce a system that would truly improve clinical information management, not just duplicate the existing paper system. One vendor went so far as to advertise that its product would make significant improvements in productivity and the quality of care for physicians' offices— without changing a thing! The fundamental lesson learned from these early projects is that improvement requires change.

Reality

Since the IOM released its first study on patient records, hundreds of vendors have been selling what they have promoted as EHR products. Many of these vendors quickly went out of business or were sold to save their investment. The lure of the "better mousetrap" still attracts new vendors, but there is a more stable set of vendors with much more robust products.

The EHR market is beginning to settle down, in part due to market forces and in part due to CCHIT certification, which requires vendors to meet a certain set of criteria for functionality, security, and interoperability. Although the market is still very segmented by acute care and ambulatory care, despite a desire for integrated systems across these environments and despite that some vendors have tried hard to bridge the gap between these environments, when organizations undertake an EHR project now, they have a far greater understanding of what it means to implement an EHR.

Installation vs. Adoption

Perhaps the biggest challenge is effecting the clinical transformation that the EHR requires.

There is considerably less information available about hospital adoption of inpatient EHR than physician adoption of ambulatory EHRs, although neither are solid. A study conducted by the RAND Corporation in 2005 (Fonkych) suggests that the level of sophistication of hospital information technology systems may range from a "basic EMR" (with an estimated upper limit of 32 percent adoption using the 2004 HIMSS-Dorenfest database) through "EMR and clinical documentation" (27 percent), to "EMR and CPOE" (9 percent) and "EMR and picture archiving and communication system (PACS) and CPOE" (5 percent). The study also reported an upper limit of 17 percent adoption of ambulatory EHRs.

An interesting element reported in the RAND study was the degree of acceleration or increasing rate of adoption. The study observed that what it identifies as "inpatient EMR" had the slowest rate of acceleration and that, in contrast, ambulatory diffusion appears more dynamic. The RAND study also includes an analysis of adoption rates as reported by different organizations conducting such studies, noting wide disparity often according to the survey respondents' predilection.

The RAND study makes another, critical distinction. It observes that there is a significant difference between a system being installed (or even implemented) versus a system being adopted. An organization may invest in a system, install the hardware and software, and expose clinicians to it that are all parts of **implementation**, but **adoption** requires acceptance and use of the system on a regular basis. The Center for Information Technology Leadership (CITL) also makes this observation, reporting on a study demonstrating that 32 percent of hospitals indicated they had a CPOE system, yet only 13.7 percent of hospitals required its use by physicians. Similar variations in reporting EHR adoption rates in general, and discrepancies between installation and adoption, are reported for clinic settings as well. A survey of close to 3,000 physicians conducted between September 2007 and March 2008 and reported in the *New England Journal of Medicine* (DesRoches et al 2008) found that 16 percent of physicians said their office had purchased an EHR, but had not yet deployed it; 13 percent said they had a basic or partially functional EHR; and 4 percent said they had a fully functional EHR. This same survey also found wide variation in EHR adoption by size or organization. In practices of 50 or more physicians, 51 percent used an EHR, whereas in smaller clinics, as few as 9 percent used an EHR.

EHR Limitations

Designing, marketing, and implementing information systems that provide access to clinical data and process data into information that contributes to knowledge for improved quality of care has been challenging. A number of major stumbling blocks are being addressed in clinical and technological areas.

Clinical Data Limitations

Clinical data are textual and contextual, but computers have been designed primarily to manipulate discrete, factual data. Computers are good at storing large volumes of data and performing mathematical formulas or clearly defined retrieval functions. However, they do not have the human capability of "thinking" or making associations or assumptions on their own. Although a lot of work is being done to program computers to perform more "reasoning" functions and to "learn" to offer decision-making support, these functions are sophisticated and still under development.

A good example of clinical data limitations may be to consider how a computer can process a simple statement such as "the patient has red skin." Interpretation of "red skin" depends on the context to define what is meant by "red." Does red describe a burned area, a rash, or an increase in temperature? What is the cause—fever, embarrassment, allergy, burn, high blood pressure, or something else? Unless we are satisfied with simply recording this information and making it available as documentary evidence of something care-givers observed, the field of computer science must learn how to structure data to associate them properly with other data for future processing.

One significant initiative that is helping with the adoption of a standard, clinical vocabulary has been the licensure of the comprehensive Systemized Nomenclature of Human and Veterinary Medicine (SNOMED) vocabulary by the National Library of Medicine (NLM). Adoption of a standard vocabulary such as SNOMED and its use in structured data will open the door for much broader use of clinical decision support systems.

In addition to data comparability that could be achieved through adoption of a standard, comprehensive vocabulary, clinical practice requires more information than it did in the past. First, there is much more to know—thousands of new drugs, new strains of viruses, and so on. The field of medicine is continually changing and expanding. Physicians have to track numerous diagnoses, procedures, diagnostic tests, clinical processes, devices, and drugs, and in many cases the payment rules associated with some of this. Just keeping up with the literature is daunting. For example, MEDLINE, an online bibliographic database of medical information compiled by the NLM, indexes nearly half a million new articles each year from biomedical literature alone. Connectivity to the Web and its resources has opened a huge opportunity to access information. Now the task is to convert that information into usable knowledge, which includes evaluating its reliability and validity.

Another factor that has presented limitations to clinical use of information systems includes the volume of patients and thus productivity concerns surrounding what typically is a more time-consuming method to record information. For example, it is not uncommon for a primary care physician to be expected to see a patient every 8 minutes. To quickly record data for this volume of patients, the way in which the caregiver enters or retrieves data needs to be perfected. Data entry performed by patients via a Web portal or kiosk in a waiting room is one way many busy clinics are addressing this issue. Such data entry can speed up the process of capturing data, as the provider only needs to validate the data during an encounter.

Data reuse also is becoming popular. This refers to the ability to "copy and paste" data from templates, previous visit documentation, or even documentation developed for use in other patients' records. In some cases, the provider literally copies content from one patient to another. In other cases, a word-processing macro, or "smart text," is used to generate a standard sentence, paragraph, or other description in which is embedded variables, the values of which need to be changed to fit the given patient. Obviously, these data entry strategies save time, but must be applied very carefully and cautiously to ensure that the same data apply directly to the current patient and episode of care. (Amatayakul, Brandt, and Dougherty 2003; Dimick 2008).

A final clinical data limitation is that many caregivers find it foreign to rely on information systems for clinical decision support. But the IOM patient safety reports highlighting medication errors, and the subsequent efforts of employer groups and major corporations to sweeten contracts for those providers using IT to improve patient safety, has led to greater acceptance of clinical decision support systems.

Technological Limitations

Technological limitations have made clinical information systems difficult to use in some cases. Even as a new generation of caregivers emerges that is accustomed to using computers and engaging patients in their use, physical limitations still abound because healthcare is such a mobile profession. The care of patients requires direct interaction between patients and caregivers. Pen and paper that slip into a pocket are easier to manage when a caregiver is making rounds and administering to patients. Wireless networks, new devices, longer battery life, and improvements in voice and handwriting recognition are beginning to address technological limitations. So, too, are efforts to redesign care processes that better incorporate use of computers.

Another technological limitation is the extent to which disparate computer systems can be made to work together and exchange data. Standard protocols have been developed to help, but vendors must adopt the standards and conform to their requirements explicitly. In some cases, vendors have developed highly proprietary systems to encourage providers to buy all components from one vendor. When the vendor does not offer a specific component, the provider is faced with doing without until the vendor creates the component or buying the component from another vendor and hoping an interface (a special program to enable data exchange) can be written that will permit the data to flow across the two different vendor platforms. The lack of interoperability between systems has sometimes meant that providers have been unable to adopt EHR systems as rapidly as they would like.

Cost and Value Limitations

A major consideration for any provider adopting EHRs is cost. Today, all healthcare providers are seeing reduced revenue and increased costs. The Healthcare Financial Management Association (HFMA) reports that providers are often strapped for cash and many have very limited access to capital (HFMA 2003). The EHR is considered an investment that must pay for itself. The systems undoubtedly cost a significant amount of money in addition to the time required to tailor them to the environment and to manage the degree of change they create. For example, it may be necessary to create interfaces enabling independent systems to communicate with one another and with the EHR. All the application templates must be populated with the provider's specific requirements, clinical practice guidelines, any unique terminology, its own formulary and charge data, and many other requirements. In addition, although it generally does not take much time to learn how to document in an EHR when it is properly designed, it does take time for the adoption process to occur and to manage workflow change.

Many have questioned whether the EHR can truly pay for itself. Part of the issue is that both costs and benefits are somewhat elusive. Because the EHR depends on the integration of all other clinical and administrative systems, sometimes some of this cost is attributed to the EHR when it should be attributed to processes that need attention anyway. Although there are many direct, monetary benefits, many benefits either cannot be quantified or are difficult to quantify—even when the effort is made to do so, which is often not the case.

A number of incentive programs, pay-for-performance, low- and no-cost loan programs, and even malpractice insurance discounts are being tried by the federal government, various health insurance programs, and malpractice carriers. Relief from restrictions on hospitals or groups making donations to physicians under the Stark Law and Anti-Kickback Statute have also helped address the cost–benefit issue. Many providers are finding that an EHR is now becoming a cost of doing business in an increasingly competitive marketplace. Still, for many small providers, and with the average cost of an EHR estimated to run between $25,000 and $60,000 per provider, it can be a cost-prohibitive investment even if the value proposition for patient safety and quality is easy to make.

Standardization Limitations

As alluded to in the preceding descriptions, the lack of standardization—to define the EHR, write interfaces, compare data, ensure data quality, and perform many other functions associated with EHRs—also has made it difficult to achieve widespread adoption.

It is not that some standards do not exist. For example, there are standards for writing interfaces, but not every vendor is required to use them and they contain a high degree of optionality. Moreover, there are standard vocabularies, although their number, until recently converged into SNOMED, has equated to a Tower of Babel.

Even though every vendor should be able to apply its own "bells and whistles" to enhance and distinguish its products, standardization would at least achieve a baseline product expectation. To some extent, the CCHIT certification process and incentives based on having a certified product is promoting such standardization. The mark of a mature industry is when it can adopt standards that achieve baseline functionality, making the products it uses commodities. For example, the automotive industry has established a standard construct for what a car is. Yet, everyone also knows the difference between a Chevy and a Cadillac. The EHR market needs to create a "car" to which vendors can apply more or less "leather and chrome."

Change Limitations

Also alluded to in the earlier descriptions of limitations is the underlying issue of the degree of change imposed by EHR systems. Although somewhat dependent on the computer skills of healthcare professionals, the immensity of change begins with our frame of reference. Today, our frame of reference is largely the paper-based record that contains a collection of paper documents, bound in a cover, with strict rules for use, and even more significant limitations on its usability. Adoption of an EHR requires a huge change in how we work with health information. Some describe the scope of this change as a clinical transformation. However, even more than the change brought about by using a computer to do many things we do today, the notion that an EHR can do more than its paper-based parent is an even greater challenge.

Many cite learning how to use a computer as a significant change management issue. Despite the prevalence of computers, many healthcare professionals currently do not routinely use a computer at home or at work and need basic computer skills. Workflows and processes in healthcare also represent enormous obstacles. Despite the fact that new procedures, tests, and drugs are constantly being developed, health professionals have an ingrained sense of process. In fact, such habits enable them to react quickly to rapidly changing circumstances. It is extremely difficult to change these processes to accommodate what many healthcare professionals still view as "only" documentation rather than information that is a source of knowledge and value.

The extent to which the health profession rejects process change has resulted in many EHR product design efforts attempting to replicate the paper environment. This can be seen in screens that have "tabs," the volume of printouts generated in a paperless environment, and, essentially, the rejection of performing work that is typically viewed as clerical (such as order entry). When considered from a cost–benefit perspective, is it any wonder that executives question the value of a system that does nothing but automate today's environment?

The issue of change is something of a catch-22 in healthcare. The EHR should introduce sufficient change so as to improve quality, cost, and access to healthcare but still reasonably reflect processes essential to healthcare delivery.

EHR Implementation Strategies

Much work remains to overcome the limitations and achieve the fullest possible vision of the EHR. However, the vision expands as each new system is developed. Each implementation of an EHR also provides insights into implementation strategies that organizations can adopt to improve their chances for success.

First, a key ingredient in ultimately achieving a successful EHR is to determine the organization's readiness for an EHR before proceeding down a migration path. Readiness for an EHR may need to be cultivated if there is resistance to computer use. Engaging those who will be users is absolutely critical. When developing its vision, goals, and migration path to the EHR, the organization should engage all stakeholders, including representatives from all groups who will be expected to use the system. Time and again, systems have failed to be adopted appropriately or yield their true results because the individuals who used the system were not involved from the start. For example, a significant failure in implementing CPOE systems is now recognized as not engaging the physician community. Without being a part of the process of identifying need, selecting the system, helping build the system, and determining its rollout, physicians have not trusted these systems or the organization's motives for installing the system.

A second critical strategy is to plan the migration path to the EHR based on a shared vision of the ultimate goal. There may not be a quick fix or instantaneous solution. Although many might like a "big bang" that goes from minimal automation to the vision of the future, it is difficult to pull off in the best of environments. EHR achievement will more likely be an evolution rather than a revolution, even though we can attempt to speed up the evolution. A major factor contributing to a lack of migration path planning is that healthcare organizations tend to be reactive rather than proactive in all their activities. In many cases this is unavoidable. An organization has to keep up with new regulations, accreditation requirements, and medical breakthroughs. Unfortunately, being reactive also has meant that information systems have been adopted to react to a new finding, a vendor sunsetting the product, or the "latest trend." For example, many hospitals are implementing CPOE systems without considering whether CPOE or EMAR should be first or even whether all clinical data are available to support the CDSS in a CPOE system.

Selecting the EHR system that is right for the organization is another strategic imperative. Many providers are firmly entrenched with one major vendor, even though the vendor may not be the best for EHR. It may be necessary to compromise timing of benefits and extend the migration path until the vendor catches up, compromise the functionality (especially the customizability) to achieve the best integration with the incumbent vendor, or "bite the bullet" and switch vendors. The organization should conduct a thorough cost–benefit analysis to look at the overall picture.

Carefully planning implementation of each EHR component also is a strategic imperative. Although any component of an EHR system will have its own specific implementation plan, certain general principles should always be applied to the components of an EHR system. These include the following:

- Complete mapping and analysis of all processes and workflows that will be impacted by the EHR component

- Review and understanding of the system's data requirements and information flow

- Review and approval by the clinician users of all decision support elements

- Thorough testing of all new processes and workflows

- Comprehensive training for all users, including education, skills building, system overviews, and direct how-to instruction

- Thoughtful chart conversion, turnover strategy, and go-live preparation that appreciates the impact on users, their productivity, and their ability to interact with their patients; and full support for users during go-live (this has been described as "swarming" users with help)

A final strategy that is often overlooked is the need to measure success. This is the ultimate feedback mechanism. Although every step in EHR planning, migration path development, and implementation requires feedback, understanding the true level of adoption and actual benefits that are resulting should be essential. These steps permit course correction (when needed), permit system enhancements, and, perhaps most important, provide the critical element of celebrating success and recognizing all who have contributed to that. A benefits realization study is key to determining the EHR system's return on investment. If this is not what was expected, it is a signal for course correction. When benefits are achieved, the results can justify further enhancements.

Conclusion

Planning and implementing an EHR system is a significant undertaking for any healthcare organization. Although the concept of the EHR is not new, the industry is only now beginning to fully appreciate the complexity of the people, policies, and processes as well as the technology required to achieve a comprehensive EHR. Indeed, many of the major stumbling blocks in the form of content, value of information, technological limitations, and even cost are being addressed. Some suggest the need exists to wait further for the various limitations to be addressed; however, the rapid rate of change in IT would only present the organization with a different set of issues to be overcome.

References and Resources

Amatayakul, M., M. Brandt, and M. Dougherty. 2003. Cut, copy, paste: EHR guidelines. *Journal of AHIMA* 74(9):72,74.

American Health Information Management Association. 2003. A vision from the e-HIM future. *Journal of AHIMA* 74(8):suppl.

American Health Information Management Association. 2007. *Vision 2016: A Blueprint for Quality Education in Health Information Management.* Chicago, IL.

Aspden, P., J. M. Corrigan, J. Wolcott, and S.M. Erickson, eds. 2004. *Patient Safety: Achieving a New Standard for Care.* Washington, DC: National Academies Press.

Carlton, F., L.S. Hotchkiss, and R.A. Sheff. 2004. *Lessons Learned: A Guide to Evaluating and Implementing CPOE.* Marblehead, MA: HCPro, Inc.

Center for Information Technology Leadership. 2003 (Nov. 21). The Value of Computerized Provider Order Entry in Ambulatory Settings. RFA Number: RFA-HS-04-012. Bethesda, MD: NIH.

Centers for Medicare and Medicaid Services. 2006. Physicians' Referrals to Health Care Entities with which they have Financial Relationships, Exception for Certain Electronic Prescribing and Electronic Health Records Arrangements, Final Rule, *Federal Register.* http://www.cms.hhs.gov/apps/media/press/factsheet.asp?Counter=3226&intNumPerPage=10&checkDate=&checkKey=&srchType=1&numDays=3500&srchOpt=0&srchData=&keywordType=All&chkNewsType=6&intPage=&showAll=&pYear=&year=&desc=&cboOrder=date

Certification Commission for Health Information Technology. www.cchit.org.

Collen, M.F. 1995. *A History of Medical Informatics in the U.S. 1950–1990.* Bethesda, MD: Hartman Publishing.

Computer-based Patient Record Institute. 1995–2004. *Annual Nicholas E. Davies Award Proceedings of the CPR Recognition Symposium.* Chicago: Healthcare Information Management and Systems Society.

DesRoches, Catherine M, et al. 2008. Electronic health eecords in ambulatory care—a national survey of physicians, *New England Journal of Medicine.* 359(1):50–60.

Dickinson, G., L. Fischetti, and S. Heard, eds. 2003. HL7 EHR System Functional Model and Standard, Draft Standard for Trial Use, Release 1.0 and EHR Collaborative Report of Public Response to HL7 Ballot 1 EHR, August 29.

Dimick, Chris. 2008. Documentation Bad habits: Shortcuts in Electronic Records Pose Risk." *Journal of AHIMA.* 79(6):40–3.

eHealth Initiative. 2004. Who We Are. www.ehealthinitiative.org.

EHR Collaborative. 2004. Who We Are. www.ehrcollaborative.org.

Fonkych, K., and R. Taylor. 2005. *The State and Pattern of Health Information Technology Adoption.* Santa Monica, CA: The RAND Corporation.

Fox, L.A., and P. Thierry. 2003. Multiple visions undermine success of EHRs. *ADVANCE for Health Information Management* 13(14):8–9.

Health Level Seven. 2007 (Apr.). HL7 EHR System Functional Model.

Healthcare Financial Management Association, in partnership with GE Healthcare Financial Services. 2003. *How Are Hospitals Financing the Future? Access to Capital in Health Care Today.* Westchester, IL: HFMA.

Healthcare Information Management and Systems Society. 1995–2005. The Annual Nicholas E. Davies Award of Excellence. www.himss.org.

Healthcare Information Management and Systems Society. 1990–1999. *The Hewlett-Packard/HIMSS Leadership Survey.* Chicago: HIMSS.

Hospitals and Health Networks. 2002. Most Wired. Available online from hospitalconnect.com.

Hughes, G. 2003 (June). Practice brief: Transfer of patient health information across the continuum (Updated). *Journal of American Health Information Management Association.* www.ahima.org.

Institute of Medicine. 1999. *To Err Is Human: Building a Safer Health System,* edited by L.T. Kohn, J.M. Corrigan, and M.S. Donaldson. Washington, DC: National Academies Press.

Institute of Medicine. 2003 (July 31). *Letter Report: Key Capabilities of an Electronic Health Record System.* Washington, DC: National Academies Press. www.nap.edu/books.

Institute of Medicine. 1997. *The Computer-based Patient Record: An Essential Technology for Health Care,* edited by R.S. Dick, E.B. Steen, and D.E. Detmer. Washington, DC: National Academies Press.

Institute of Medicine. 1991. *The Computer-based Patient Record: An Essential Technology for Health Care,* edited by R.S. Dick and E.B. Steen. Washington, DC: National Academies Press.

National Alliance for Health Information Technology. 2008 (April 28). Report to the Office of the National Coordinator for Health Information Technology on Defining Key Health Information Technology Terms.

National Committee on Vital and Health Statistics. 2002 (Feb. 27). Letter to Secretary Thompson, U.S. Department of Health and Human Services, on Recommendations on Uniform Data Standards for Patient Medical Record Information.

National Committee on Vital and Health Statistics. 2001. *Information for Health: A Strategy for Building the National Health Information Infrastructure.* Washington, DC: NCVHS.

National Library of Medicine. 2003. Fact sheet: Integrated advanced information management systems (IAIMS) grants. www.nlm.nih.gov/pubs/factsheet/iaims.html.

Rhodes, H., and M. Dougherty. 2003. Practice brief: Document imaging as a bridge to the EHR. *Journal of AHIMA* 74(6):56A–G.

Rhodes, H., and G. Hughes. 2003. Practice brief: Redisclosure of patient health information (updated). *Journal of American Health Information Management Association* 74(4):56A–C.

Shortliffe, E.H., and L.E. Perreault, eds. 2001. *Medical Informatics: Computer Applications in Health Care and Biomedicine,* 2nd ed. New York: Springer-Verlag.

The Leapfrog Group for Patient Safety. 2004. About Us. www.leapfroggroup.org.

Chapter 2
Information Systems Theory and Systems Development Life Cycle

Information systems theory relates to the fact that an information system is considered a set of components that work together to achieve a common purpose. In science, *theory* refers to a comprehensive explanation of an important feature of nature that is supported by many facts gathered over time. Theories also allow scientists to make predictions about as yet unobserved phenomena. From a practical perspective, the **systems development life cycle** is the embodiment of information systems theory. It is used to ensure that following a formal methodology will enable the information system to be more valid and reliable.

Every information system is described, at a minimum, by its inputs, processes, and outputs. In planning any information system, from the simplest to the most complex, it is necessary to appreciate and anticipate the impact of these components on the desired outcome of the system being planned.

There are various types of information systems. For example, in healthcare there are laboratory information systems, pharmacy information systems, patient accounting systems, disease registry systems, online purchasing systems, automated instrumentation systems, and many others. Although all these information systems have inputs, processes, and outputs, their purpose is generally limited in scope to either the department's operations in which they exist (for example, laboratory, pharmacy) or their primary function (for example, claims processing, supplies procurement, or vital signs monitoring).

An electronic health record (EHR) is also an information system, and as such has inputs, processes, and outputs. However, it is typically much broader in scope than an application designed for one department or for one function. Instead, an EHR depends on many other systems for its input, performs many different types of processes, and generates a wide array of outputs. The scope of change brought about by an EHR is often described as a clinical transformation. This chapter:

- Introduces general systems theory in order to emphasize the importance of planning for the components that comprise an EHR

- Presents general information theory to establish a baseline understanding for developing data infrastructure requirements

Key Terms

Attributes	Human systems	Objects
Closed systems	Information systems theory	Open-systems
Cybernetics		Outputs
Data quality	Inputs	Processes
Electronic systems	Knowledge	Systems
Health information exchange (HIE) organization	Man–machine systems	Systems development life cycle
	Manual systems	Templates
	Mechanical systems	

- Addresses information systems theory to effect the clinical transformation brought about by using EHR technology and functions, which requires significant information resource and change management

- Explains the systems development life cycle within the context of health information technology (HIT) and the EHR

General Systems Theory

Systems theory is an interdisciplinary field of study that analyzes and describes how any group of objects work together to produce a result. Systems theory generally grew out of biology and the notion that systems are open to, and interact with, their environments, and that they can acquire qualitatively new properties through emergence, resulting in continual evolution.

Rather than reducing an entity (for example, the human body) to the properties of its parts or elements (for example, organs or cells), systems theory focuses on the arrangement of and relations between the parts that connect them into a whole. Thus, the same concepts and principles of theory organization underlie different disciplines. The concept of general systems theory is shown in figure 2.1. Systems concepts include: system-environment boundary, inputs, outputs, processing, and goal-directedness.

General types of systems with which you are most likely familiar include:

- **Mechanical systems** are developed by humans but can operate without human intervention. Heating and cooling systems are examples of systems where external temperature, barometric pressure, humidity, and other inputs process adjustments to maintain a constant desired environmental goal.

- **Human systems** are organized relationships among people. The political system in the U.S. is one in which the input is the alignment of many citizens with one of

Figure 2.1.   Concept of general systems theory

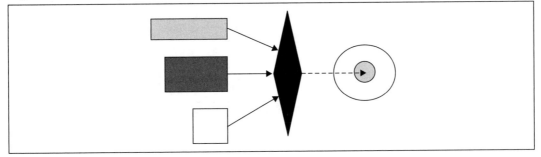

two major parties to carry out a process by which voting results in persons being elected to offices where they govern for the good of all. Healthcare is a human system. Its **inputs** are individuals seeking healthcare services. The healthcare delivery system's **processes** are the providers, payers, oversight agencies, and so on that deliver healthcare-related services; its **outputs** are the cures of or improvements on the illnesses and injuries in the human inputs.

- **Man–machine systems** are any form of supportive operations that assist humans in the performance of their work. **Manual systems** are those that entail humans performing certain processes; **electronic systems** are those aided by electronic computing devices. A filing system where paper charts are pulled and filed in accordance with specific policies and procedures is a manual system designed to enable easy retrieval of charts. An information system where humans enter data into a computer to be stored and later retrieved to support patient care is an electronic health information system.

Sometimes systems also are characterized as being either deterministic or probabilistic. A deterministic system is one where the parts function according to a predictable relationship. Most mechanical systems are deterministic. A probabilistic system is one where all the relationships among the parts cannot be defined in advance. These systems are subject to fluctuations in use and certainly describe human systems and man–machine systems.

Finally, systems may be closed or open. A closed system is one where all parts operate together without external influences. An open system is one in which the parts of the system are impacted by the environment. These basic differences are illustrated in figure 2.2.

In general systems theory, a closed system is frequently described as one that will eventually cease to function as a system because it does not have the feedback necessary to adjust to changes in the environment. This is an interesting observation because in information systems theory, **closed systems** are those in which specifications are kept proprietary. This results in making it difficult to use third-party software in association with the proprietary software. It also makes the organization dependent on the proprietary vendor to update the software given trends in the industry. Alternatively, IS vendors that apply an **open-systems** philosophy build software to conform to open, or readily available, standards. They encourage organizations to use the software and enhance it with whatever functionality appears to be needed at the time.

Figure 2.2.   Closed vs. open systems

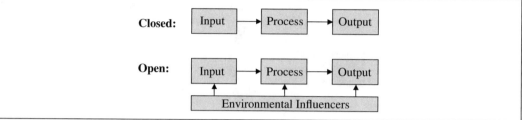

It must be noted that "readily available" does not necessary mean "free." It simply means that the vendor who has created an open system is willing to sell the software to others who, because it is standards based, may modify it to work with other information systems. Many healthcare IS vendors have chosen the closed-system approach, believing that their customers will be forced to buy all components from them and hence keep them in business. Proponents of open-source software often note that in the commercial world, useful software may be abandoned if it does not generate sufficient profit compared to other products. This may, in fact, be why many EHR vendors have struggled to survive. Because EHRs are essentially a system of systems, they depend on being able to connect with many systems.

The result of the closed-system approach to designing healthcare information systems has been a lack of interoperability among systems. *Interoperability* refers to the ability of one IS to exchange data with another IS. In the past, many providers accepted this lack of interoperability for several reasons, including:

- Providers were adopting information systems slowly, needing to prove their value. These systems were often limited in scope to single departmental functions, where sharing data with other systems was not a particular concern. For example, the laboratory does not have a great need to share data with radiology.

- If a single proprietary vendor were interested in having internal systems communicate with each other, it often could provide almost everything it needed for its basic operations. For example, in a hospital, patient demographic data from an admitting system were shared with other component systems. Charges captured in each system then were sent to a patient accounting system.

- Providers have been slow to adopt EHRs because of their cost, complexity, and need for a fully developed infrastructure. As a result, what information systems they used were aids to operations. For example, a pharmacy information system primarily helps the pharmacy to maintain an inventory of drugs and dispense them to the nursing unit. These are not clinical systems because they do not automate clinical information needs. Thus, the pharmacist, not the computer, evaluates the drug's potential efficacy and identifies any contraindications that would be communicated (verbally) to the provider.

- Providers want to ensure the confidentiality of their patients' health information. Many providers found it easier to manage confidentiality in a paper world than in an electronic world, where sophisticated access and audit controls meant added cost and effort, even when they were available in products, which was often not the case. Until only recently, standard practice was to print any information from operational systems that was needed for documentation in the medical record and from which release of information could be carefully controlled. In the "collegial" environment of healthcare, physicians wrote referral letters to provide other physicians with information about their patients, as needed, or permitted copies of documentation to be sent to other providers at no cost to the patient. Currently, under the Health Insurance Portability and Accountability Act of 1996 (HIPAA) regulations that permit providers to disclose information for treatment purposes without authorization (§164.502[a][1][ii]), many providers require authorizations because of a lack of trust and to protect themselves against complaints of wrongful disclosures.

- Providers often viewed the collection of health information about their patients as proprietary. Despite access controls that can block attempts to gain access to confidential data (and which are also required under HIPAA, §164.312[a]), many providers still are concerned about the potential for such access and prefer to retain the paper records or not use a remote site to store their electronic data.

Much is changing in healthcare. It is now recognized that readily exchangeable information across the continuum of care cannot depend on manual system processes to support patient safety and quality. As a result, the need for vendors to adopt open standards to achieve interoperability has finally been recognized, although not fully accepted even yet.

Information Theory

To further the pursuit of EHRs in an interoperable environment where their use will generate more than merely improved access to the paper documents, general information theory needs to be understood. The expectation is that EHRs will not only increase availability to records but also support clinical decision making at the point of care, provide the foundation for real-time public health surveillance, and contribute data for predictive modeling to develop better treatment protocols.

The current paper world results in the capture, storage, and retrieval of documents. These documents contain primarily data points as recorded by persons or generated from operational systems. Data points would include the patient's chief complaint, history of present illness, past history, results of physical exam, vital signs, medications administered, procedures performed, and observations about the patient's response to treatment. Rarely do clinicians document their rationale for their actions. There is little attempt to explain the process used to draw certain conclusions or describe what clinical practice guidelines, if any, were being applied. Because the data points are largely handwritten in a nonstandard manner with nonstandard terminology, it is extremely difficult to

Figure 2.3. Information theory

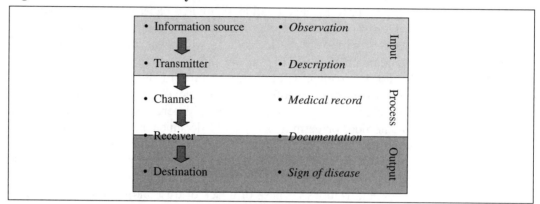

abstract data from medical records for meaningful research. In fact, most researchers retain "shadow records" or "research databases" to enable them to capture more specific data on a cohort of patients they are treating in order to be able to process these data into useful information.

Data Flow

Basic *information theory* describes the flow of data from an information source to its ultimate destination. (See figure 2.3.) In general, data are input into a system for the purpose of being processed and output as useful information. From a practical perspective, data flow must be understood to ensure that data needed to create useful information are indeed supplied and do indeed generate the desired information.

Data Sources

Input requires a *source* of data. In the case of health data, the source is generally an observation about a patient or a response to a question asked of the patient.

There must also be a *transmitter*, which is often a clinician, although it may also be a monitoring device or autoanalyzer. The clinician records a description of an observation, the response, or summary of the two. This may be strictly objective, such as "the patient is observed to be short of breath" or "the patient complains of shortness of breath for the past 2 days." In some cases, some judgment as to the accuracy of the patient's response also may be recorded, such as "the patient states that she has been short of breath for the past 2 days, although she also appears confused about what day of the week this is."

Processing raw data into useful information is performed by a *channel*. In the manual world, the channel would be the paper-based medical record. Obviously, processing is very limited in this case. At best, there is a process of forms that guide the capture of data. Sometimes these are color coded for ease of retrieval. Some forms may be formatted, which provides direction about where content should be recorded on the forms. For instance, many forms have boxes for recording the patient's name and medical record number. Some forms contain a list of data and the sequence in which the data should be dictated, such as for a history and physical examination, operative report, or discharge summary. A small number of forms may contain preprinted checklists or graphics for recording data, such as a standard order set, a nursing assessment, or a vital signs record. Organizations planning adoption of an electronic document management system may start to design their forms with bar codes. Organizations thinking about acquiring an EHR as the channel, which is heavily dependent on standardized and structured data, would do well to introduce more standardization in their forms to accustom their clinicians to the use of templates.

Information theory next recognizes that the channel is not the ultimate goal of the system. The goal of an EHR is patient safety, quality of care, productivity improvement, and so on. To achieve these goals, there must be a *receiver*. In the case of the medical record, the receiver is documentation, the direct output of the process. However, in the case of an EHR, the receiver has much enhanced utility beyond documentation—including expanded communication capabilities and knowledge generation.

The ultimate *destination* of the information flow is the goal of the system. There must be value to the information processing. The EHR has many goals. Some are global, such as "improve quality of care;" others are more specific, such as "alert the provider to a medication contraindication" or "provide a differential diagnosis." The destination is the information gleaned from processing the data so that the multiple data points captured during the history and physical taking, for instance, what points are related to the disease conclusion? In the manual world, the clinician records the data points, draws the conclusion in his or her mind based on his or her clinical training, and then records the information, essentially as another data point. In an electronic world, although the EHR should never be a substitute for clinical thought, the processing of the data could aid the clinician in making a diagnostic decision, especially where a complex set of data points is captured over time. A good example of this might be use of an EHR in a busy emergency department. A child seen several times for apparent accidents may actually be a victim of abuse, which may not be apparent at any one episode of care or even within one care setting. An EHR that can retrieve the data from all previous encounters, and from other emergency departments, might help a clinician more quickly spot the potential for such a situation. This is an example of the importance of a **health information exchange (HIE) organization**, which is an entity that oversees and governs the exchange of health-related information among disparate care delivery (and other health-related) organizations according to nationally recognized standards.

Data Uses

Information theory, then, recognizes not only the flow of data, but also how data are used, how they may be converted to information, and how experience may be applied to the information to support the creation of knowledge. A data–information–knowledge continuum is often described as part of information theory. (See figure 2.4.)

In the data–information–knowledge continuum, data are the discrete variables that can be processed by the computer. This is an important distinction for those planning an EHR.

Figure 2.4.   Data–information–knowledge continuum

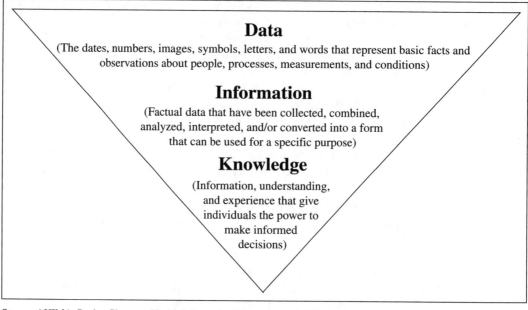

Source; AHIMA, Pocket Glossary: Health Information Management And Technology,
Chicago: American Health Information Management Association, 2006.

Although "data" can have a broad meaning and may be recorded in any number of forms and formats, for data to be processed into information by a computer system, they must be in discrete, or structured, format. Table 2.1 distinguishes unstructured from structured data and provides examples of each.

Information is the result of processing data. For example, when entering a birth date in a specific field designated to contain birth date, the computer can compare the data in the birth date field with the current date to calculate age.

Data Quality

It is important to note that data quality becomes an increasingly important element of computer use. As stated in Appendix C.1, **data quality** relates to the accuracy, completeness, timeliness, precision, currency, granularity, relevancy, definition, accessibility, and consistency of the input (AHIMA 1998). For example, if someone entered a patient's admission date in the field designated to contain birth date, the computer can only carry out the processing as specified, calculating age based on whatever date is entered.

To overcome errors, **templates** designed for data entry often have predefined parameters that are checked as data are entered. However, such edits can address only the most logical errors and too many such checks can be distracting for users. For example, if a medication dose field for a given medication could only logically contain a value between 0.1 and 1.0, the computer can check for any entry out of these bounds and alert the user. However, short of comparing previous entries for a birth date field or whether the admis-

Table 2.1.   Structured vs. unstructured data

Unstructured Data	Structured Data
Definition: Textual objects and images that can be stored and accessed in a computer, but not processed by a computer	Definition: Discrete facts and figures that can be encoded and processed by a computer. The value of variable able to be processed by a computer.
Examples: • Narrative notes • Print files • Video and voice files • Scanned images of documents • Pictures	Examples: • Data entered into templates • Coded data (for example, ICD, CPT, SNOMED) whether coded by a person or encoded by the computer • Bar codes, radio frequency identification (RFID)

sion service is newborn, there are probably few logical ways to check for errors in a birth date field that calculates age.

The potential for data-entry errors also is a reason why computer systems are designed for fixed data to be entered only once and used in all subsequent processes. For example, when a person's birth date is as positively identified as possible, such as from checking a driver's license or asking the patient his or her age and doing a mental check of the birth date, this date is not going to change. Whenever the patient's birth date or age needs to be used elsewhere in the system, it should be used from its original source.

Determining whether data are fixed or variable, however, can sometimes be tricky in healthcare. For example, a patient may have a recorded allergy to penicillin, yet another physician querying the patient more fully may decide that the patient's reaction is only a hypersensitivity. Although an allergy initially would appear to be a fixed, rather than a variable, data point, it does not necessarily mean the data point could never be changed.

Knowledge Creation

Knowledge is the application of experience to information. This is an area of healthcare computing that is only just now being explored. A good example is the case of the allergy described earlier. If capturing allergy data is found over time to be excessive to human users, a query could be run on the data to determine how often an allergy field is changed or an allergy alert is overridden. If these events appear to occur frequently, this knowledge could be used to construct additional fields that should be used to confirm that a reaction is probably an allergy.

Although the allergy example used to describe the creation of knowledge is legitimate, there is a cost to adding data in cases where human knowledge may be applied more readily. The cost entails not only a computer programmer's time to develop the instructions, but also, more important, the effort it requires a clinician to perform data entry on what may appear to be a trivial matter, considering his or her level of education and experience. Most organizations reserve knowledge creation for quality improvement, outcomes management, and research activities.

Information Systems Theory

Information systems theory, then, is the explanation that information is generated by data that are processed in ways that contribute value. An information system:

- Uses devices to capture data in multiple formats that are converted to a machine-processable state

- Applies instructions, also converted into a machine-processable state, to index, store, calculate, compare, and perform other functions on the data

- Uses devices to display the original data at another time or place and present the results of calculations, comparisons, and other functions to users in various formats

Just like the human body, which is a system of many components (nervous system, musculoskeletal system, integumentary system, and so on) integrated into the human form that allow people to function (to walk, talk, think, and so on), an IS requires data and instructions for processing to produce results. Unlike the human system, however, ISs are often designed for specific purposes that can—and frequently do—stand alone. The body's musculoskeletal system cannot stand alone; instead, it must be integrated with the nervous system to detect pulses from the brain that direct movement, with the integumentary system for protection, and so on. Alternatively, a laboratory IS can manage specimen collection, report results, and generate charges, all based on paper input and output without ever having any connection to any other IS. Of course, it is helpful for the laboratory IS to have a connection to an admitting or practice management system so that patient demographics do not have to be reentered into the laboratory IS. Once an order-entry system is adopted, a connection to a laboratory IS becomes necessary so that the request for a specific test can be directed to it automatically.

These distinctions are made between the human body and IS because an EHR is more like the human system than other ISs because of its dependence on multiple systems. The EHR is a system of systems, much like the human system. It is a means to capture data from multiple source systems and to process the data into many forms for many purposes. As information technology (IT) advances, information systems can be programmed with instructions to perform many information management functions the human system can perform tirelessly and sometimes more accurately.

However, no matter how well the programmatic instructions are written for an IS, there are always changing requirements and changes in the external environment that may not have been anticipated at the time the original instructions were written. Information systems have been programmed to "learn" and "predict" through complex pattern analysis. Those that are highly sophisticated may be able to respond to some changes, but most information systems require changes to their instructions to continue to be useful in the face of external change. Information systems also are incapable of heuristic thought, or generating "gut instincts" that something could be wrong or needs attention.

Hence, EHRs truly represent a clinical transformation impacting many people who have never been impacted by information systems previously. They are much more inte-

Figure 2.5.   The role of technology in healthcare

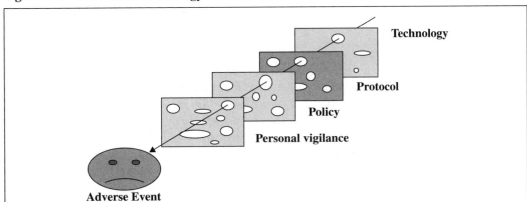

Adapted from Reason, cited in Valusek, JHM, 16;1: 34-39

grated than the departmental or operational systems with which they interact. However, EHR systems are still only tools and not substitutes for human interaction. Figure 2.5 illustrates the importance of human thought (personal vigilance) as a key element of the EHR system.

Characteristics of Information Systems

It has been noted that the fundamental elements of an IS are inputs, processes, and outputs. These fundamental elements are accomplished through the adoption of hardware (equipment) and software (computing instructions), but an IS is more than just hardware and software. One way to describe all the elements of an information system is to consider not only the hardware and software, but also people, policy, and process.

- *People* are the key reason for ISs to exist—and also how they exist. ISs have been characterized as man–machine systems because people design them and people use them. Interestingly, both components of the people equation can be troublesome. In the grand scheme of things, people have only begun to use computers to help process data into information fairly recently. Early computing efforts started just about half a century or so ago. This may seem like a long time to some, but it is very short when considering that early records of human existence date back thousands of years.

    The result of the "youthfulness" of computing versus the age of mankind often results in a disconnect between how we can actually design a computer and what we might like it to do. *Star Trek* is still a popular movie series because it continues to capture our imagination. Yet, some people have never used a computer and fear the use of one. Virtually every implementation of EHR systems currently is accompanied by some people who believe they will lose their jobs or who absolutely refuse to use the system. And because computer design is not yet perfect, even those who use computers regularly for some part of their work or play may find that computers are not yet suitable for other aspects. Taking people into consideration when designing an IS requires attention to detail and management of change.

- *Policy* refers to directives or principles upon which people perform their work or other activities of their lives. An individual's policies may center on their business practices, social interactions, use of drugs, frequency of watching television, or myriad other things that direct how they live their lives. When a person becomes a member of a group, the group may establish policies. In informal groups, these policies may more likely be normative behaviors. In communities, the policies may be codified by local ordinances, state statutes, and federal laws and regulations. In social organizations, bylaws or codes of conduct may be the policy directives that provide guidance. In business organizations, policies may be written or unwritten, formal or informal. There may be formal, written policies on who may access what information; there may be informal, unwritten policies on acceptable dress.

  Interestingly, in healthcare organizations, there are frequently many policies because of the highly regulatory nature of healthcare, yet few, if any, policies relating to use of information systems, other than acceptable use of the Internet and e-mail. In an EHR environment, where so many intended users are new to computers and where the EHR itself is a new construct, it is not surprising that there are not more policies, but that makes them no less important for their adoption.

  For example, policies on what information should or should not be entered into the EHR may seem unnecessary when data entry is so structured, yet many healthcare organizations are struggling with whether to require a rationale for overriding a clinical decision support alert. Policies also may be needed to direct whether printouts will continue to be provided to some users, whether some users will be permitted to continue dictating instead of directly entering data, and so on. Such policies may have a huge economic and risk impact on a healthcare organization, as multiple and parallel processes always add operational costs and are frequently error prone.

- *Process* is the manner in which a task is performed. A simple example is a process a provider uses to write an order for a medication. In the past, an order may have been handwritten on an order sheet or called in to an individual qualified to accept a verbal order, even possibly without referencing the patient's chart. When an IS is available for order entry, the provider is expected to look up the patient, key in the various components that comprise an order, and respond to any alerts or reminders for contraindications. These are different processes for performing essentially the same task.

  Process change is one of the most significant factors in the success or failure of EHR adoption. Even where people may be willing to use a computer or where policy dictates that they must use it, process changes can have a significant impact. They need to be well designed, accurate, kept up-to-date, and provide as intuitive use as possible. Current processes must be understood so that both control points can be retained and workarounds and bottlenecks can be eliminated.

Austin and Boxerman (1998) similarly describe complex ISs as having relationships, unity of purpose, and a feedback mechanism.

- *Relationships* between objects and attributes help an IS achieve its purpose. **Objects** are the component parts of a system; **attributes** are the properties of those objects that describe what they do and how they work. Relationships tie the component parts together in accordance with their characteristics. The goal is to achieve a purpose or function equal to, or better than, any individual object could achieve. Relationships may be planned or unplanned, formal or informal, but they must exist if the collection of components is to constitute a system. A key lesson for designing an EHR system is that many disparate systems and their respectively disparate stakeholders must come together to form new relationships.

- *Unity of purpose* causes the collective parts of an IS to have integrity. A system must have an identity and describable boundaries. Interestingly, ISs are becoming so vast in scope with so many potential relationships that unity of purpose is becoming less clearly defined, or at least less proscriptive. One only needs to consider the Internet as a vast IS. Although the Internet's purpose is to exchange information globally, its integrity is subject to many factors. Closer to home, the EHR system must be designed around well-established policies that set the boundaries not just for where the system starts and ends, but also for the adoption and realization of benefits. Too often, such systems are implemented and not fully adopted and result in less-than-expected value.

- *Feedback* mechanisms provide information about environmental factors that interact with the functioning of the system. Feedback includes a number of factors. Social factors are characteristics of individuals and groups of people involved in use of the IS. Social factors may dictate how a system is designed, what input devices are used, and how users are trained to use the system. They are important determinants of EHR adoption, requiring significant human-factors engineering of the IS as well as change management for the intended users. Economic factors are well-known determinants of whether and what information systems are acquired. Unfortunately, economic factors are often directly in conflict with social factors, where highly sophisticated, intuitive systems are more readily adoptable, but much more expensive. Political factors are the competing demands that influence both the social and economic factors. Political factors may promote incentives for use of an IS over disincentives or may cause a provider organization to use its financial resources to build a parking structure rather than acquire an EHR. Physical environmental factors also may affect IS decisions. An organization may not have the space to install a data center and so will use an application service provider (ASP) or may be located in an old building where it is difficult to use a wireless network effectively.

  An EHR system represents a level of change that has been described as a clinical transformation. This level of change can be neither created nor maintained without a constant feedback mechanism that both celebrates success and identifies where course correction is needed.

Cybernetics Applied to Information Systems Theory

Early IS theorists described a special case where the systems incorporated self-regulation. This special case was identified by Wiener (in Austin and Boxerman 1998) as **cybernetics**. Cybernetics is derived from the Greek word for "pilot," as in "auto pilot" or "pilot light." It is a theory of control systems based on communication (transfer of information) between systems and environment and within the system, and control (feedback) of the system's function in regard to the environment. Austin and Boxerman summarize Weiner's work as adding three elements to the general systems components of inputs, outputs, and processes. These elements include a sensor, a standards monitor, and a control unit where modifications can take place (1998). Austin and Boxerman have applied cybernetics to health ISs. They describe a clinical laboratory as a cybernetic system, where:

- *Inputs* are the scheduled lab tests, stat orders, and various professional, technical, and material resources.

- *Processes* are the specimen collection, testing, and results reporting.

- *Outputs* are the test reports, patient charges, and statistical reports.

- *Sensors* are the number of tests by category, quality control data, and resources consumed. The outputs are used to capture these data.

- *Standards monitoring* is performed by comparing the sensor data to various standards and cost/efficiency goals.

- *Control processes* are then instituted when standards monitoring detects variation in the sensor data from the standard data. Control processes may include continuing education, retraining, revised policies and procedures, staffing changes, recalibration of equipment, and so on.

The feedback loop created by cybernetics is a powerful concept that ensures integrity among the basic elements that have relationships comprising an IS. This feedback loop can be easily applied to the model of open systems, as shown in figure 2.6.

Cybernetics should not be forgotten in designing an EHR system. All too often, EHR systems are treated as yet another stand-alone system, assuming that another part of the overall healthcare delivery system will sense a potential error and take corrective action. However, in fact, people, policy, and process often converge in the EHR system with the result that there is no other feedback mechanism.

Figure 2.6.   Cybernetics

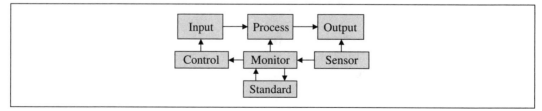

Systems Development Life Cycle (SDLC)

The purpose of reflecting on general systems theory and general information systems theory is to appreciate the steps necessary to develop, or at least plan for implementing, an EHR system.

The **systems development life cycle** (SDLC) is often cited as the primary resource for managing complex IS projects. As a conceptual model for project management, the SDLC has been around for as long as computerized applications have been built. In general, the SDLC focuses on development of the software to be used in the IS being designed. The primary purpose of the SDLC is to ensure that software is developed correctly, and within time and budget constraints. However, the SDLC has additional, important practical applications beyond the development of software. The SDLC is useful to consider in describing an organization's migration path to EHR. It is also a useful approach in undertaking an EHR system selection. Finally, the SDLC guides project planning for implementation of the EHR in general and workflow and process redesign in particular.

Traditional SDLC Methodology

In general, traditional SDLC methodology includes the following steps, as illustrated in figure 2.7:

1. *Feasibility*: The existing (manual) system is evaluated and deficiencies are identified. The result is the determination as to whether it makes sense to proceed with the project.

2. *Analysis*: New (automated) system requirements are defined. In particular, deficiencies in the existing system are addressed with specific proposals for improvement.

3. *Design*: The proposed system is designed. Plans are laid out concerning the physical construction, hardware, operating systems, programming, communications, and security issues.

Figure 2.7.   Traditional SDLC

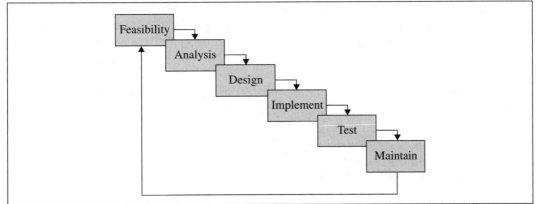

4. *Implement*: The new system is developed. The new components and programs are obtained and installed. Users of the system are trained in its use, and all aspects of performance are tested. If necessary, adjustments are made at this stage.

5. *Test*: The system is put into use. This can be done in various ways. The new system can be phased in, according to application or location, and the old system gradually replaced. In some cases, it may be more cost-effective to shut down the old system and implement the new system at the same time.

6. *Maintain*: When the new system is up and running for a while, it should be exhaustively evaluated. Maintenance must be kept up rigorously at all times. System users should be kept up-to-date about the latest modifications and procedures.

New Models for Software Development

The traditional SDLC methodology has been named the "waterfall" methodology because it describes a linear set of phases. Because such a methodology is probably more theoretical than practical, over the years, several alternatives have been created to guide the processes of software development. These have included methodologies-dubbed phrases such as "adaptive project framework," "agile software development," "build and fix," "dynamic systems development model," "feature-driven development," "lean development," "rapid application development," "spiral," "synchronize-and-stabilize," and others. As suggested by these names, every effort is being made to improve on and speed up the process of software development. Frequently, several models are combined into some sort of hybrid methodology, especially when the model is used to guide project management.

SDLC for EHR Project Management

As noted, the SDLC's primary focus has been on software development. The basic concepts and fundamental steps associated with the SDLC, however, are important to apply even when an organization is acquiring the software and implementing it, rather than developing it. Most healthcare organizations currently approach EHR from the strategy of acquiring software rather than building it themselves. The basic tenets of the SDLC then are frequently adapted for project management.

In addition to a greater focus on implementation rather than development, because most EHR systems are systems of systems, the traditional SDLC's linear approach is generally replaced with a more "spiral"-type of model where steps are repeated for each component implemented.

In general, when the SDLC is applied to project management where software is acquired and not developed, the following phases are included:

1. *Initiation* often addresses both the feasibility and analysis aspects of project management. In fact, because an EHR now is viewed as a cost of doing business that will ultimately have to be addressed at some point in the organization's near future,

"feasibility" may actually be turned into "readiness assessment." Components of the initiation phase often include:

—Setting a strategic business goal

—Defining expected benefits

—Anticipating potential organizational changes regarding facilities, staffing, and so on

—Identifying budgeting, scheduling, and personnel constraints

—Assessing attitudes and beliefs

—Assessing computer skills

—Performing communication planning, including what messages should be provided to whom, by whom, and when

—Performing change management to address the human factor elements

—Doing a cost-benefit analysis and financing feasibility

2. *Planning* is potentially the most important, most often shortchanged, phase. It entails:

—Executing a project overview for all stakeholders involved in the project, including creating a migration path for the various components of EHR system implementation

—Delineating staff roles and responsibilities and appointment/acquisition

—Performing process mapping and specifying functional requirements

—Specifying technical requirements

—Identifying project and risk management methodologies

—Defining deliverables, based on the migration path

—Identifying control requirements and standards

—Charting a conversion strategy and implementing any bridge technologies

—Documenting planning for everything from requirement specifications to a code of conduct for vendor selection to project issues, job descriptions, and policies and procedures for use of the new system

—Performing staff development, from education to skills building to training

3. *Acquisition* or *design and development* involves numerous steps. If the project entails software development, an overall design specification is created from the various requirements identified in the initiation and planning phases and then development is the conversion of the design specification into executable software programs or computer instructions. Because most healthcare organizations will

acquire an EHR rather than develop it themselves, the steps in acquisition are described as:

—Performing market research to understand the products that are available and how they match with the organization's functional requirements

—Submitting a request for proposal development that includes functional and performance requirements

—Submitting a request for proposal distribution, receipt, and analysis

—Performing due diligence to verify proposal content and further explore product and vendor features

—Negotiating the contract

—Obtaining approval to acquire the product

—Financing the acquisition

4. *Implementation* is the phase in which the product is installed, customized to meet the organization's requirements, and turned over to the users for adoption. It is important to recognize that implementation is more than just installation. A common misconception relating to EHR implementations is often that software can be installed and used directly thereafter. Even the simplest EHR for a small clinic or solo practitioner requires some system building, training, and testing. Steps include:

—Establishing an issues management and change control process

—Scheduling project tasks, milestones, and resources, including budgeting project expenditures over the life of the project

—Developing a turnover strategy

—Planning training

—Planning for testing

—Installing hardware and software, including storage components

—Reconfiguring communications and network components, as needed

—Implementing security controls

—Training "super" users who assist end users in learning the system

—Building the system, including data modeling, tables and files creation, template building, report development, unit testing, and system testing

—Developing an interface and testing integration

—Converting data

—Performing stress testing

—Performing end-user training

—Providing documentation

—Providing go-live management and support

—Performing acceptance testing

5. *Operations/maintenance* relates to the ongoing support needed to keep the system current and accurate. For an EHR, this is where the spiral model of the SDLC comes into play. Because most hospitals and even some (especially large) clinics implement their EHR in components, operations and maintenance will necessarily include looping back to readiness, planning, and, in some cases, selection—and certainly implementation of new components. In general, operations/maintenance includes:

—Performance measurement

—Benefits realization: Return on investment (ROI), provider and patient satisfaction, outcomes, celebration, and course correction

—Software maintenance, including patches, routine modifications, major upgrades, emergency changes, keeping subscriptions current

—Hardware upgrades and maintenance

—Hardware and software inventories and license agreement maintenance

—User preference changes

6. *Disposition/disposal* relates to the orderly removal of surplus or obsolete hardware, software, or data, and including the potentiality of change in vendor control or software obsolescence. Although most healthcare organizations are just in the process of acquiring an EHR and are not anticipating any immediate change, it is conceivable that obsolescence will occur more rapidly, at least for some of the equipment and potentially some of the bridge, or interim, components.

Conclusion

Armed with general systems theory, information theory, and ISs theory, managing information resources should take on a systems approach, ensuring an organized approach to managing what can literally be thousands of tasks for a large EHR project. The level of detail in acquiring, implementing, and maintaining an EHR, especially because the EHR is a system of components, can be daunting if there is not a logical process. The SDLC lends a structure to this process. The nature of system should reassure the information resource manager that an EHR is a complex, but manageable, undertaking.

References and Resources

Alexandrou, A. 2006. Systems Development Life Cycle. www.mariosalexandrou.com/methodologies/systems_development_life_cycle.asp.

AHIMA Data Quality Management Task Force. 1998. Practice Brief: Data quality management model. *Journal of AHIMA* 69(6).

American Health Information Management Association. 2006. *Pocket Glossary of Health Information Management and Technology*. Chicago: AHIMA.

Austin, C.J., and S.B. Boxerman. 1998. *Information Systems for Health Services Administration,* 5th ed. Chicago: Health Administration Press.

Chisholm, M. 2004 (June 23). Business rules evangelist: Do business rules fit the systems development life cycle? *DM Review.* www.dmreview.com/article_sub.cfm?articleID=1005616.

Cummings, et al. 2006. *Management Information Systems for the Information Age*, Toronto, McGraw-Hill Ryerson.

Degoulet, P., and M. Fieschi. 1997. *Introduction to Clinical Informatics.* New York: Springer-Verlag.

Developers View. 2006. Software Development. www.startvbdotnet.com.

Developers View. 2006. System Development Life Cycle. www.startvbdotnet.com.

Federal Financial Institutions Examination Council. 2004 (Apr.). Systems Development Life Cycle. *Development and Acquisition.* www.occ.treas.gov/efiles/disk2/booklets/d_a/d_and_a.pdf.

Government of British Columbia, Information Management Branch. System Development Life Cycle (SDLC) Standards.

Open Source Initiative. 2006. www.opensource.org.

Chapter 3
Challenges to EHR Adoption

Electronic health records (EHRs) hold great promise, with increasing numbers of providers recognizing that EHRs are becoming essential for providing high-quality healthcare services. Yet, there are still challenges to their adoption. Anticipating these challenges early in the adoption cycle helps to overcome them or at least to reduce their intensity. This chapter:

- Addresses the legality of the EHR

- Offers suggestions for overcoming clinician resistance

- Addresses issues associated with patient/consumer acceptance and use and privacy and security concerns

- Identifies business challenges and how to address them

- Recognizes the primary role that leadership plays in EHR adoption

- Describes the convergence toward a nationwide health information network

The Nature of Challenge

Challenges to any change are many and varied. They also may be real or perceived. Often they are a combination. Many of the early challenges to EHRs were real. For example, design limitations were very real and the efforts to overcome them were likewise real. This has led to the current level of sophistication. However, the early limitations may have resulted in lingering concerns. In some cases, overcoming bad experiences can be a greater challenge than overcoming the initial hurdles themselves. For example, many clinicians believe that data entry into an EHR takes longer and executive managers often believe that the cost of EHRs is prohibitive, even though they may not have studied the actual time or cost savings.

Key Terms

Admissibility	Encryption	Nationwide health information network
Audit controls	Informatics	
Authentication	Information access management	Nonrepudiation
Case law		Outsourcing
Contingency plans	Integrity	Redundancy
Conversion strategy	Metrics	Servers
Digital signature	Minimum necessary use standards	Wet signature
E-Discovery		
Electronic signature		

Another challenge is that of overcoming uncertainty. Many care delivery organizations have fears about the legality of an electronic record and the implications of the Health Insurance Portability and Accountability Act (HIPAA) in an electronic environment. Clinicians, and especially physicians in their office practice, perceive their patients may not want them using the computer in the examining room—even though this is more likely to be an issue for the physician who is not very computer savvy than for the patient. Actually such fears, while largely unfounded, can spur organizations toward taking proactive steps in better managing their legal health records, privacy, security, and interactions with their patients.

Challenges to EHR adoption have been particularly great because the stakes are high and the change they bring about is great. The direct cost of EHR adoption can be large. This is especially apparent when access to capital financing is difficult for many organizations in a time of decreasing reimbursement and revenues. In addition, many observers question caregivers' willingness to fully use the EHR and, therefore, whether the expenditure of limited funds is appropriate. The technology to properly implement EHRs is highly sophisticated. As a result, the expected benefits are great. When the benefits are not achieved or are not perceived to be achieved, the disappointment is immense. This can easily cast doubt for any future endeavors; when other providers do not see the benefits being achieved, they may not undertake EHR.

The cycle of vendor hype and disappointment that characterized early EHR efforts may have contributed more to the challenge of EHR adoption than any other factor. Early in the development of EHRs, many vendors hyped products that were not real or did not fully deliver on their expectations. Uncertainties also arise about vendor capabilities and stability when so many vendors enter and leave the marketplace. This is changing, both as healthcare delivery organizations are getting smarter about asking the right questions and as standards and certification criteria for EHR functionality have come into existence.

Uncertainty is the hallmark of immaturity. It may be that the many different terms and intermediary implementations have come about because the challenges were too great.

However, many of the challenges currently are eroding and the view of the EHR as a migration path is emerging.

Legality of the EHR

One of the earliest concerns for EHR adoption centered on legal issues, especially with respect to the admissibility of records compiled electronically and their authentication. Updates in state laws and other legal and regulatory initiatives have lessened this concern somewhat, although there are new laws relating to e-discovery and for reporting security breaches, and new laws are increasingly being created, especially impacting health information exchange (HIE) services requiring more active consumer consent for release of their information. Laws, with respect to technology, usually lag behind, but laws for health information technology (HIT) are starting to catch up and must be monitored closely.

Sources of Law

It is state law that primarily provides the legal basis for health records, whether paper based or electronic. In addition to differences among states, many different laws that address or pertain to health records sometimes exist within a single state. For example, legal directives for health records or medical documentation are embedded in hospital and professional licensure laws. Laws pertaining to general business records also are a source of law relating to whether health records are admissible in a court of law. Because many of these laws were enacted before computers existed or became commonplace, they do not address electronic records, leaving **case law** to decide the legal issues. The good news is that many states are updating their laws pertaining to electronic records in general, EHRs in particular, as well as for release of information within a HIE environment.

Some examples of newer state laws include:

- New Jersey Admin. Code tit. § 8:43G-15.2(b)(1)(1998) requires hospitals to "develop a procedure to assure the confidentiality of each electronic signature and to prohibit the improper or unauthorized use of any computer generated signature." The New Jersey Board of Medical Examiners and the Board of Physical Therapy require their respective licensees to have systems that are designed to protect the integrity, authenticity, and confidentiality of the patient records maintained in electronic medical records.

- New York amended its hospital medical records regulations in 1998. 10 NYCRR § 405.10(c) requires hospitals to provide assurances with respect to authenticity, security, and confidentiality. They must adopt internal criteria and procedures for the use of computerized medical records. The regulations explicitly make electronic signatures and computer-generated signature codes acceptable as **authentication** when used in accordance with hospital policy. In addition, the date, time category of practitioner, mode of transmission, and point of origin must be recorded in the medical record for each electronic or computer entry. New York also requires hospitals to ensure that electronic communications and entries are accurate, providing two examples of acceptable ongoing verification processes:

—Protocols for ensuring that incomplete entries, reports, or documents are not accepted or implemented until reviewed, completed, and verified by the author

—A process implemented as part of the hospital's quality assurance activities that provides for the sampling of records for review to verify the accuracy and integrity of the system

Other Sources Supporting Electronic Records and Signatures

When state law has not been updated recently or is otherwise silent on EHRs, the clear trend is toward acceptance with appropriate controls. In addition, other sources of guidance can be applied.

Case law typically provides precedence. There is not a lot of case law with respect to EHRs, which is a good sign. In some of the cases that have reached the courts, there is only peripheral application, although these cases can still be used as indicators of acceptance. Following is an example of one case that supports electronic signature:

Walgreen Co. v. Wisconsin Pharmacy Examining Board, No. 97-1513, 217 Wis.2d 290, 577 N.W.2d 387, 1998 WL 65551 at 4 (Wis. App. Feb. 19, 1998). In this case, the Wisconsin State Court held that computer-transmitted prescriptions were similar to prescriptions transmitted orally by telephone, which Wisconsin statute expressly allows to be filled without being signed by the physician.

In addition to state law and case law, the Medicare *Conditions of Participation* address issues relating to the safe storage of records. The Joint Commission (formerly JCAHO) holds hospitals responsible for ensuring that they have a mechanism in place to safeguard records and information against loss, destruction, tampering, and unauthorized access or use.

Although HIPAA does not explicitly address the legality of protected health information (PHI) in electronic form, it does promote the use of information systems and provides for the privacy and security of PHI in electronic media. HIPAA also called for recommendations on uniform data standards for patient medical record information that set the stage for many of the standards being adopted now.

Even more explicitly, the Medicare Prescription Drug, Improvement, and Modernization Act of 2003 (MMA) called for adoption of standards to support e-prescribing (e-Rx) and also provided for safe harbors and exceptions to the Stark Law and antikickback statutes that enable hospitals to donate certain e-prescribing and EHR arrangements. Regulations concerning the donation arrangements set forth the specific provisions under which these arrangements can occur.

Finally, precedence can be inferred from the acceptability of electronic records and signatures from other industries or general laws. The following establish a framework for the legality of electronic signatures in general:

• The Federal Electronic Signatures in Global and National Commerce Act of 2000, also known as the E-SIGN bill, contributes to making electronic signature legal. It declares the validity of electronic signatures for interstate and international commerce. Additionally, it prohibits denying the legal effect of certain electronic documents and transactions signed by electronic signature. Further, the act clarifies broad circumstances in which an electronic record satisfies any statute or regulation that mandates a record in writing, requires inquiries into domestic and foreign impediments to commerce in electronic signature products and services, and embraces all technologies. Exclusions are clearly spelled out in the act. These are limited to certain testamentary instruments, matters of family law, defined sections of the Uniform Commercial Code, specific judicial documents, defined credit-related proceedings, the Uniform Anatomical Gift Act, and the Uniform Health-Care Decisions Act.

- The Department of Health and Human Services (HHS), Food and Drug Administration (FDA), 21 CFR Part 11 Electronic Records; Electronic Signature, March 1997, provides criteria for FDA acceptance of electronic records and signatures under certain circumstances. It states that electronic records, electronic signatures, and handwritten signatures executed to electronic records are equivalent to paper records and handwritten signatures executed on paper. These regulations apply to all FDA program areas and are intended to permit the widest possible use of electronic technology, compatible with the FDA's responsibility to promote and protect public health.

- The Uniform Electronic Transactions Act (UETA) was approved in July 1999 at the National Conference of Commissioners on Uniform State Law and recommended for adoption in all 50 states. This is a model act relating to the use of electronic online communications and contracts, electronic records, and online signatures. Although not all states have enacted this model as law, the framework is referred to specifically as the implementation guide in the E-SIGN Act.

- The MMA sought recommendations for regulations allowing federal preemption of state laws that are either contrary to the federal standards or that restrict the ability to carry out e-prescribing. This is an important issue because there is wide variation among state laws regarding the extent to which e-prescribing can be done, what information e-prescriptions must contain, how the information is worded and represented, and whether and how the information can be received into or transmitted from that state.

  A particular concern relates to electronic signature on prescriptions for controlled substances. Current Drug Enforcement Administration (DEA) regulations require a **wet signature** (that is, signed with a pen on paper) for controlled substances, representing about 10 to 13 percent of all prescriptions written. As a result, prescriptions for such substances are either handwritten or printed from an e-prescribing device and signed and handed to the patient. At press time, the DEA proposed regulations to allow e-prescribing of controlled substances as long as there were additional controls on the provider's e-prescribing system for identity proofing, two-factor authentication, reporting of security incidents, and other elements pertaining to the content of the prescription; and on the pharmacy's system for access controls, auditing, logging, archiving, and processing. It is important to watch for the final regulations, as e-Rx can significantly improve patient safety and has accounted for considerable cost savings, where physicians may be reminded of lower-cost generic equivalents to brand name drugs and where considerable time savings are achieved in the refill and renewal process.

Legality of Records Issues

A common theme can be identified throughout all sources of law and standards with respect to the legality of EHRs: There must be demonstrable evidence that the records are retained as they were created and are not altered. This addresses their admissibility in a court of law, affords consumer protection, and guards against professional liability. Five major issues that all laws and regulations address in some form relate to retention and durability, storage, signature, accuracy of entries, and transmission integrity.

- *Retention and durability* ensures that electronic data follow required retention schedules and can be retrieved from the electronic media on which they are stored. There have been concerns in the past that some electronic media failed to last for long periods of time because they were so new. Optical disks were of particular concern. However, simulations have been performed on optical disks to determine and correct any untoward effects of the aging process. By now, most current electronic media have passed the test of time, but new forms of media may emerge that also must have appropriate testing and **contingency plans** to ensure durability. Contingency plans with respect to media durability often include recopying data onto new media. Reliable evidence of the chain of copying must be preserved.

- *Storage* refers to safeguarding data against loss, destruction, tampering, and unauthorized use. These are the same principles that the HIPAA privacy and security rules espouse. Obvious safeguards would include everything from data backup plans, emergency mode operation plans, and disaster recovery plans to workforce and physical security, device and media controls, workstation use and security, access control, audit controls, authentication measures, integrity controls, and transmission controls. Not as obvious, but just as important, are the administrative security requirements of risk analysis and management, having an information security official, performing clearance checks on members of the workforce, ensuring that incident reporting and response mechanisms are in place, having a means for ongoing monitoring and evaluation, and ensuring that a chain of trust has been established contractually with one's business associates so they adhere to the same standards. Providers should establish **minimum necessary use standards** that are supported by **information access management** processes and technical access controls as well as **audit controls** to provide the ability to examine activity in their information systems. Policies and procedures and workforce training need to be in place to ensure that uses and disclosures are made only as permitted or required by federal and state law.

Figure 3.1.   Forms of signatures in the EHR

- **Digitized signature**—Scanned image of a "wet" signature. This is considered weak because someone could acquire a copy of the image and use it without the person's knowledge.
- **Electronic signature**—Application of a password to an electronic document. This is often used for signing transcribed dictation or orders in a CPOE system. It can be strengthened by using two-tiered authentication (for example, password and token) or biometrics.
- **Digital signature**—Cryptographic signature that authenticates the user, provides nonrepudiation, and ensures message integrity.

Source: Adapted from Cohen and Amatayakul 2003, p. 16.

- *Signature issues* are of major concern for EHRs because many healthcare actions rely on an order being signed, not only by an individual authorized to have access, but one also credentialed to issue the order. Documentary evidence of action depends on the signature's authenticity. In some respects, EHRs make authentication easier: Entries can be stamped automatically with date, time, and user identification. This provides the elements of an **electronic signature**. Added to that can be **encryption** and **nonrepudiation**, which would create a **digital signature**. (See figure 3.1 for types of signatures in EHRs.) Whatever form of signature is used, controls must be in place to ensure that the signature elements are not altered or deleted. Additionally, controls must be in place to ensure that the individuals using electronic or digital signatures are actually who they claim to be. This is the intent of authentication measures such as passwords, tokens, and biometrics. It also is the intent of nonrepudiation controls in a digital signature. No state or federal laws pertaining to health information requires a digital signature, but some providers are evaluating their use in certain situations.

- *Accuracy of entries* has always been a concern, whether in paper or electronic forms. Several states require ongoing verification of accuracy, although none has specific technical requirements. In general, documentation accuracy has been a function of quality reviews often performed retrospectively. State and federal laws and regulations have tried not to require specific information technology associated with checking accuracy because of how rapidly technology changes. However, EHR systems are being built with significant edit checking and reminders about proper documentation, which can only enhance compliance with such requirements.

- *Transmission integrity* refers to controls placed on data when they are sent to another entity. HIPAA's Security Rule defines *electronic transmission* as "the exchange of information in electronic media that may occur through the Internet, an extranet that is accessible only to collaborating parties, leased lines, dial-up lines, private networks, and the physical movement of removable/transportable electronic storage media" (45 CFR 160.103[2]). Each means of transmission affords greater or lesser protection of data. The Internet is considered the least protected; physical movement of media is considered the most protected. HIPAA requires transmission controls, including that providers address **integrity** and encryption as they may be needed for the means of transmission involved. The Centers for Medicare and Medicaid Services (CMS) has an Internet policy that does not permit the transmission of PHI to it through the Internet without encryption.

- *Admissibility*, evidence, and discoverability are important legal concepts that are essentially the result of the five key measures laws and regulations require of any form of health record. **Admissibility** refers to the fact that health records are business records. Because business records are a compilation of many different persons' recordings, they are hearsay. Although there is some variation in how states treat business records, all have some way to except the hearsay rule and allow the records to be used in court. In general, a record custodian must testify that the record was compiled in the normal course of business. This is as true in an electronic world as a paper or hybrid world.

- *Evidence* refers to the matter of producing the original or other readable output of a record placed into evidence in court. Microfilm or any other form of miniaturization or electronic storage are deemed equivalent to the original by most courts today. What may dismay some who would produce a paper copy of an EHR for court is that the EHR may not look exactly like the paper copy did in the past, or may need to be generated from multiple locations. As a result, some hospitals continue to print all documentation from source systems and then scan that material back into an electronically accessible EDMS. Although this is not necessary from a legal perspective, each hospital should evaluate all factors to determine a best practice for its own environment. A completely paperless record all contained in one location can be very convenient. However, many physicians do not like accessing scanned documents and so may prefer to access original results from the source systems. Alternatively, they may do neither in the hospital, relying on staff to print out what is needed from whatever source in which it resides or relying on a discharge summary as a means to review previous admission data for a readmission.

  It also must be remembered that the EHR is more than a paper chart because it provides clinical decision support, access to knowledge bases, and other utility not provided by its paper parents. There is still controversy surrounding just exactly where the "record" ends and other functionality begins. AHIMA's concept of the legal health record may serve as guide for preparing the record for court. It is a good idea for each organization to have its own policy and procedure to support this process, which is likely to change several times along the migration path to the EHR (AHIMA 2005; Servais 2008).

- *Discoverability* is another important concept. **E-Discovery** refers to Amendments to Federal Rules of Civil Procedure and Uniform Rules Relating to Discovery of Electronically Stored Information, which many states are also adopting. Although a healthcare organization may carefully produce such screen shots or reports from the EHR or even a mix of such along with paper copies from a hybrid record that it believes represents the "legal record," there may be other components, especially in the EHR, that could still be discovered and required, through a court order, to be brought to court. For example, an EHR's metadata, audit trails, decision support rules, clinical practice guidelines from which templates are developed, and other such information may be subject to discovery. E-discovery is also not limited to information associated with the EHR, as all records of how information systems in general are maintained may be subject to discovery. For example, a case settled out of court rested on the fact that the hospital could not produce evidence, such as a maintenance log, of a claimed crash of its dictation server that was associated with potential spoliation of evidence.

Overcoming Clinician Resistance

Although health records are certainly maintained for legal purposes, the primary purpose of maintaining health records is to support patient care. Key to EHR success, then, is that clinicians use the records directly in the course of providing patient care. At the risk of oversimplification, overcoming clinician resistance to this new technology involves two strategies. The first is to engage clinicians in the process from conception through benefits realization, and the second is to effect change in their health record use and documentation such that the EHR becomes more comfortable and trusted than the paper chart. (See figure 3.2.) Clearly, both represent huge challenges.

Recognizing Similarities and Differences

Differences exist in the settings in which physicians and other healthcare clinicians and professionals use the EHR. These settings must be considered when applying the two strategies for overcoming resistance to the new technology.

Physicians may view the EHR in their office differently from the way they view it in the hospital in which they have medical staff privileges. In the office, the physicians are the primary decision makers regarding when an EHR is implemented and how it is used. Although the majority may rule in a large office or group practice where pockets of resistance may still exist, by and large such a setting can offer more direct involvement in decision making and design as well as more direct benefits to the physician. However, such groups should recognize that nurses and other staff members also are major users of the system and, as such, should not be left out of the decision-making process. Considerable

Figure 3.2.   Tips and rationale for changing work patterns

Change should not occur solely for the sake of change.
But if current methods and processes are burdensome, error prone, or do not advance organizational goals, they warrant evaluation and potential change.
When making a major investment where significant benefits are expected, something must change to achieve those benefits.
EHRs support a number of inherent benefits, such as legibility of entries and access to data by multiple people at multiple locations. Even greater benefits are in store for those who use EHRs to help them make changes that support those benefits.

resentment can build up when nurses or other clinicians are expected to adapt rather than adopt. Administrative functions should not be negatively impacted by the system. Physicians may be interested primarily in their user interface, screen customizability, and other data use and documentation issues, but they will be unhappy in the end if the office cannot function properly and the revenue cycle is affected.

For physicians to use the EHR in the hospital, they need to be involved in system selection and design as well as accompanying process improvements and workflow changes. The EHR is predicated on capturing data at the point of care, thereby immediately supporting caregiver decision making. A system that does not include physician use in its design may be a bridge to further information system development, but it is not a comprehensive EHR.

Without a clear vision of the future and a migration path toward that end, interim systems may turn into temporary systems that last forever. If such systems are designed initially not to support physician use, and later the expectation is for physicians to use them, they will have less chance of success. The reason is that the designers will not have paid attention to the two primary ways to gain physician support, which are to engage the physicians in the decision making and to help them effect change in their processes and workflow.

Gaining Clinician Involvement

Of the two primary strategies for overcoming clinician resistance, gaining clinician involvement is key to managing change. Although engaging clinicians in developing a vision and making a selection may take more time up front, the time will be well spent. The time is as useful for educating clinicians about what an EHR is, how it can be achieved, and the functionality it offers as it is for obtaining clinician input.

Just as clinicians are expected to be the primary users, they also should be the primary drivers. This is not to suggest that they may not need their involvement facilitated and supported or that they are the only voice, but if they detect that their participation is only superficial, it will be lost. Some specific steps to managing clinician involvement include:

- *Seek active involvement of all types of clinicians and create teams that are both focused and cross-cutting.* In many cases, physicians need and want to work separately from other clinicians. Even certain physician specialty groups may need to work independently of others. This can be equally true for nurses, therapists, pharmacists, and others who must use and document in the EHR. However, healthcare is a team process, and eventually these focused teams need to interact with one another to ensure that their interactive practice needs are addressed.

- *Recognize that time is perhaps the most precious commodity any clinician has.* Clinician input will best be gained when support personnel truly provide support for the EHR project, making the time clinicians spend highly focused on key issues. An important factor in getting voluntary involvement is the history of the organization's culture. An organizational culture that has not been one of team decision making and involvement may need to be overcome before true involvement can be achieved. It may be necessary to place authority for the EHR project with the executive most open to such a process or to use a formally appointed project manager. However, whoever heads up the project must have the authority to be effective, have strong project management and communication skills, and clear lines of communication to executive management. As the process unfolds, and if it is highly effective, willingness to participate will likely occur even beyond the minimum.

- *Engage sufficient numbers of clinicians so that all points of view are represented (the inherent educational process is also spread to all).* It is good to have clinician champions, but if they are viewed as not representative of mainstream interests, other clinicians will not participate. One provider with an exemplary EHR implementation has suggested that an effort be made to solicit the curmudgeons whose passion for negativity can be turned into passion for optimism.

- *Compensate clinicians for their participation.* The jury may be out on the extent to which clinicians should be compensated or cajoled for their participation. Mealtime meetings are popular among physicians. However, if the expectation is to gain full cooperation from all clinicians and others are asked to take their mealtime to participate as well, it seems appropriate to provide the meal. If certain clinicians are expected to have extensive involvement, it will be necessary to evaluate a partial or temporary reassignment of their duties, and for physicians, some direct compensation. It is not uncommon for organizations to hire a medical director of information systems (MDIS) or a chief medical informatics officer (CMIO), or to compensate the physician project leader(s) for a percentage of his or her time. Medical informaticists, nursing informaticists, and health informaticists may be brought on board to support the project as well. **Informatics** is a field of study in which the use of technology to improve access to and utilization of information is studied. Informaticists help care delivery organizations make better use of EHRs. Still, grassroots involvement will be necessary to achieve overall support. Finally, although appropriate forms of compensation are important, cajoling clinicians can backfire and should be avoided as a tactic to gain participation.

Gaining Clinician Acceptance of Change

As noted in the preceding section, clinician acceptance of change will be smoother when the clinicians are involved in the design from the beginning. However, part of the design will be to overcome resistance to change and part of the implementation will be to gain acceptance of change en masse. Some suggestions for effectively managing change, in addition to encouraging involvement, are discussed in the following subsections.

Determine the Environment's Degree of Readiness

It is important to determine the environment's degree of readiness for EHR change. There will always be some resistance to change, even among the most committed participants. Understanding the extent of exposure to and knowledge of EHR, measuring the degree to which clinicians have experience using an EHR (at another hospital, in their office, or during their training), and learning about expectations and concerns can provide information that will be useful in structuring the participation and implementation processes. However, such information must be carefully interpreted. For example, clinicians experienced in using an EHR may have had a positive or negative experience. If the experience was negative, try to capitalize on the lessons learned and use those individuals to help avoid making the same mistakes. Unrealistic expectations also may have to be tempered. Although EHRs hold great promise, reality must prevail. In fact, some physician office or clinic EHR products are so sophisticated that physicians using them may become frustrated with less at the hospital. Finally, the physician's age is not necessarily an indicator of acceptance. Younger physicians may take their lead from their mentors, feel time pressures more acutely than older, well-established physicians, or be more frustrated with inadequate, older technology.

Establish a Clear Vision and Migration Path

Establishing a clear vision and migration path will require considerable education about what is currently available, how others may overcome some of the current limitations, and what might be possible in the future. Some clinicians may have had minimal exposure to EHR concepts. As difficult as it may seem, some clinicians still have limited exposure to computers in general. Thus, their vision of an EHR may be limited to something that would overcome their most immediate pain points. They may not recognize the full scope of potentiality or appreciate the potential benefits. Management of either the hospital or the office and any vendors they engage or use to showcase their products should be careful to focus on describing benefits that are both personal and organizational. Productivity improvements should help the individual clinician save time and do a better job. Even patient safety, which is a current focus of many EHR projects, may not "sell" well to clinicians if they do not believe in the magnitude of the problem or if they see it as someone else's problem.

Establish Expectations

A vision and a migration path are important for planning. They define the current scope of what can be accomplished and the time period over which a more comprehensive vision can be achieved. Part of visioning is to anticipate benefits and part of laying out the migration path is to prioritize adoption of functionality to achieve those benefits over time. But establishing specific, measurable expectations of benefits is one step beyond the vision and migration path. This process helps achieve a commitment on the part of all participants to making the EHR work. However, just as gaining participation depends heavily on the culture of the organization, expectation setting must be done in an environment of trust and support. The organization must be willing to commit sufficient resources to achieving the specified goals and support users in achieving those goals in a nonpunitive manner. Moreover, expectations must be truly measurable and measured. Vague descriptions and generalities will not provide the **metrics** necessary to really determine whether there has been a change. Not measuring against the metrics will not help define course correction steps that may be necessary to help achieve the goals (Wesner et al. 1995).

The right metrics also must be used to determine that expectations are met. A good example of meeting expectations is the time it takes to enter data into the EHR. The perception is that it takes longer than it does to enter data into the paper record. However, the reality is that the time is variable, depending on the system, whether the data are simple or complex, and the degree of dexterity and comfort the user has with using the system. Some data entry into an information system actually may take 30 to 60 seconds longer than data entry performed via pen and paper, whereas other data entry may take less time than documenting on paper.

Because this perception has been so strong and is so objectionable to users, ways to reduce data-entry time are continuously being sought. Some include improvements in voice and handwriting recognition that would permit data entry at the same speed as a normal conversation. Handheld data-entry devices reduce the time it takes to get to and log on to a workstation. Many different kinds of data processes that permit quick data entry and even data reuse, as appropriate, also are used to reduce data-entry time. Some physician offices are starting to use automated history-taking applications where their patients can submit data via a secure Web portal in advance of a visit or via a kiosk in the waiting room. If structured appropriately, the data entered only need to be validated, saving considerable data-entry time. However, another measure should be factored into the equation. Because the data entered are more complete and legible, the time spent answering phone calls about what was written should be reduced. Add to the complete and legible benefits the result of decision support, and any additional time to manage the data entry at the back end is virtually eliminated. Many suggest that a more appropriate measure be whether the EHR reduces the time clinicians have to stay late to finish charts or the number of interruptions at home by calls about form documentation issues.

Commit the Necessary Funds

The organization must commit the funds needed to achieve the identified goals or cut back on the project and its expectations. When a decision is made to go forward with an EHR, executive management and the board of directors must be committed to supporting it over the long haul. A major disaster may have to result in EHR cutbacks, but routine budget prioritization is unacceptable. A classic example is the case of an organization that decided to invest a large sum of money in an EHR project that was not as effective as it could be because the organization shortchanged itself in the number of workstations deployed. The inadequate number of workstations initially resulted in queues to use them, which eventually went away only because many refused to use the system at all. In another example, a document-imaging EHR system was actually well liked by clinicians, except for the fact that it was constantly experiencing downtime. Because the system was viewed as "bridge" technology to an EHR, full **redundancy** and fail-over measures for the **servers** that ran the system were not considered necessary or made part of the initial implementation.

The old axiom "Do it right or don't do it at all" definitely applies to EHRs. This is not to say that an organization should not start down the path but, rather, that it should be careful about defining its vision, migration path, and expectations.

Addressing Patient and Healthcare Consumer Issues

Gaining acceptance and use by those who are the subject of the EHR is a growing issue in addition to clinician acceptance and use, which actually is diminishing, especially in communities where there are younger physicians who have trained at locations with EHRs. Even though many healthcare consumers want greater access to providers and to health information in general, and many have access to and use the Internet and e-mail, they still have a number of issues regarding the privacy and security of health information.

Figure 3.3. Consumer Awareness and Perceptions of EHRs

Findings	2008	2007 (Where available)
Number of respondents who have gone online to learn about a medical condition	65%	Not available
Respondents who have used their insurance company's online tools to learn about their care	38%	29%
Respondents who have "seen, read, or heard about electronic medical records"	57%	43%
Respondents who have a preference for doctors who use EHRs	47%	Not available
Respondents who have a preference for insurance companies that employ EHRs	61%	69%
Respondents who believe the value of EHRs outweigh associated risks	61%	73%

Source: Survey Conducted by StrategyOne for Kaiser Permanente, May 8–11, 2008.

One point to clarify is that the individual who is the subject of the EHR may be a patient, a resident, or a client when he or she is consuming healthcare services at a hospital or physician office, in a long-term care facility, or from a home health agency or behavioral healthcare provider. Persons who are healthy and want to document information about their health status also may use an EHR or a personal version of one, referred to as a personal health record (PHR). For purposes of this discussion, the terms *patient* or *healthcare consumer* are used interchangeably to include anyone who is the subject of an EHR in any location.

A second point to clarify is that, although an increasing number of consumers are aware of EHRs and do believe in their value, addressing the issues associated with health information from a consumer perspective is broader than any form of health record. Kaiser Permanente has been conducting nationwide surveys on consumers' awareness and perceptions of EHRs. Figure 3.3 shows the results of their most recent survey conducted in May 2008. George Halvorson, chairman and chief executive officer of the Kaiser Foundation Health Plan observes that "data is a cornerstone tool for transforming care delivery and a critical driver in reforming our nation's healthcare system. Doctors should have access to information about all of their patients all of the time. And patients should be able to take a more active role in tracking and managing their own health information online. But if we do not empower both patients and doctors to use these tools, then their great benefits may not be fully realized." He also called on the healthcare industry to better educate the public about the benefits of EHRs and ensure that all Americans can use EHRs and other digital health management tools with confidence. Other leading healthcare organizations are also following in the footsteps of Kaiser, as Cleveland Clinic's CEO, Dr. Toby Cosgrove, a heart surgeon, recently announced that in addition to providing its PHR system for its patients, it would make patients' entire EHR available to them at all times.

A final issue to clarify is that not all consumers have access to EHRs, electronic PHRs, information from Web sites, or any other form of automated information. This issue has been coined the "digital divide." Although the gap between those who have access and those who do not is narrowing, it will take a long and sustained effort to achieve total access to computers and the Internet, let alone to applications such as EHRs.

As noted, the automation of health information raises privacy and security issues. Many patients appreciate the value of sharing information among their care providers; however, for various reasons others do not want their information to be shared or at least want to control how and when it is shared. A Harris-Interactive poll conducted in 2007 found that as many as 17 percent of all patients (and 21 percent of those in poor health) had withheld information from a provider over privacy and security concerns. (It is for this reason that HIPAA includes standards not only for the ability to share information for treatment, payment, and health-care operations [TPO] purposes among providers without a patient authorization, but also to require verification of the identity and authority of any individual requesting such access and to afford patients the right to request restrictions on who may have access.) Some states have gone further than HIPAA, initiating legislation that would require a consumer to opt in or opt out of HIE services. Consent management has become a major function of newly forming RHIOs and other HIE organizations. Privacy and security issues are also impacting the architecture of HIE services. Many consumers are concerned that a centralized repository would make their PHI less secure, even though a number of security experts in the industry suggest that a centrally managed security system could afford greater protection than relying on different levels of security at each and every organization that connects to an HIE.

Security concerns may be being fueled by the recent enactment in 44 states of legislation requiring notifying individuals whose personal data have been exposed in a security breach and in California, where even more recent laws make it a misdemeanor to negligently disclose confidential health information (AB 211 and SB 541, January 1, 2009). "Personal data" in this case is not just health information, but all forms of personal data, including financial and others. Identity theft is one of the fastest growing crimes in the U.S. and medical identity theft also is becoming a concern.

Healthcare consumers also are concerned about the quality of the information they are able to access on the Internet, although many may not even be aware that they should be concerned. Several organizations have emerged to filter and qualify the information available to consumers on the Internet. The most widely recognized organization is the Health on the Net Foundation. (See figure 3.4.)

Figure 3.4. Health on the Net™

This symbol has become recognized internationally as a symbol that the health information Web site agrees to the HON Code of Conduct for medical and health Web sites and addresses the principles of:

Authority	Justifiability	
Complementarity	Transparency of authorship	
Confidentiality	Transparency of sponsorship	
Attribution	Honesty in advertising and editorial policy	

Source: Health on the Net Foundation 2004. Copyright Health on the Net Foundation. Reprinted with permission. The HON Code is a formal and proper certification.

Addressing Business Challenges

Healthcare faces many business-related challenges, including economic issues, reduced reimbursement, staffing shortages, escalating costs for all aspects of operations, and limited access to capital. Funding an EHR project is a major concern. Historically, EHR projects have taken more time and money than originally budgeted. But just as legal issues are waning and clinician resistance can be overcome, business challenges also are being addressed in many ways. Following are three examples:

- *Technological advances are making EHR systems more cost-effective.* However, the lower cost of technology is often offset by the adoption of more complex systems and more comprehensive deployments. On balance, the benefits are still greater with lower-cost technology configured with more expensive complexity. However, to achieve these benefits, implementations must actually work as intended. An interesting scenario frequently happens: The vendor describes a cost savings from a paperless environment, but the organization is unwilling to go paperless and hence is unable to achieve the full benefits expected. Weaning an organization off paper that has always totally relied on paper is a huge challenge. There are legal concerns, researcher hesitancy, and clinician resistance to change. Sometimes fears exist about job loss. Thus, an entire infrastructure may develop over protecting the paper and making it readily available. The same situation is true for other aspects of EHR implementation. The amount of physician dictation commonly increases after an EHR is implemented because dictation is used as a means to avoid key entry of data. Often this is the result of poorly designed screens, lack of sufficient numbers of workstations, or use of cumbersome devices for data entry. Overcoming these issues must be part of the system's design, and management must take a firm position with respect to its **conversion strategy**.

- *Vendors realize they must meet on-time and on-budget commitments.* In their desire to make sales, vendors often used to describe a rosy picture. Now, realizing this strategy is backfiring, many vendors are more realistic about costs and benefits. CCHIT certification has also helped vendors describe their product's functionality with accuracy. Some vendors have even gone further, establishing strict requirements for implementation time lines and staff support the providers must meet in order to receive discounts—recognizing that it is not only product but people, policy, and process within a provider setting that influences successful adoption of an EHR. Unfortunately, not all vendors are able or willing to make such commitments. Some vendors still underestimate the level of effort required to create interfaces, install all components, debug programs, and tailor screens and clinical decision rules, and so on. However, the organization must take an active role in managing this situation. The better educated that management is on the extent of its EHR undertaking, the better able it is to ensure that the vendor has anticipated all the organization's requirements in terms of price and time line. Moreover, management must ensure that the team managing the project has clearly articulated its vision, migration plans, and expectations to the vendor.

- *Providers are finding innovative ways to fund an EHR.* For example, the organization might tie the EHR project to another capital project, such as a new center of excellence, new construction, or a merger or acquisition. In some cases, funding for an EHR may be considered a component of the larger project for which bonds have been issued. Another way to justify the use of capital funds might be to link the EHR to major projects such as HIPAA requirements (perhaps as an updated claim standard [ASC X12 5010] may introduce ICD-10-CM), managed care–contracting incentives, or changing standards from The Joint Commission. In other cases, an application service provider (ASP) may be a solution, where the extent of capital funds required is not as great and the cost of the EHR is borne through operations. This tends to be more popular for physician offices or for hospitals that use **outsourcing** for their information technology support.

- *Other potential sources of funding include private or public grants, especially when linked to the formation of an HIE organization.* A number of federal grants have been available from the Agency for Healthcare Research and Quality (AHRQ) and Health Resources and Services Administration (HRSA) and states also are starting to create e-health initiatives that afford funding, low-cost or no-cost loans, or incentives. Additionally, private foundations sometimes support a portion of EHR implementation if it represents a unique process or special area of interest to them. There might be opportunities to pair up with health plans, employers, or other related entities where there would be mutual benefit. Health plans have started giving providers e-prescribing systems that promote patient safety and reduced cost of drugs when used to prescribe fewer brand name drugs. Previously mentioned as a potential sources of funds include the safe harbors and exceptions to the Stark Law and Anti-Kickback Statute that were promulgated by the Centers for Medicare and Medicaid Services (CMS) and Office of Inspector General (OIG), respectively, where hospitals may be able to donate e-prescribing and EHR arrangements. Cooperative arrangements, such as afforded by HIE organizations, may be a potential source of funds, and they are excluded under the Stark Law and Anti-Kickback Statute.

Involving the Organization's Leadership

Throughout this discussion of the challenges facing EHR implementation has been a common theme—the significant involvement of management. In studying exemplary EHR implementations, an element common to all is the shared conviction, starting at the top of the organization, that healthcare is an information business and that executive management involvement and leadership in managing that information is critical to the success of the EHR project.

Executive management in provider settings with exemplary EHR implementations view the EHR with strategic importance and do not subject its implementation to classical cost–benefit or return-on-investment (ROI) analyses. One awardee's chief executive officer (CEO) is known to have likened an EHR to plumbing, a vital infrastructure element that does not have to be separately justified when building a building. Value has not been assumed, however. In fact, exemplary implementations more often than not study the impact, or value, through careful measurement of achievement of goals. Even in one organization established as a research institute where significant EHR studies have been conducted, the chief architect of the EHR indicates there is "unremitting pressure to show value."

Another common theme in organizations with exemplary EHR implementations is that not only does strong executive management commitment exist, but so does continuity of leadership. Despite the varied backgrounds of the EHR project leader, including physicians, informaticists, pharmacists, chief information officers (CIOs), nurse administrators, and system engineers, all demonstrated lengthy tenure with the organization. This is quite unique because the average tenure of many CIOs is just 2 or 3 years.

Some of the results of strong management support have been strong project management, a commitment not to automate what is not working in a manual environment, and sustained investment.

Executive managers also recognize the importance of a customer service and end-user orientation of the project staff and approach. Attention to detail is critical. An understanding of healthcare processes and the information systems that support them is important. But the ability to engage the ultimate users of the systems in design, implementation, and continual feedback is critical to ongoing success.

Another recent and important phenomenon is the leadership roles taken by professional medical societies in promoting the use of information systems. Several medical societies have been issuing all their communications via the Web to encourage their members' use of the Internet. Many have developed instructional materials and provide educational sessions on EHRs, and several participate in EHR standards-setting activities.

Converging toward a Nationwide Health Information Network

Individual provider leadership is essential for successful EHR implementation within an organization. However, federal leadership is seen by many as critical to the overall health of the nation's people. There has been a growing number of federal initiatives and more federal government support for private-sector initiatives for standards setting, through the Healthcare Information Technology Standards Panel (HITSP), state law harmonization through the Health Information Security and Privacy Collaboration (HISPC), product certification (by CCHIT), HIE development, and prototyping and trial implementations of a **nationwide health information network** (NHIN) that would connect HIEs and other special purpose networks together, as a network of networks. In fact, there has been so much activity recently in the area of HIE and NHIN that a new chapter was added to this book in its third edition and has been greatly expanded in this edition to address these projects. (See chapter 18.)

Conclusion

Adoption of EHR systems faces a number of challenges, many of which are being overcome by clinicians themselves and with the support of the key stakeholder in the EHR—the patient. Indeed, bearing the patient in mind as the key stakeholder may help focus a vision and move individual organizations along a migration path that one day may help achieve not only the EHR, but also the vision of the NHIN.

References and Resources

AHIMA e-HIM Work Group on the Legal Health Record. 2005. Update: Guidelines for defining the legal health record for disclosure purposes. *Journal of AHIMA* 76(8):64A–G.

Amatayakul, Margret and M. Cohen. 2008. The legal health record, *ADVANCE for Health Information Executives* 12(7).

American Health Information Management Association. 2002. Practice Brief: Maintaining a legally sound health record. *Journal of AHIMA* 73(8):64A–G.

American Health Information Management Association. 2001. Practice Brief: Definition of the health record for legal purposes. *Journal of AHIMA* 72(9):88A–H.

Assembly Bill 211 adds Cal. Health & Safety Code §§ 130200-130205 and Senate Bill 541 revises Cal. Civil Code § 56.36.

Blasingame, James. 2003 (Mar.). Patients as clinical data entry partners. Presentation at Sixth National HIPAA Summit, Washington, DC.

Cohen, M., and M. Amatayakul. 2003. HIPAA corner: Electronic signatures. *ADVANCE for Health Information Executives* 7(8):16.

Department of Health and Human Services. 2003 (Feb. 20). Final rule: Security standards. *Federal Register*, 45 CFR Parts 160, 162, and 164.

Department of Health and Human Services, Office of Inspector General, 2006 (August 8). Final Rule: Medicare and State Health Care Programs: Fraud and Abuse; Safe Harbors for Certain Electronic Prescribing and Electronic Health Records Arrangements Under the Anti-Kickback Statute. *Federal Register*. 42 CFR Part 1001.

Department of Health and Human Services. Centers for Medicare and Medicaid Services. 2006 (August 8). Final Rule: Medicare Program: Physicians' Referrals to Health Care Entities With Which they Have Financial Relationships, Exceptions for Certain Electronic Prescribing and Electronic Health Records Arrangements. *Federal Register*, 42 CFR Part 411.

Department of Justice, Drug Enforcement Administration. 2008 (June 27). Proposed Rule: Electronic Prescriptions for Controlled Substances. *Federal Register*. 21 CFR Parts 1300, 1304, et al.

HarrisInteractive. Many U.S. Adults Are Satisfied with Use of Their Personal Health Information, March 26, 2007. www.harrisinteractive.com/harris_poll/index.asp?PID=743.

Healthcare poll. 2005 (Oct. 14). *Wall Street Journal*.

Health Data Management. 2003 (Sept. 26). Payers unload MedUnite. www.healthdatamanagement.com.

Health on the Net Foundation. 2004. HON Code of Conduct. www.hon.ch/HONcode/Conduct/html.

iHealth Beat. 2008 (June 20). DEA to Propose Rule to Allow E-Rx of Controlled Substances.

Institute of Medicine. 1997. *The Computer-based Patient Record: An Essential Technology for Health Care,* edited by R.S. Dick, E.B. Steen, and D.E. Detmer. Washington, DC: National Academies Press.

Kingsbury, Kathleen, Medical Mouse Practice, *Time.* 171(24).

Medem's Products and Services for Physicians and Patients. 2004. www.medem.com.

Medicare Prescription Drug, Improvement, and Modernization Act of 2003. P.L. 108–173, enacted 2003 (Dec. 8).

Metzger, J.B., M. Amatayakul, and N. Simpson. 1998. Lessons learned from the Davies program: The first four years. *Fourth Annual Nicholas E. Davies Award Proceedings of the CPR Recognition Symposium, Computer-based Patient Record Institute, Inc. Healthcare Informatics Executive Management Series.* Bethesda, MD: HIMSS.

National Committee on Vital and Health Statistics. 2001. *Information for Health: A Strategy for Building the National Health Information Infrastructure.* www.aspe.os.dhhs.gov/sp/nhii/Documents/NHIIReport2001/default.htm.

National Committee on Vital and Health Statistics. 2005 (Mar. 4). Report to the Secretary on Electronic Prescribing. www.ncvhs.hhs.gov.

National Research Council, Committee on Enhancing the Internet for Health Applications: Technical Requirements and Implementation Strategies. 2000. *Networking Health: Prescriptions for the Internet.* Washington, DC: National Academies Press.

Pulley, John. 2008. EHR Awareness Can Cause Wariness. *Government Health IT.* www.govhealthit.com/online/news/350425-1.html.

Quinsey, Carol Ann. 2004. Developing e-health standards for Web sites. *Journal of AHIMA.* 75(1):56–57.

Servais, Cheryl E. 2008. *The Legal Health Record,* Chicago: AHIMA.

The big payback: 2001 survey shows a health return on investment for Infotech. 2001 (July). *Hospitals & Health Networks.* www.hospitalconnect.com.

The most wired. 2001 (July). *Hospitals & Health Networks.* www.hospitalconnect.com.

Wernick, Alan. Data 2006. Theft and State Law: When Data Breaches Occur, 34 States Require Organizations to Speak Up, *Journal of AHIMA,* 77(10).

Wesner, J.W., et al. 1995. *Winning with Quality.* Reading, MA: Addison-Wesley.

Chapter 4
EHR Project Management: Roles in Design and Implementation

Project management is a carefully planned and organized effort to accomplish a specific mission, such as implementing an electronic health record (EHR) system. Although a **project manager** is often assigned to aid an organization in identifying the myriad tasks required to achieve the project goals and objectives, determining what resources are needed, associating budgets and timelines for completion, and then managing to the project plan, it takes many different people to create an effective EHR. All stakeholder groups must be directly involved. This chapter:

- Identifies the prerequisites for a successful EHR project

- Describes the scope and characteristics of an EHR project

- Identifies human resources requirements, organizational structure, and team building characteristics for a successful project

- Addresses project planning and management techniques useful to an EHR project

- Discusses strategies for change management and the cultural transformation needed for the clinical transformation of an EHR

- Characterizes changes and identifies opportunities for change in information management roles

- Helps an individual assess potential interest in and skills at being a project manager and gaining EHR project involvement

Prerequisites for EHR Success

Virtually every healthcare organization is in some stage of planning for an EHR, if only to recognize some very early steps or bridge strategies. However, whether the organization has started down a migration path toward an EHR or is concerned that an EHR is not feasible, the fact is that an EHR remains in nearly every healthcare organization's vision.

Key Terms

Balanced scorecards	Gantt chart	Project management
Benefits portfolio	Information silo	Project manager
Change control	Issues management	Risk management
Change management	Key performance indicators	SCODF typing model
Critical path		Strategic plan
Dashboards	Milestones	Task
Data analysts	Program (or Project) Evaluation and Review Technology (PERT)	Work breakdown structure
Dependencies		Workflow analysts
Domain teams		
EHR steering committee		

This situation calls for strategic planning wherein the EHR itself is not the goal but, rather, the means to other goals. This approach recognizes the value of the EHR and helps assign appropriate resources for the EHR project.

As a result, executive management, including clinician leadership, must be clear in their understanding and commitment to EHR and carry that message to all users. Hence, the prerequisites to an EHR are planning, executive management support, medical staff ownership, user involvement, and resource allocation.

Planning

Despite the fact that virtually every organization will develop a **strategic plan** that carves out a goal for information technology (IT), such as an EHR, and constructs a separate budget for IT, an EHR project should not be viewed solely as an IT project or be totally isolated as a separate strategic initiative. In fact, it probably should not be viewed, either, as a project, but the start of an ongoing program that requires multiple projects over time. A process that tightly aligns EHR to the organization's corporate strategic initiatives and incorporates it into an ongoing information management program in no way diminishes the importance of the EHR but, rather, places it as an integral feature of virtually every initiative.

Strategic alignment of the EHR also achieves other important goals, including:

- The EHR derives its purpose from benefits expected to be achieved through the various initiatives with which it is aligned. This ensures integration across the organization's initiatives.

- The benefits of the initiatives have been anticipated and potentially quantified; hence, the benefits of the EHR are clearer.

- The initiatives have been appropriately resourced and have the attention of executive management; hence, the EHR receives its share of resources and attention.

Executive Management Support

Support from executive management has been described as the characteristic most commonly found among providers with successful EHRs. EHR projects are long-term, expensive undertakings. Their payback period often extends well beyond the 3 years that most chief executive officers (CEOs) look for in making investments. Clearly, obtaining executive management support is a critical prerequisite to a successful EHR and one that cannot be accomplished overnight. Several factors can influence the level of management support, including:

- Many members of the "C suite," including CEOs, chief financial officers (CFOs), and even chief information officers (CIOs), as well as many members of the board of directors, do not fully understand the concept and purpose of the EHR. In fact, one chief medical officer (CMO) observed that although many of his colleagues understood an EHR at the *intellectual* level, it was not until they would actually use the EHR that they would understand it at the *intestinal* level—that they would fully appreciate the level of change it brought about, not just in documentation or accessing information, but in the way they would practice medicine. Education is a key element in gaining leadership support. Educating executive management entails building trust and benchmarking. It may be necessary to find multiple venues and multiple supporters over time to persuade leaders that an EHR is an appropriate undertaking that will support the organization's corporate strategic initiatives.

- CEOs may legitimately question whether the medical staff will use an EHR to achieve maximum benefit. Providing benchmark data on physician use in other organizations can be helpful. (However, the organizations must be comparable. An organization that has many house staff or hospitalists is not the same as one whose physicians are primarily community based.) Even more critical is gaining the direct support of the organization's medical staff in planning and implementing activities.

- CEOs become more comfortable supporting an EHR project when the organization is able to build a business case for the EHR. However, the business case must be realistic. It is unnecessary to attempt to determine the monetary value of every benefit. The **benefits portfolio** can include both monetary and qualitative benefits, but qualitative benefits must be quantified in order to be supported.

Medical Staff Ownership

Medical staff ownership is essential in adopting the EHR. Executive management must support the EHR to provide the appropriate resources and demonstrate its importance to the organization, but the medical staff will be one of its primary users. One important reason that EHR systems have not been adopted as widely as desired is that physicians have not valued information in the same way that persons in other industries have valued it.

For example, pilots will not fly planes without information about weather, load, and other key factors. On the other hand, physicians have been taught to at least initiate emergency treatment for a patient without any information other than what is available from rapid obser-vation. Even in nonemergency situations and with a complete health record, physicians tend to rely on their powers of questioning and observation to reach diagnostic and therapeutic decisions. It is a rare physician who does not ask a new patient, or one not seen for some time, questions that are already answered in the health record. Unfortunately, such an approach takes time, relies on the probability of matching responses to recalled knowledge, and sometimes causes patients to doubt their physicians' knowledge and judgment. This is often explained by physicians as concerns about others' data collection abilities, the age of the information (and therefore potential changes), or reasons for the patient to have been confused or even less than completely truthful. These are certainly legitimate reasons for reviewing the data with the patient, but not necessarily the need to reenter the data or to act as though they do not exist unless there is a compelling reason to do so. Sometimes it is the perceived need to document that the information was reviewed with the patient that causes this requestioning. An EHR, however, could track the viewing of this information or prepopulate new entries for validation. This is just a different process that needs to be used to reduce the data-entry burden.

Today's healthcare environment is truly information based, and members of the medi-cal staff are coming to that realization and recognizing better ways to use information. Again, education and communication with the medical staff are critical to helping them identify the benefit of such changes and to gain their support.

Physician Champion

Another important ingredient in a successful EHR project is the physician champion. The phy-sician champion must understand **change management** and be willing to apply change man-agement techniques with colleagues who may be less inclined to support an EHR project.

In their zeal to promote EHR systems, some physician champions have been viewed more as mavericks out of touch with reality than as true leaders seeking to improve the lot of their colleagues. In such a case, it is best to cultivate other physicians in successful leadership roles to become champions in their own right and so support (and temper) the maverick champion. This may require a heart-to-heart talk with potential physician cham-pion candidates or with someone who can influence potential candidates to persuade them that there is safety in numbers. The more physicians behind an EHR, the more likely others will become involved.

User Involvement

User involvement from the start is another prerequisite of successful EHR projects. Users include the full spectrum of clinicians as well as administrative, financial, and other per-sons who rely on the health record to carry out their responsibilities. Examples of such functions include assessing quality of care, managing healthcare risk issues, providing patients access to services (scheduling, registration, wayfinding), obtaining reimbursement (eligibility verification, coding, billing), identifying potential product lines for the organi-zation, and many other functions.

User involvement in EHR planning does not mean simply a committee composed of selected potential users but, rather, a groundswell of users who are seriously interested in EHR implementation. Again, as with executive management commitment, a groundswell of user interest does not happen suddenly. Much peer work must be undertaken to develop a climate of interest in the user community. Much has been written about gaining physician support, but the EHR has a huge impact on nurses and others. Nurses adopting an electronic medication administration record (EMAR) implementation may need coaching with respect to process improvement and communication with patients. Without such coaching, nurses have reportedly found all sorts of ways to work around perceived problems with bar-coded medication administration, only creating new work for themselves and not really ensuring the "five rights" for safe medication administration (right patient, right drug, right time, right dose, right route). It may seem surprising how limited many users are in their knowledge of computers in general, let alone EHR systems. If these users have no reason to use a computer on the job now, it is unlikely they have had much other experience. Some potential users, for example, will comment that their children have more experience than they do. The most common misperceptions frequently result in clinicians tuning out information about EHR features, functions, and benefits. The following example illustrates this point:

> A physician in a clinic had heard that EHR systems often generated significant revenue by making it more efficient to conduct clinical trials. It was explained that patient candidates for clinical trials could be selected at the time the physician entered visit notes. This would decrease the nursing time required to review records for potential candidates, improve candidate participation because the physician could answer questions directly and immediately, and, ultimately, increase the number of participants in clinical trials. When asked how physicians would keep track of the criteria and then match them to the visit notes, it became apparent that the physician did not know how this was done. Obviously, the physician had never seen an EHR system with alerts triggered from embedded rules. Interestingly, after this was explained, the physician identified an entire set of desired activities and became "hooked" on the concept of the EHR.

Users need to understand they are not being replaced or necessarily expected to "do more work" but, rather, that the system will enhance their ability to deliver high-quality, cost-effective services. An EHR that saves 1 hour per day of nursing time is not going to result in the loss of a job or lowered pay but, instead, will free nurses to spend their time providing better patient care and patient instruction. When computerized provider order entry (CPOE) systems first became available, pharmacists expressed concern that they might lose their jobs. However, CPOE systems have only enhanced the pharmacist's job. Physicians who frequently dictate records after hours or on weekends will find that the EHR gives them more time to spend with their families or to pursue other interests. A fully automated health record may permit a coder to work from home. Even the stress of a job can be somewhat relieved by an EHR. An enterprisewide master person index (EMPI) can help assure registrars that they are not overlooking existing records and registering a person twice.

One way to help educate users is to distribute literature and demonstration disks, inform users of Web sites with demonstrations, or schedule a series of EHR product demonstrations so that users can begin to learn about the systems. Many larger organizations like to take contingencies of users to trade shows where it is easy to gain an overall understanding of system potential. When these activities are performed as an educational activity, however, care should be taken to communicate to both users and vendors that this is not a selection process.

One-on-one networking may be necessary to identify and address each person's fears and hot buttons. Physicians, especially, do not like to appear uninformed within their peer group. One EHR implementer observed, "you cannot overcommunicate." Multiple, short meetings with key naysayers may clarify issues that can turn them around to support of an EHR.

The result of an educational process will be a better-informed set of users who are not only more interested in pursuing an EHR project, but also who are better able to contribute to informed decision making about the type of product to purchase and how it can best be implemented.

Resources

A final major prerequisite for EHR success is appropriate and sustained resources for which there is accountability. Clearly, one major resource is funding and several innovative ideas for funding an EHR project were identified in chapter 3. However, resources also include people, policies, and processes.

Project managers, physician champions, informaticists, health information management (HIM) professionals, IT support personnel, other clinician users, and many others are all necessary to achieve success. In addition to the time commitment, people with the appropriate skills for the various jobs must be available. When the healthcare organization does not have people with the right skills, it may have to bring special expertise in-house by either hiring people with certain skills (many of which will be needed long term) or bringing in consultants for temporary, specialized assignments. When bringing in consultants, however, someone in the organization should learn about the tasks being performed. This is important for oversight purposes as well as to ensure ongoing continuity of processes.

Alternatively, an organization may decide to train certain staff members who demonstrate interest and related skills. Organizations should be aware that their staff members might have expertise the organizations are unaware of. For example, an engineer may be studying wireless technology unrelated to the job. HIM professionals may be tapped as **data analysts** and **workflow analysts**. Protective services personnel are greatly enhancing their information security knowledge and expertise. Using the knowledge and skills of internal staff can be especially rewarding for the staff members, although care must be taken not to overburden them with new responsibilities. Many organizations find that such responsibilities evolve into new, full-time jobs. It is also important to recognize one other caveat—now that an organization has trained staff in new responsibilities, the staff may be lured away by other care delivery organizations or vendors, so training may be supplied with employment agreements that require new trainees to stay on the job or repay the cost of their training.

Organizations also should establish and enforce clear policies and business rules. It is one thing to be creative and innovative, but it is clearly inappropriate to jeopardize a project or the organization itself by stepping out of applicable standards of practice. Policies may include anything from requiring use of standards recognized by the federal government where they exist for IT applications to using standard medical vocabulary, formulary, or practice guidelines. Business rules dictate how an organization will carry out its functions. For example, one organization implementing the HIPAA transactions and code set standards had a business rule that it would not seek copayments in advance of providing services. Although many organizations see the HIPAA eligibility verification process as one way to enhance their collection process, this particular hospital viewed it as a way to plan financial counseling for patients after care services had been delivered. Business rules also encompass determining who can access patient-specific information, what level of signature is required on an order, the content to include in a history and physical exam, the required components for a medication order, and many other issues that must be addressed in an EHR.

Finally, well-defined projects and system development life cycle (SDLC) processes should be utilized. A disciplined approach to managing the project and steps needed to see systems through their life cycle from conception, through planning, selection, acquisition, installation, testing, training, and implementation, to ongoing maintenance, upgrading, and enhancements will help ensure that the EHR is implemented on time, within budget, and in the most effective manner.

In addition to finding the people to provide project management as noted earlier, the processes themselves must be agreed on and adhered to. Some people are uncomfortable following a formal process or uneasy requiring others to follow formal structures. Time and again, however, projects waste time and cause frustration because formal processes are not in place. When everyone recognizes that formal project management processes are valuable, there will be no turning back.

EHR Project Scope and Characteristics

The characteristics of most projects, in general, are that they:

- Have a defined beginning and end, usually follow a standard SDLC, and have a defined budget

- Are a line function, though with special staffing often through volunteerism from many parts of an organization

- Concern something new and therefore involve uncertainty and change

- Require great attention to detail, while maintaining the ability to see the big picture

Most EHR projects have these characteristics, except for the first. This is not to suggest that an EHR project should not be completed on time, standardized, or held accountable to a budget; however, most EHR projects follow a spiral life cycle that, in reality, never ends, as many new components and modules are implemented over potentially many years. In addition, the EHR requires ongoing maintenance, as the EHR will change as the practice of medicine and health services change. Because of the complexity of an EHR, each new upgrade or maintenance requirement may be considered a miniproject in its own right.

While recognizing that the EHR becomes an ongoing program is important to ensure that it is properly maintained, the programmatic nature can also be problematic. Sometimes the result is lack of project-type accountability for a budget, with overexpenditures and

Table 4.1.   Project vs. program

	Project	Program
Activities	Many short, performed once	Variable, performed repetitively
Sequence	Defined pathway	Repetitive
Connectivity	Dependencies among activities	Independent or possible pass-off
Purpose	Single, well-defined goal	General objectives
Time	Defined start/end, intense pressure	Ongoing, pressure ebbs and flows
Money	Fixed costs avoid overruns	Budget, focus on profit and loss
Specification	Vision	Mission
Scope	Boundaries of project	Limitations of authority/responsibility
Quality	Continual assurance tests	Quality improvement projects
Resources	Variable, multidisciplinary	Dedicated
Organization	Matrix	Line and staff

a difficult-to-calculate return on investment. Another issue is that when an EHR project becomes a program composed of a series of projects, the repetition of performance typical of any programmatic work can set in and result in a lack of focus on milestones and completion of each of the components of the project. As an example, this happened to an academic medical center implementing an EHR in each of a dozen or so clinics. It found that after implementing about half of the clinics, everyone seemed to lose interest. The result was that the remaining clinics did not get implemented, and in those that were implemented, over half had virtually no utilization by physicians because no one considered it a project on which to conduct follow up or return on investment analysis. Table 4.1 lists the differences between a project and a program.

EHR Project Management Resources

Most projects follow a fairly standard pattern of human resource allocation. There is a project manager who typically reports to a project sponsor. However, many other individuals are involved in carrying out the work of the project, with the project manager providing oversight, facilitation, and coordination. Some of the individuals work for the organization in other capacities and also work on the project because they either have been assigned to do so or have volunteered to help. These often become members of the **EHR steering committee** or other subcommittees or **domain teams**, which are groups of people that work on special aspects of the project. Other individuals may be hired as new employees to help implement and maintain the project, or may be temporary employees or consultants primarily available to help during implementation and go-live.

EHR Project Organizational Structure

Most hospitals will construct a fairly structured organization to undertake their EHR project. This includes an EHR steering committee composed of all stakeholders that will guide the process of visioning and product selection, at a minimum, and often are involved in high-level implementation activities. This steering committee may be aided by subcommittees and/or domain teams that focus on specific aspects of the project and report back to the steering committee. Some organizations not only create such a committee structure, but also assign specific decision-making authority to the structure. This can be helpful because clarity about who can make what decisions improves the chances for the project to stay on task, on time, and on budget.

A steering committee, however, is essentially a "volunteer" group of individuals who carve out time from their normal day to participate or who may be assigned a small number of hours from their routine tasks. As such, a project manager, or even a project management office, is necessary for ongoing coordination and support. This project manager usually resides in a matrix reporting structure—perhaps reporting to the CIO or chief operating officer (COO), but accountable to the EHR steering committee and its executive sponsor, who may well be the CMO or vice president of patient care services.

EHR Steering Committee

Although an **EHR steering committee** may go by different names, virtually every organization that undertakes an EHR project forms a steering committee of some type to initiate the project and gain representation from all stakeholders in product selection and implementation. In some organizations, the steering committee is composed of senior managers or even executives. In this case, there will be a number of specific domain teams. Although it is advantageous to have executive management engaged in the EHR project, their myriad commitments may make it difficult to attend meetings and substitutes may not be given the same level of authority to make decisions. The result is often delays in making forward progress. In addition, the domain teams that form to do the nuts and bolts work are then often homogeneous and continue the **information silo** effect that an EHR is intended to overcome. Another, often better, way to lend executive support is for an executive sponsor to be committed to the EHR steering committee that is composed of more representative users. The composition of such an EHR steering committee is described in Table 4.2, with some variation based on the size and type of organization. Subcommittees or domain teams may still be needed in this structure because of the volume of work. Some of these may focus on nursing, physician, or other specific clinician interests, but where feasible should focus on interrelated sets of functions such as medication management, care planning, or quality improvement. During the vendor selection process, there may be a small group that reviews technology and another that studies the cost effectiveness of the products; there may be a large group that reviews demos and a small group that goes on a site visit. All such groups, however, need to either come together as the steering committee or provide representatives to the steering committee on a regular basis.

Table 4.2. Composition of the EHR steering committee

Members	Purpose
EHR Project Manager	Provides EHR project direction and support
User Representatives (from major functional and business units, including their informaticists, as well as Medical Staff, Research, Quality Improvement, and other major clinical data users or suppliers)	Understands current data requirements and work flows, evaluates functionality of new systems and ability to implement new work flows and processes, gains buy-in for EHR adoption
IT Professionals (e.g., Applications, Operations, Network, Telecommunications)	Understands and evaluates technical capability of current and proposed systems and level of "fit"
HIM Professionals	Perform data analysis, ensure data quality, support operations and data flow, oversee data sets, act as data brokers
Internal Consultants (as needed, e.g., financial analyst, contracts manager, human resources, labor relations, legal, etc.)	Provide probability and criticality estimation, offer ways to implement controls, represent customer interests
Trainers	Gain insight into creating training and programs
Corporate Compliance Official Information Privacy Official Information Security Official	Coordinates with compliance activities
Executive Sponsor	Represents executive management, can help interpret message for executive management

EHR Project Manager

A **project manager** supports the steering committee and is responsible for overseeing that all aspects of the EHR project are completed. A project manager requires skills much like a general contractor for a building project. A general contractor hires the mason, plumber, electrician, painter, and so on. He or she may not be technically skilled in any one of these roles but can read a blueprint and understands the skills needed to perform each role. Thus, the general contractor knows when to bring an individual on board to perform a particular job and how to evaluate the end product.

Like a general contractor, the EHR project manager should have a good understanding of what an EHR is, have some healthcare background, and have knowledge of project management tools and techniques. Above all, however, the project manager should have strong leadership skills to work with many different people, provide compelling direction, build trust, manage conflict, and use influence to get things done (Doll 2005).

Frenette (2003) suggests that a project manager needs to possess "extra magic" to accomplish the project goals. Many are beginning to recognize that an EHR is not a typical IT project and that IT skills or even strong technical project management skills are less important to the EHR project manager role than vision and leadership. The projects are sufficiently large in scope that IT skills, ability to use project management software, and even clinical knowledge can all be achieved by the team members the project manager leads.

Table 4.3.   EHR project manager checklist

❏ **Are you entrepreneurial? Do you care what's next?**
(If a project should have a defined end, that may also mean an end to the job, or at least a shift to a different project. Some people thrive on such constant change; others prefer a more stable environment.)

❏ **Do you generally get tasks done on time?**
(Some individuals always are procrastinators, have "hope creep" where they believe they can get the work done even though they cannot, or have "effort creep" where they are working very hard but not producing the desired work. A proven track record of getting project done early or on time—and correct—is essential.)

❏ **Do people respond well to your requests?**
(An internal candidate for EHR project manager sometimes carries "baggage" that is difficult for others to see past. If you are viewed as a nag, servant, geek, or having other negative characteristics, these may be difficult to overcome even with the best of skills. In addition, because the project manager does not have line authority over the members of the project team, influence must be used to get team members to complete tasks they agree to undertake.)

❏ **Do you like to share the spotlight?**
(An EHR project requires a team effort. While the project manager should get credit for a job well done, others must also be recognized. The chair of the EHR steering committee, for example, may have the spotlight while the project manager is the force behind the scenes.)

❏ **Are you comfortable communicating with all?**
(Individuals with limited experience in communicating to large groups, persons with authority, or highly technical individuals may find it difficult to be as assertive in communications as necessary. A project manager must be able to build trust and interpersonal relationships to achieve project goals.)

❏ **Do you see "all sides"? Value opposing viewpoints?**
(A project manager needs to be able to present alternatives clearly and without bias, but also to steer a group to make unbiased and objectives decisions. If you carry personal biases or always play devil's advocate, it may be more difficult for you to be neutral.)

❏ **Are you a diplomatic "straight-shooter"?**
(In some cases, a project manager must convey bad news or take tough stands in order to move the project along. This must be done, but done with diplomacy or respect can be quickly lost.)

❏ **Do you see the big picture, while attending to detail?**
(EHR projects can include hundreds if not thousands of tasks, many of which have dependencies and all of which must be managed. However, the project manager must also motivate the team to keep it moving forward and be mindful of the overall project purpose and goals.)

❏ **Are you comfortable with change?**
(A project manager will face not only the end of the project as a change, but must be able to help others with process improvement and a truly clinical transformation that brings enormous change to users.)

❏ **Do you delegate appropriately?**
(A project manager must delegate the work of the project to individuals who have the knowledge and skills to perform the work. Taking on tasks others can and should perform leaves the project manager with no time to manage the project.)

Table 4.3 provides a checklist to help you evaluate a project manager's potential. For those aspiring to become an EHR project manager, figure 4.1 may be a useful tool. Likewise, a sample project manager job description is provided in figure 4.2.

Figure 4.1.   HIM checklist for EHR project involvement

I. Make yourself an expert.
  A. Keep up to date. Scan as many health information management and systems trade publications as possible. (See references at the end of the chapters for suggestions of resources.) Review Web sites for trade publications you do not get in hard copy. Monitor government and association Web sites for news and information. At a minimum, keeping up to date should include keeping track of revisions in the following types of materials:
    1. Standards (for example, ASTM E31 standards for security, EHR content, and EHR system functionality)
    2. Regulations (for example, HIPAA administrative simplification rules)
    3. Accrediting agency requirements (for example, The Joint Commission's ORYX requirements and NCQA HEDIS requirements)
    4. Applications (for example, Web-based messaging systems and voice recognition correction systems)
    5. Market conditions (for example, current events on Wall Street)
  B. Acquire some new basic skills. For some skills, you may want to take a class or attend a seminar; for others, you may be able to do some formal independent study or literature review. You may even consider acquiring an advanced degree, such as in health informatics. Here are some examples of new skills that are easy to obtain on your own:
    1. Internet research
    2. Project management
    3. Development of use cases
  C. Develop an understanding of information technology. It is not necessary to become a technological wizard. But just as you learned the language of medicine, you need to speak some of the technology language if you are to become the liaison among disparate members of your healthcare community. For example:
    1. Clip and file articles to use when called on for special expertise. You never know when you will be asked to lead the effort in developing a data dictionary or to explain the differences among a data repository, a data warehouse, and a data mart.
    2. Ask questions of your IS staff and others. (A well-placed question does not make you look less informed but, rather, triggers a relationship with the other person, who might ask you a question within your expertise.)
    3. Compile a set of glossaries. These are everywhere and are designed for various knowledge levels. Everyone is trying to learn as much as possible about new technology because it affects everyone's life. Glossaries are invaluable as you begin to learn your new language.
  D. Initiate required changes brought about by new regulations or new technology. To be prepared, address changes before required deadlines or implementations. Changes may be required for:
    1. Bylaws (for example, on updating signature requirements to incorporate digital signatures)
    2. Procedures (for example, for changing passwords)
    3. Systems (for example, for new identifiers required under HIPAA regulations)
  E. Learn about other types of organizations and how they must manage information in order to extend your expertise across the IDS. You may be called on to assist various other entities and will need to know:
    1. What physician practice management systems are
    2. How home health agencies operate
    3. With what requirements nursing homes must currently comply
    4. What reporting requirements corporate headquarters are imposing
    5. How data flow to external databases
    6. How nursing documentation systems work (or do not work)
    7. What systems can support capitated managed care

(continued)

    F. Monitor the progress of other organizations toward an EHR. Sometimes the most convincing argument for getting the attention of top management is to compare your situation with that of other organizations. Healthcare is a highly competitive environment, and it would not be unheard of for an EHR project to be initiated because the organization "down the street" is thinking about such a project. Keep in touch by:

       1. Calling fellow HIM professionals/former classmates/colleagues in other professions
       2. Becoming involved in local HIM associations, HIMSS, HFMA, and other associations
       3. Scanning trade publications to see what other organizations are doing
       4. Participating in list serves

    G. Come up with your own ideas for becoming an expert:

       1. _____

       2. _____

II. Help others gain expertise.

    A. Identify key individuals, the types of information they need, and the modalities they will use to learn about EHR.

    B. Copy articles (preferably as many as possible from the *Journal of AHIMA*) and highlight key points for physicians in leadership positions, IS staff who have specific knowledge requirements, and selected others who will read and benefit from more than a paragraph of text. You may even want to write a brief summary sentence or note on the copy describing what implications the content has for your organization.

    C. Refer IS professionals or others who are Internet fans to interesting Web sites for information.

    D. Summarize information into a short, "punchy" e-mail message for those who have little time to read. Draw attention to the message by using an intriguing subject line. Avoid giving away the punch line in the subject, however, or you will not get the rest of the message read.

    E. Circulate information about conferences. Sometimes these are useful not for the suggestion of attending the conference but, rather, for getting across the level of attention being placed on a new technology, issue, impending regulation, or the like.

    F. Offer to show videos, conduct demonstrations, provide tapes, or bring guest speakers to meetings, especially when you feel you are not as believable as you would like to be or when pictures are worth more than words. AHIMA has a wide range of multimedia products for use in such situations. Vendors are more than happy to do demonstrations. Keep all such activities relatively short. Make sure there is time to discuss the content.

    G. Benchmark your institution continually against others in your area, state, and category. You may want to maintain a spreadsheet or small database on key competitors and their systems. Apply some market research to gather your intelligence. Report findings as you find something of interest but do not make this a regular part of your reporting because it will get lost in the routine.

III. Make sure you receive credit as the expert.

    A. Write your name, credentials, and department directly on articles you circulate as a permanent reminder of who supplied the article; a separate piece of paper attached to the article can get lost.

    B. Document in a memo to your boss, with appropriate copies, any ideas you have discussed in meetings or informal discussions. This ensures that you will get the credit and provides a second opportunity for visibility. A classic dictum of education is "Tell 'em what you are going to tell 'em, tell 'em, and then tell 'em what you have told them." This holds true for every idea you have that appears to have support. If your idea is not well received, hold it until either you also decide that it is not a good idea or the idea may generate better support. Be wary, however, of people who downplay an idea only to raise it again as their own. If you are in an environment where this might happen, test your idea on colleagues you can trust to get their feedback before you present it at a key meeting. Then, if its value is recognized, document it in such a manner as to remind people that it was your idea.

(continued)

Figure 4.1.   (Continued)

    C. Identify minutes you take, drafts you prepare, and so on as "prepared by." Better yet, have someone else take minutes so that you can be more actively involved. Just be sure your name gets in the minutes as the generator of an idea, contribution, or whatever.

    D. Write articles about your achievements in your department or, when instituting new policies, about meetings you have attended and so on for any communication tool or Web site your organization may have.

    E. Make demonstrable changes in your department. "Show 'em you can do it!"

    F. Change your job description to not only encompass new areas of responsibility, but also broaden your role for today and the future.

IV. Take on volunteer assignments.

    A. Serve on a committee.

    B. Start a committee.

    C. Provide a presentation to a committee you would like to be on.

    D. Start a list serve.

    E. Update the Web site.

    F. Provide a biweekly fact sheet about EHRs.

    G. Do anything that will legitimately promote your knowledge and expertise. However, if you volunteer, you must be prepared to follow through. As with everything else in life, respect is earned. HIM professionals are generally characterized as detail-oriented, well-organized people who follow through. Do not disappoint. One misstep is often worse than no step at all. If you cannot produce as promised for a specific task, delegate it (and give joint credit) or find a replacement (and share credit). It is not necessary to do everything oneself, but it is necessary to assume one's responsibilities.

V. Educate, educate, educate.

    A. Yourself.

    B. Your staff: Your staff needs to learn about EHRs and what you are doing. They need to understand what their future may be like. Also prepare them to take over your routine responsibilities to free yourself to do more of the EHR project support. They need to begin to move into new roles.

    C. Physicians and other caregivers: This is best done one on one. Physicians, more than most other people, do not like to expose their lack of knowledge. A recent survey is a good example. A large physician practice was considering the purchase of an EHR product. To help the practice understand the type of product it wanted, a survey was conducted of physicians, nurses, and other potential users. The survey listed some 30 functions an EHR could perform. In some cases, the functions were conflicting. For example, chart tracking and paperless system were both functions on the list. But chart tracking is an unnecessary function in a paperless environment. Invariably, physicians checked either every possible function or nearly every function. No other annotation was made. However, nurses and other potential users went through the checklist and frequently added a question mark or note indicating they were not certain what a specific function meant. In interviewing physicians after the surveys had been collected, it was found that many who said they wanted all the functions did not know what some of the functions were.

    D. Administration: Not all administrators are knowledgeable about EHR systems. Unless administrators have a specific interest, they will not necessarily have current knowledge of EHR functionality, price, alternatives, and so on.

    E. Vendors: Vendors also need education about your organization's requirements, what the organization is capable of implementing, and its knowledge level of systems. When vendors understand your position, they are better able to help your organization.

(continued)

Figure 4.1.   (Continued)

F. Patients: Although computer savvy varies by community, patients in general are becoming much more computer literate. They expect to find computers managing information on their financial records, school reports, and so on. Moreover, patients seek information on their symptoms and diseases from the Internet. Many physicians find their patients to be more knowledgeable about current treatments of some conditions than they themselves are. Some organizations have begun to collect information directly from patients through secure Web sites or kiosks in physician offices, waiting rooms, and so on. Alternatively, patients are very concerned about the confidentiality and accuracy of their health information. An entire field of consumer health informatics has grown up around the concept of merging consumer health education with patient health information from health records.

EHR Project Manager Skills

The Project Management Institute (PMI) is an organization that provides guidance to those interested in becoming more knowledgeable about project management, perhaps even making it their professional career. The PMI's *Project Management Body of Knowledge* is an important resource for any project manager. It identifies five critical skills for a project manager to possess: leadership, communication, negotiation, problem solving, and influence. As special considerations in communications, one might also add team building and meetings facilitation.

Leadership
Leadership skills involve establishing direction, aligning people, motivating and inspiring people, and building consensus. These skills are distinguished from management knowledge and skills. Management of an EHR project may require general management knowledge of finance and accounting principles; research and development; strategic, tactical, and operational planning; organizational structures, organizational behavior, and personnel administration; work relationships, including motivation, delegation, supervision, team building, and conflict management; and self-direction through time management and stress management. Management of an EHR project also would include knowledge of EHR concepts, although detailed technical skills are not required.

Although the EHR project manager is expected to manage and lead, he or she generally—and ideally—shares the leadership tasks with others. It is hoped that a physician champion, other clinician leaders, executive management leadership (including the CIO), and others who are needed will head up teams and assume responsibility for project tasks.

Communication
Communication involves the ability to convey information in a clear, unambiguous, and complete manner. The schematic in figure 4.3 illustrates the scope of communication requirements for an EHR project manager. The scope is very broad. There are internal and external communications, from communicating specific tasks to, and receiving reports from, team members to potentially preparing media releases with the organization's public relations staff and creating informational materials for patients. The project manager must be as much at ease communicating with peers as with those individuals engaged in specific tasks who may be anywhere within the organization's hierarchy and with executive management

Figure 4.2.   Project manager job description

Position: EHR Project Manager

Reports to: Chief Science Officer

Key Functions and Responsibilities

Integrated Healthcare Information

1. Using an evidence-based approach, facilitate culture of having integrated healthcare information by screening clinical systems for appropriate fit, integration potential, and timing of projects based on EHR architecture. This will be done in partnership with the chief information officer and person(s) championing the specific clinical system.

Electronic Health Record System

2. Direct selection and implementation of EHR components to include:
   a. Enterprisewide master person index
   b. Clinical data repository
   c. Document imaging to include medical (for example, PACS) and administrative images
   d. Physician order-entry and electronic signature capabilities
   e. Patient care documentation
   f. Clinical decision support tools to include:
      (1) Clinical alerts and reminders
      (2) Care management protocols
   g. Other information systems and emerging technology as necessary and feasible

3. Lead breakthrough project team to deliver the following:
   a. Longitudinal record of patient care across the organization's continuum of care sites
   b. Clinician utilization of EHR that facilitates and enhances patient care delivery processes at the point of care and remotely as appropriate
   c. Patient interaction with clinicians, access to their personal health record of care at the organization, and quality education
   d. Tools that facilitate cost-effective care management and respond to a growing number of managed care contracts
   e. Capacity to perform large patient database searches and studies without impacting the performance of the EHR in day-to-day activities
   f. Support for the organization's training and research programs

Business Process Redesign and Information Protection

4. Coordinate reengineering of work flows and patient care documentation with clinical users to leverage and maximize organizational and personal productivity to improve patient care delivery processes.

5. Ensure that systems selected are compliant with all applicable laws, regulations, and standards, and that their storage, retention, authentication, accuracy, and transmission integrity support admissibility.

6. Develop processes for determining who has access to specific health information; how users will be educated, trained, and kept continually aware of patient privacy and security requirements to provide data confidentiality, integrity, and availability; and ensure that ongoing auditing of access is performed and supported by appropriate sanctions and disciplinary processes.

Budgetary/Operational Responsibility

7. Develop and account for operating and capital budgets for above processes.

8. Determine appropriate staffing and resource requirements for the EHR project.

9. Establish appropriate metrics and monitor benefits realization.

Skills/Experience Required:

- Knowledge of health information management and technology, clinical user needs, and healthcare work flow
- Extensive and progressive healthcare management experience
- Experience with the selection and implementation of healthcare information systems
- Ability to enroll and build strong relationships with all levels of management, physicians, and staff
- Ability to lead a project team through uncharted territory, shift paradigms, take risks, and bring ideas from concept to reality
- Relentless focus on outcomes

Adapted from Job Description for Director, Integrated Healthcare Information, Central DuPage Health System, Ann Ogorzalek, RHIA.

Figure 4.3.   Management communication skills

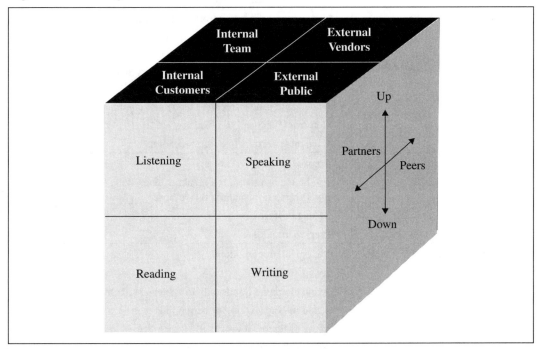

and the board of directors. Written and oral communication skills are a given, but the art of listening and the ability to quickly gain knowledge are possibly even more important.

The project manager must have not only general communication skills, but also the ability to manage project communications. Project communication skills are listed in table 4.4. Effective communications for an EHR project should begin with not only an effective communicator at the helm of the project, but also a communication plan. Figure 13.2 (in chapter 13) provides a sample communication plan for use at the start of an EHR project implementation. Key elements of that plan include a variety of messages, messengers, and media to convey the messages.

Team Building

Team building is an important subset of communication skill. As noted, every EHR project will have a steering committee, and large EHR projects will likely involve several additional teams. Teams also may form and disband as the need arises. Some common teams used in the EHR project are described in table 4.5. For whatever teams may be required in the EHR project, including the steering committee, the ultimate goal is problem solving and decision making to achieve the success of the project. However, good results from teams do not happen automatically. Team building encompasses selecting the right team members and understanding and managing group dynamics:

- *Selecting the right team members:* Organizational culture determines how individuals come to be part of an EHR team. Some organizations simply appoint people

Table 4.4.   Project communication skills

Project Needs	Communication Skills
Instruction	• Select appropriate medium: Oral, e-mail message, informal memo, demonstration, formal procedure. • Use appropriate communication style: Active versus passive voice, sentence structure, word choice, body language.
Feedback	• Understand sender–receiver models of communication. • Construct feedback mechanisms. • Recognize barriers to communication.
Meeting Management	• Prepare agenda. • Facilitate discussion: Ice-breaking, energizing the group, gaining input from all, managing the verbose. • Manage conflict. • Prepare minutes.
Building Consensus	• Be logical, not emotional. • Avoid "win–lose." • Avoid changing minds only to achieve harmony. • Avoid majority voting or bargaining. • Value different views. • View initial agreement as suspect. • When individuals understand and accept the logic of a different point of view, you have reached consensus.
Follow-up	• Select appropriate aids to manage schedules, calendars, and communication among team members. • Select appropriate time frame: Regular, intermittent, key milestones only, based on exception reporting. • Select appropriate medium: Oral, e-mail message, informal memo, formal request. • Document follow-up.
Data Collection	• Determine scope of required data: High-level, detailed; identified; deidentified; quantitative, qualitative; anecdotal, trend, or benchmark. • Select appropriate collection tools: interview, observation, questionnaire, survey.
Reporting	• Understand the audience and scope of required report: Executive-level, general, specific, exception reporting, status reporting. • Select appropriate medium: Oral, written; informal, formal. • Use appropriate presentation techniques: Body language, visual aids, written report binder.

Table 4.5.   Types of EHR teams

Type of Team	Purpose
Steering committee, or project team	Provides oversight and represents the broadest number of stakeholders in the EHR
Vendor selection team	May be a subset of the steering committee or project team, responsible for using the functional specifications and request for proposal (RFP) to narrow down vendor candidates, conduct site visits and reference checks, and make recommendations for approving a vendor of choice with which to begin negotiating a contract
Negotiation team	May be a special team of individuals with experience in large procurements, consultants, and legal counsel who negotiate the contract to acquire the EHR and its components
Implementation team(s)	Responsible for the installation of hardware and software, following domain team specifications for system build and testing
Domain teams, perhaps with names like "nursing IS team," "ancillary services EHR team," "cardiology team," and so on	Provide special expertise and represent direct users in building the system (templates, decision support rules, reports, and so on) to meet specific needs of the organization
Training team and/or super users	May be a separate (existing) group that learns the system well and supports users throughout rollout
Ongoing maintenance team and/or clinical advisory team	May be created as a way to ensure clinical aspects of the EHR are kept up-to-date and ongoing users' concerns are addressed

Copyright © 2008, Margret\A Consulting, LLC. Reprinted with permission.

Figure 4.4.   Myers-Briggs Type Indicator questions

Guiding Question	Types	
Where do you direct your energy?	Outer world (**E**xtroversion)	Inner world (**I**ntroversion)
How do you process information?	Through known facts (**S**ensing)	Through possibilities (i**N**tuition)
How do you make decisions?	On the basis of logic (**T**hinking)	On the basis of personal values (**F**eeling)
How do you organize your life?	In a way that is structured (**J**udgment)	In a way that is flexible (**P**erception)

based on their knowledge, skills, and perceived or expressed interest. Others call for volunteers to form teams and will generally accept anyone who volunteers. For an EHR project, it may be necessary to have some control over team composition, although volunteers can help achieve buy-in that is critical for adoption. During team formation, it is important to consider the personalities of the team members. One well-recognized measure of personality is the Myers-Briggs Type Indicator. The questions in figure 4.4 are used to characterize an individual on four scales (for example, ESTJ), with the result being 16 different personality types.

Sometimes the Myers-Briggs personality typing is too much to introduce into an EHR steering committee or other team. A smaller, more manageable number of characteristics that may help distinguish roles in a group is the **SCODF typing model** (created by the author). This model identifies traits that individuals may have relative to their project contributions. Each SCODF type has both positive and negative characteristics and each person usually displays one predominant trait:

—**S**tarters are those who are anxious to get started, even when planning may not yet have been finalized. Their strength, however, is to push and not let projects languish.

—**C**reators are those who are constantly generating ideas throughout the project, but may never succeed at carrying any of them out. Their strength is to ensure that new ideas do not get lost and to instill innovation in a project.

—**O**verseers are those who promote decision making and delegate well but may be seen as manipulative. Overseers can be natural leaders if they learn to be discerning and diplomatic.

—**D**oers are those who can turn good ideas into reality. They are not innovators, but they are cooperative and get the job assigned to them done.

—**F**inishers are conscientious and deliver on time, but may be too painstaking and anxious to complete the project, potentially putting it at risk for not ensuring that all control points have been tested or new ideas considered. Teams may also need and want advisors, occasionally, who are knowledgeable about a specialty area but do not know or care about the big picture.

Regardless of the professional backgrounds of the team members, it is a good idea to have as broad a mix of personality types as possible on a team.

• *Understanding group norms, managing group dynamics, and valuing diversity:* Understanding personalities may not only ensure that a balanced group is involved but can help individual members relate to each another, manage conflict, and negotiate to achieve consensus. Another important aspect of team building is diversity. Many organizations are beginning to recognize that not only is there diversity within their organization (or not), but that there may be disparity between the diversity that exists in the organization and those served.

Understanding how formal teams work and facilitating this work is also an important task for the project manager. Tuckman (1965) describes five stages of group development (table 4.6) that the project manager may find useful to understand and address as the EHR steering committee forms and starts its work. A common challenge in an EHR steering committee is that, although healthcare delivery requires teamwork, the healthcare team is quite different from a project team. The healthcare team has a specific leader (the physician) who directs other specialists (nurses, therapists, technicians, and so on). Everyone understands the structure of the healthcare team and his or her position in it. The healthcare team does not undergo the stages of team building. In some respects, the fact that healthcare is so dependent

Table 4.6.   Five stages of group development

Stage	Description	Aids to Move to Next Stage
Forming	Stage where personal relations are characterized by dependence on other group members for guidance and direction. Group members desire acceptance by the group and so attempt to keep things simple and avoid controversy.	Formal orientation processes, potentially including "fun" break-the-ice exercises or formal member characterization activities, such as Myers-Briggs personality assessments. Each team member must relinquish the comfort of nonthreatening topics and risk the possibility of conflict
Storming	Stage characterized by competition and conflict in personal relations. Because of fear of exposure or failure, team members seek structural clarification and commitment. Typically some members will become completely silent and others will attempt to dominate.	Group members need to move from a "testing and proving" mentality to a problem-solving mentality. Listening and conflict management techniques are essential. To manage the natural conflict, the project manager needs to be firm about setting goals, communicate frequently, encourage team members to be open and honest about concerns and differences, let team members create something, and emphasize the importance of following project management techniques.
Norming	Stage where group members demonstrate cohesion and are engaged in active acknowledgment of all members' contributions. This is when team members experience trust and the sense of group belonging and even relief as a result of resolving interpersonal conflicts. Data will flow freely and creativity is high.	The major drawback of the norming stage is that members may begin to fear the inevitable future breakup of the group and may resist change as a result. No one will own up to this concern, but the project manager should suspect this is occurring when the group cannot settle down and make decisions. Change management techniques must be employed to get the group to the next stage.
Performing	Stage where the team genuinely solves problems leading toward optimal solutions. In this stage, members can work independently, in subgroups, or as a total group with equal facility. Individual members are self-assured and no longer need group approval but respect other members' contributions.	This is the ultimate goal of team building. Unfortunately, experts report that many groups do not achieve this stage. The project manager must be skilled in advancing the group through the earlier stages as quickly as possible, while recognizing that each stage is unavoidable and must be managed to get to the next stage. Once in the performing stage, however, the project manager must also prepare the team to adjourn.
Adjourning	Stage that terminates the task and members disengage from the group's relationships. Sometimes this creates apprehension and may be regressive.	The most effective interventions in this stage are celebration and recognition. Individual members can also be recruited for ongoing monitoring activities, trainers for new staff, and subsequent projects. However, promises for such activities should only be used when they advance the disengagement process and are real.

Source: Adapted from Tuckman 1965, 384–99, and Tuckman and Jensen 1977, 419–27.

on a specific type of teamwork may make creating effective EHR project teams more difficult. Physicians, who are always in the position to direct, may find themselves in other roles on teams, and those who typically take direction may be called on to direct. Any tools the project manager can use to convey the nature of a project team, how individuals can be valuable and equal members of project teams, and what to expect on a project team can help work the team through the team-building stages.

Some organizations or members of teams find it "uncomfortable" or believe it unnecessary to participate in team-building activities, especially where they may be required to adhere to a special methodology, game playing, or other activity with which they are unaccustomed. Instead of avoiding the activities and missing their value, however, team leaders should find ways to overcome concerns. Team members uncomfortable with such activities may find it even more difficult to change processes and adopt new technology.

Managing Meetings

With teams generally comes the requirement for meetings. Meetings are both the most universal part of work life and the most despised part of work life. So many meetings are unproductive that individuals who may make great team members and have significant contributions to make to an EHR project may be reluctant to volunteer or agree to participate simply because they do not want yet another set of meetings to attend. Even despite new collaboration software that allows communications with many individuals without meetings or to hold virtual meetings, meetings continue to be the primary form of achieving project work. In 1996, Eric Matson wrote a treatise on meetings he called "The Seven Sins of Deadly Meetings." Figure 4.5 provides a summary of these "sins" and their salvations.

Figure 4.5.   The seven sins of deadly meetings and their salvation

Sins	Salvation
1. People don't take meetings seriously. They arrive late, leave early, and spend most of their time doodling.	1. Adopt the mind set that meetings are real work; have an agenda, know your role, and follow the rules for minutes.
2. Meetings are too long. They should accomplish twice as much in half the time.	2. Track the cost of your meetings; use technology for providing feedback.
3. People wander off the topic. Participants spend more time digressing than discussing.	3. Get serious about agendas and store distractions in a "parking lot."
4. Nothing happens once the meeting ends. People don't convert decisions into actions.	4. Convert from "meeting" to "doing" and focus on creating a document.
5. People don't tell the truth. There's plenty of conversation, but not much candor.	5. Consider anonymity through technology—but avoid gamesmanship through facilitation.
6. Meetings are always missing important information, so critical decisions are put off.	6. Get data, not just furniture, into meeting rooms (maybe remove the furniture).
7. Meetings never get better. People make the same mistakes.	7. Monitor meetings and apply quality improvement techniques.

Source: Matson 1996.

Communicating with End Users and Others

In addition to communicating with those actively engaged in the EHR project, building teams, and managing meetings, communicating with the ultimate end users, among many others, is important.

Without communication about the EHR project, potential end users may think they are left in the dark and become concerned for their jobs, sometimes even leaving or taking early retirement, with the organization losing valuable employees. Some important points to bear in mind concerning the ultimate users of the EHR include:

- Engage users in all applicable project phases to the extent possible. This might include period surveying or forming subdomain teams for educational purposes.

- Communicate regularly with users concerning project status and needs through newsletters, posters, and agenda items in standing meetings.

- Listen to potential user needs and concerns; be patient with user reticence and manage the "squeaky wheel."

- Respond actively to user needs and concerns.

- Work with users to develop trust in the system.

Others with whom it is important to communicate (obviously at varying points in the EHR project) include those in the organization who may not become users but who may think they will lose their job or be required to do something for which they are not being prepared, those outside the organization who may have a need to know and from whom the organization may actually gain benefit (for example, suppliers who may be able to link into the new automation capability, malpractice carriers who may be willing to reduce increases in insurance rates, employers who may see opportunities for pay for performance, and so on), and patients. In fact, some organizations are recognizing that clinicians may not fully understand how to communicate with patients while using the new EHR tools. There are now consulting firms that provide training in clinician–patient communications in an electronic environment.

Negotiation

Another skill needed by a project manager is negotiation. Negotiation involves trying to reach consensus on an issue. Consensus is collective judgment or belief, not necessarily 100 percent agreement. Many projects struggle because team members think they must reach absolute agreement from all parties on all issues before proceeding. Because the EHR is a complex project involving many components and stakeholders, reaching a position where at least a majority is comfortable with the direction or accepts a single position is the best that can be achieved.

To achieve consensus, some parties give up something to gain something in return. Negotiation is to be expected in dealing with vendors. When negotiating with external parties, cost is often the primary issue, although scope, schedule, changes, and other terms and conditions are important issues as well. Figure 4.6 illustrates the notion of moving from total agreement, which is generally unattainable, to acceptance by many and thus consensus by all that they are willing to accept the compromises necessary to proceed.

Figure 4.6. Consensus building

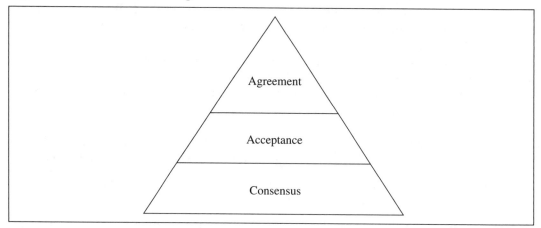

Problem Solving

Problem solving combines problem definition and decision making. Problem definition requires distinguishing symptoms from root causes. Like weeds, problems rarely are resolved by getting rid of the symptoms without addressing the root cause.

Problem definition is rarely easy. It may be necessary to thoroughly study the flow of an operation, conduct various tests on processes, or undertake surveys and analyze results to determine root cause. Decision making includes analyzing the problem to identify viable solutions and then making a choice from among the solutions. Again, this is no easy task. Identifying solutions requires creativity and the willingness to be innovative and inventive. A noncritical setting must be used to identify a potential solution set and then to select the solutions that are most viable. It may even be necessary to develop a prototype or test a process before making a decision.

Selecting the best solution requires attention to that which is most effective. "Effective" means the solution achieves the goals with the fewest resources. Effectiveness is not achieved by applying the most costly measure if a lower-cost solution achieves equal results. Moreover, effectiveness is not achieved when the solution is the lowest cost but only rarely produces the desired results. Project managers must be able to lead their teams in defining the problems and making the best decisions.

Influence

Influencing means the ability to get the job done. Some suggest that this is the "power and politics" of being a project manager. The *Project Management Body of Knowledge* (PMBOK) cites Pfeffer in defining power as "the potential ability to influence behavior, to change the course of events, to overcome resistance, and to get people to do things that they would not otherwise do" (PMI 2000, 26).

Power often has a negative connotation because it suggests asking people to do something illegal, immoral, or inconsistent with their personal beliefs. This should never be the case in an EHR project. Rather, positive power helps people change their behavior patterns in ways they may not have considered before but are for their own and the organization's betterment. In conducting a project, power should never rest with one or a few people. All members of a project team should feel empowered. The *PMBOK* also cites Eccles et al.

Figure 4.7.   Rate of IT project failure in Canadian hospital survey

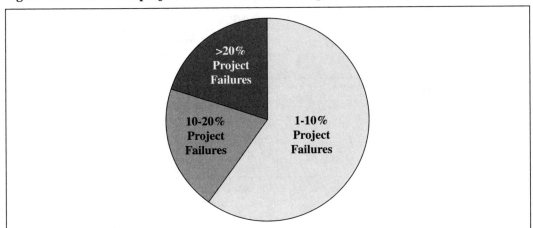

Source: Knight 2005, 59.

when defining politics as being "about getting collective action from a group of people who may have quite different interests. It is about being willing to use conflict and disorder creatively" (PMI 2000, 26). Eccles et al. also note that the negative connotation of politics "derives from the fact that attempts to reconcile these [different] interests result [in] power struggles and organizational games that can sometimes take on a thoroughly unproductive life of their own." The project manager should understand the formal and informal structures in the organization and be able to use the positive aspects of power and politics where influence is appropriate. They also should guard against the negative aspects of power and politics rearing their ugly heads.

Project Management Office

Because of the large, multidimensional, and continuing scope of many EHR projects, hospitals and very large clinics are starting to create a project management office (PMO), sometimes referred to as a standing operational implementation team (Morrison 2006). PMOs can establish a relationship between IT and organizational business units that focuses projects on user needs and removes the notion that the project is "just an IT project" or "IT is to blame" (Isola et al. 2006). Additionally, they can better coordinate a project portfolio, or the collection of all projects to be planned, given sufficient resources and managed for the organization (Pickens and Solak 2005).

Knight (2005) reports on a Canadian study conducted in 2004 of 262 hospitals that reported 50 percent of respondents had one to four major IT projects in process at one time and 16 percent had 17 or more major projects underway at one time. The rate of project failure, where the project was not on time, within budget, or met functional requirements, reported in this survey is depicted in figure 4.7.

In addition to the fact that a PMO can serve as a team of experts with various skill sets, it can manage the project with appropriate project management techniques and progress measures. Knight also identifies nine mistakes IT managers make when managing projects. These are listed in table 4.7.

Table 4.7.   Typical project management mistakes

Mistake	Cause/Effect
Not having a project portfolio	Complexity of many projects results in unclear priorities, overallocated resources, and misaligned implementations
Projects not prioritized	Prioritization of project often results from a reactive acceptance of perceived need rather than proactive ranking using objective scoring to determine appropriate need and logical sequence
Lack of project sponsorship	Lack of sponsor or lack of commitment from sponsor reflects lack of organizational commitment to success
Lack of project ownership	Project sponsors should pass authority to project leader so that public ownership is acknowledged. Project leaders without authority will fail.
"Accidental" project leader	Awarding an already overburdened staff member with another project because of the success of a previous project will ultimately lead to inability to attend to all projects assigned
Not using a methodology	Some organizations do not like the formality of any methodology, but are then unlikely to have an objective way to assess success
Not using project management software	IT projects are becoming more mission critical as they are focused on clinical processes and need to be managed to successful completion
Misuse of project management software	Adopting the project management software only for identifying tasks and not managing the plan is not much better than a paper–pencil plan
Not investing in project management training	Lack of training in project management often continues the cycle of poor project success

Source: Knight 2005, 59–61.

EHR Project Management Techniques and Tools

Whether a professional project manager is used or an individual who is well organized and well respected in the organization assumes this role, formal project management techniques are essential for ensuring that the EHR project engages all applicable parties and stays on time and on budget.

Project Management Standards

Project management is the application of knowledge, skills, tools, and techniques to project activities to meet project requirements. Formal project management is often required when a project competes with other projects or day-to-day activities for scope, time, cost, risk,

Table 4.8. Project management knowledge areas

PMBOK® Guide Areas	Summary of Key Tasks
Project Integration Management	• Project planning • Change control
Project Scope Management	• Project authorization • Scope planning
Project Time Management	• Activity definition, sequencing, and duration estimating • Schedule development and control
Project Cost Management	• Resource planning • Project cost estimating, budgeting, and control
Project Quality Management	• Evaluating overall project performance and monitoring specific project results
Project Human Resource Management	• Organizational planning • Staff acquisition and team development
Project Communications Management	• Communications planning and distribution channels • Project performance reporting • Administrative closure on key phases or project completion
Project Risk Management	• Managing adverse events that may stall or derail project
Project Procurement Management	• Planning solicitations • Source selection • Contract management

Source: Adapted from Project Management Institute 2000.

and quality. Formal project management also helps bring convergence among stakeholders with different needs and expectations. The field of project management has a formal "body of knowledge" that is approved as an American National Standard by ANSI. The Project Management Institute, based in Newton Square, Pennsylvania, with a worldwide membership of more than 100,000, oversees development and maintenance of the standard, which is in its third edition (the first being published in 1987). The Project Management Institute also offers certifications as Project Management Professional (PMP®) and Certified Associate in Project Management (CAPM®). The standard offers generally accepted principles of project management adaptable to fit any project needs (Hughes 2000).

Table 4.8 lists the project management knowledge areas and excerpts of key tasks from the ANSI/PMI 99-001-2000, *Project Management Body of Knowledge* (PMBOK Guide).

Project Phases and Life Cycle

By their nature, projects are differentiated from day-to-day work activities because they are unique undertakings, generally with a specific start and finish. The start-and-finish aspects of a project are qualified by the word "generally" because some projects start before formal project management begins. This is often the case with EHRs, where various IT projects that constitute the early stages of the EHR migration path have been ongoing for many years. Eventually, however, the next major hurdle is recognized as a significant project. Even then, formal project management techniques may not be used until the project appears to be in trouble. For example, adequate progress is not being made, competing interests are difficult to resolve, there are cost and time overruns, or project goals are not being met.

Projects also should have a specific finish. This is often difficult to achieve with an EHR project because the journey is long and winding and new components are continuously being identified. The organizations that are considered "most wired" or have exemplary EHR implementations frequently state that they are nowhere close to achieving the EHR (even though those with far less technology and functionality sometimes declare themselves to have an EHR). However, all projects should have an ending point so they become stable enough to begin to evaluate their results. It may be necessary to break up the EHR project into phases where key milestones signify the end of a given phase. Not only is it difficult to sustain a project for too long a period of time, but at some point the project must be folded into the day-to-day activities and enter a maintenance mode. The maintenance mode should include the ongoing monitoring and evaluation of results with course correction as necessary. The course correction itself may entail an entirely new project.

In addition to defining the EHR project's boundaries and potential phases that can be treated as separate projects, each project has phases within it that are important to be recognized. Taken together, these phases are referred to as the project's life cycle. Figure 4.8 illustrates the major, generic phases within a project's life cycle as described by the Project Management Institute.

Initiating Processes

Initiating processes include project formulation, feasibility studies, and strategic design and approval. This is the phase in which the EHR vision for the organization is conceived and an overall migration path for achieving that vision is described. Feasibility studies

Figure 4.8.   Phases of a project's life cycle

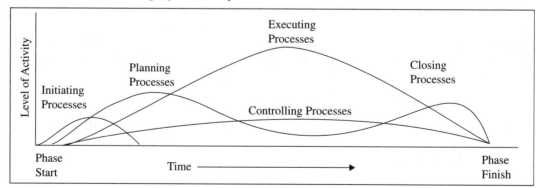

Project management institute, *A Guide to the Project Management Body of Knowledge (PMBOK Guide), 2000 Edition,* Project Management Institute, Inc., 2000. Copyright and all rights reserved. Material from this publication has been reproduced with the permission of PMI.

might include a readiness assessment, general ROI analysis, and technical assessments of various parts of the EHR infrastructure.

The purpose of this phase of the project's life cycle is to scope out the project, estimate its general cost, and gain executive management approval. In this phase, concepts are described, but specific details are not yet defined. The initiating processes are generally performed by a relatively small group of people but should include representatives from all major stakeholders. Conceiving the EHR within the IT department or in a clinical department will not achieve the broadest goals for adoption.

Planning Processes

The planning processes phase begins to focus on the specifics. After the EHR project is approved, a specific migration path is developed, with goals and timeline parameters. Some EHR project planners may use a term other than *migration path,* such as IT strategic plan. The concept of a migration path, further discussed in chapter 6, however, is to recognize that there are several stages of technology, functionality, and user adoption toward the ultimate EHR. This is not an implementation plan, where very detailed tasks of acquiring, installing, testing, and training are performed. Such tasks are performed for any information system implementation. Rather, a migration path considers the sequence and prerequisites for each module or component of an EHR. Chapter 1 describes a continuum of such technology, functionality, and user adoption for the EHR. Not all organizations will include all the components outlined in chapter 1 or may not sequence them in the same manner, but most will find they have been following—and will continue to follow—some form of path toward their ultimate vision of the EHR. This phase also includes establishing formal project management, committing people to teams and teams to tasks, selecting vendors and negotiating contracts, and developing a highly detailed implementation plan.

Executing Processes

Executing processes are the actual implementation steps. This is what is plotted on a detailed implementation plan. If not done in the initiating phase, this phase also should include defining the metrics for benefits realization to ensure that goals are met when the EHR or one of its components is up and running. Although the metrics may need to be fine-tuned throughout the process of system implementation, early definition ensures that value is considered throughout the project. Of course, the typical executing processes also include taking delivery of the hardware and software, designing screens, creating tables and rules, revising work flows, installing hardware and software, testing, implementing new procedures, and training. Multiple iterations of these processes may be performed before all components of the EHR project are implemented.

Many organizations phase in the EHR by clinical department or function. The various teams that worked on planning processes may be directly involved in implementation or somewhat reconstituted with others that have skills associated with the executing process tasks. New teams may form and others may go away. However, the project manager and the executive sponsor should remain throughout the duration of the project, and the executive sponsor should commit to ongoing monitoring and evaluation of results.

Closing Processes

The closing processes phase should include implementation of benefits realization studies using the metrics defined earlier. This phase supplies the feedback mechanism to correct course, fine-tune, or prepare for the next major phase of the EHR migration path. Closing processes also should ensure that team members are given appropriate recognition and are returned to their day-to-day activities. Finally, this phase ensures operational and production support for ongoing use of the EHR.

Controlling Processes
Controlling processes are the project management functions of identifying teams and their members throughout the project life cycle, facilitating and supporting teamwork, appropriately sequencing steps, ensuring that the steps are achieved within the resources allocated, educating and providing feedback, managing change, recognizing and celebrating success, and reporting on progress. As illustrated in figure 4.8, the controlling processes are performed throughout the project's life cycle.

Project Management Tools

In addition to the knowledge and skills that give a project manager unique techniques for managing complex projects, several tools are available to aid the project manager in project planning. The project plan is the project's manager's roadmap. A good outline of the elements of a project plan is provided by Hughes (2000) and listed in table 4.9.

Project Charter, Scope, or Deliverables and Approach
An EHR's migration path provides a good way to appreciate an EHR project's charter. Within that migration path, the component or set of components that is the current focus should provide the project's scope. Whereas a given IT project's deliverables tend to be an installed information system, an EHR's deliverables may be more tied to key milestones in implementation, adoption by users, or even achievement of goals. A project manager should understand what the deliverables are because they define the scope of the project.

An organization's culture and the vendor's culture both determine the project approach. Evaluating the vendor's standard implementation plan should have been a part of the EHR

Table 4.9.   Project plan outline

• Project charter, scope, or deliverables
• Description of project approach
• Work breakdown structure
• Cost estimates
• Start dates
• Controls
• Performance measurement baselines
• Major milestones and target dates
• Risks, constraints, assumptions, and responses to each
• Open issues
• Supporting detail

Source: Hughes 2000, 72.

selection process in order to ensure that the two organizations' cultures do not clash over the implementation. It is not unusual for a vendor to want to come into an organization, take over the project management, implement the project, and quickly leave to go to the next project. If the healthcare organization prefers a more staged approach or more active involvement by its own project manager and team or has other ideas, these need to be reconciled before a contract is signed and may be one element that keeps a specific product from being acquired.

Work Breakdown Structure

The **work breakdown structure** refers to the specific tasks within the project and how they are divided into various phases of the project. A **task** is work to be performed. Highly complex projects, such as EHR implementations, may have several major project goals, each with several activities and each activity with several tasks, as illustrated in figure 4.9.

Cost Estimates

Some healthcare organizations are interested in assigning cost to each task or activity. Although this certainly provides information about the total cost of ownership, many of the human resources used to accomplish the tasks involved in the project have already had their time allocated to their primary work function. The value of the human resource time spent on a project may be of interest to a healthcare organization, but it is not commonly tracked. Alternatively, the time vendor resources are spent on each task is essential for the vendor to know because implementation time may be billed on an hourly basis. Additionally, there may be contractual limits to the amount of overall time a vendor spends to accomplish the project or specific activities and tasks over which the vendor will charge. Healthcare organizations should understand their contracts and track their usage of the vendor's human resources accordingly.

In general, a healthcare organization is more concerned about an overall budget and managing to the budget instead of managing to cost estimates on a project plan.

Figure 4.9.   Portion of a project work breakdown structure

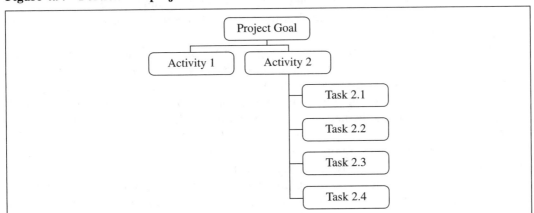

Start Dates

A start date should be identified carefully for each task. Start dates are important not only because each initial task should be scheduled, but also because the start dates of subsequent tasks may be dependent on completion of previous tasks. Such **dependencies** are critical to identify. In fact, when plotting tasks and their start dates on a project plan, the tasks that have dependencies are often the most critical to be accomplished in order to keep the project on time. A project's **critical path** is the sequence of the tasks where there is no slack. In other words, if one task cannot start on time because another has not been completed, there is no slack and the project will be delayed. If a task can be performed at any time, or if there is some range of time within which a task can be completed, there is some slack in the schedule.

Controls

Several types of controls should be built into a project plan. These include work authorizations, change controls, and testing.

Work Authorizations

A *work authorization* is the formal process that enables the project and each activity or task within the project to start. Although not every task necessarily needs permission to be undertaken, certainly any task that has a dependency should at least have some oversight showing that it has been sufficiently accomplished. The level of authorization depends on the criticality of the activity or task.

In managing a project plan, the project manager should maintain control over the start and end dates of each task. Although most project tasks will be delegated to someone else, the individual or team responsible for completing a task should report to the project manager, who, in turn, will verify completion and post an end date. Groupware or collaboration software and access to the project plan are important tools for all stakeholders in the project, but access should not include the ability to make changes to the master plan.

Change Controls

One important reason for managing project task completion is obviously to avoid "hope creep," where someone posts completion of a task knowing that the work is behind but hoping it will be accomplished "before anyone notices." This does not help the project manager ensure that the plan is being carried out, and someone authorized to start a task as soon as the previous task is completed may inadvertently attempt to begin too early. Another reason for maintaining control of the project plan is that any problems with tasks can be identified.

Beyond control of the project plan, **change control** also refers to the requirement for determining what changes can be made and by whom, when, and for what reason. Change control, sometimes called configuration management, is a formal process of tracking every request for a change in a system, determining its impact on other elements of the project or the system itself, obtaining the necessary authorization for the change to be made, keeping track of the change in the event a future action is dependent on understanding what has been changed, and then carrying out the change with the necessary resources. During project implementation, changes may result in scope creep. In an EHR project, a change to the system can have a profound effect on another part of the system. For example, a change to a data element may impact a clinical decision support process. On an ongoing basis, it may be necessary to remember that a change has occurred so that its impact can be determined on any future system release.

Finally, change generally involves additional resources. Some IT departments get so many requests for change that they cannot accomplish them all at once and need to prioritize them. They also should recognize that a change without appreciation for its impact can be disastrous to the overall project or use of the system in an ongoing program.

Testing

Tests may be considered tasks within the project plan, but because they so frequently are not performed as thoroughly as they should be, treating them as control points in addition to tasks can help ensure the system is thoroughly tested.

Performance Measurement Baselines, Major Milestones, and Target Dates

In many cases, implementation of controls depends on understanding a baseline and desired performance measures. For example, if an organization plans to have all its end users trained on computer navigation prior to training them on the EHR system, it can be helpful to have a baseline measurement of how many people have such skills, what skills others need, and when training has been accomplished.

Performance measurement baselines also help establish major milestones. A **milestone** is a work product or the accomplishment of a deliverable as opposed to a task that is an action or work package. Milestones should be plotted on the project plan to both recognize the need to achieve them as part of the overall project dependency schema and celebrate their accomplishment.

Tasks generally have duration, with a start and an end date. Completion of a task is not necessarily a milestone. A milestone does not have duration, but is an event. In some cases, the event is the start or end of something, such as go-live day, and in other cases, a milestone is progress toward a goal. For example, if training is set to occur over a 2-month period from one date to another, that is the training task's duration. On the other hand, achievement of 95 percent of staff trained is a milestone.

Risks, Constraints, and Assumptions

As previously described, risk refers to the probability that a threat will exploit a vulnerability and do harm. A project manager should understand the probability that a task may not be completed on time, resulting in other tasks being delayed, which may result in cost overruns and project delay. Contingencies may need to be built into the project plan where risk is high for some harm to occur. It may be necessary to develop some if-then scenarios or assumptions and potential responses to them as part of the contingency planning.

In addition to time and cost factors, risk also relates to the quality of the deliverable. If it is necessary to shortchange performance of a task, what impact will that have not just on time and cost, but also on later use of the system? Because an EHR is a tool that supports clinical care, the risk of inaccuracies or lack of task completion can be very serious. A clinician may not trust such a system and therefore be unwilling to use it so that patients do not get the benefit of information that may not necessarily be available to the clinician or available on a timely basis. A clinician also could rely on erroneous information in such a system to make a decision that could be detrimental to the patient.

Open Issues

Issues management is yet another part of overall project management. There will always be issues during the course of a project, from a minor event such as someone taking an extra day to accomplish a task that does not have a dependency associated with it to an interface that that does not work the first time it is tested. Issues may be related to many different factors. Most project managers keep an issues log for this purpose. When the project manager is satisfied the issue has been resolved, he or she can indicate it on the issues log. Open issues, however, need to be tracked and their completion managed.

One reason it is important to understand the reporting relationships among all members of the project's human resources, as well as the reporting relationships among the members of the vendor's implementation team, is in the event issues must be escalated beyond the authority of the project manager.

Supporting Detail

In order to manage the myriad tasks and other project elements, a project manager will frequently use project planning software. Microsoft Project is one of the most widely recognized software tools for planning. Although only basic components of the software can be used, it has many sophisticated features, including resource leveling and budgeting features. The basic component is a **Gantt chart.** A Gantt chart is used to illustrate project tasks, phases, and milestones, and their start, end, and completion dates. It helps to illustrate where more than one task must be performed simultaneously. Figure 4.10 illustrates a portion of a simple project plan Gantt chart using Microsoft Project. If Microsoft Project or other such specialty software is more than needed for the project, a spreadsheet often works as well for simple tracking.

More sophisticated components of project planning software permit showing dependencies among tasks (where completion of one task depends on the start, specific progress, or finish of another) as well as actual completion dates for each task, which can help the project manager estimate whether the entire project will be completed on time. Determining the overall impact of dependencies is performed using a **Program (or Project) Evaluation and Review Technology (PERT)** chart (or view in the software). A PERT chart helps to evaluate the entire schedule and to make adjustments based on dependencies, criticality of tasks, and minimum, maximum, and average duration time of tasks.

Project planning software can be coupled with document sharing and collaboration software, such as Microsoft's SharePoint, which permits the exchange of project information with team members and others so that various task alerts and files can be shared.

Some project managers may also find it helpful to use **balanced scorecards**, **key performance indicators**, and **dashboards** in addition to project management software. Balanced scorecard is a system that measures and manages defined metrics derived from institutional sources and aligns the metrics with the strategic goals of the organization (Schade and Gustafson 2003). Key performance indicators (KPIs) are quantifiable measurements, previously agreed on, that reflect the organization's critical success factors. A dashboard is a tool that collects data from multiple sources to unify a variety of metrics into a single view (Wyatt 2004).

As the project manager works through the issues in the plan, supporting detail should be documented. This might be in the form of an e-mail or formal report saved in a file associated with the plan. Communication with the vendor also should be maintained. If the vendor indicates it can start later with no impact on cost or overall project completion, but

Figure 4.10. Project plan Gantt chart

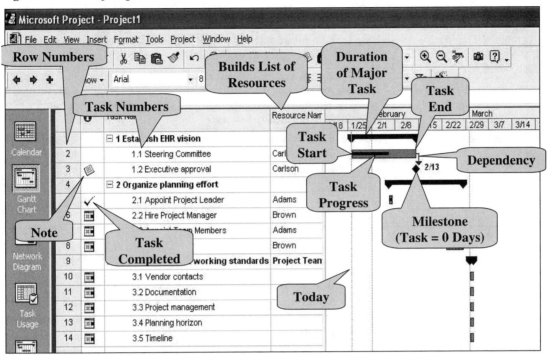

Copyright © 2008, Margret\A Consulting, LLC. Reprinted with permission.

later claims the loss of time was to blame for additional costs, the project manager would need to have supporting documentation. Most documentation deals with issues, meeting agendas and minutes, invoices, testing results, training scores, progress reports to executives, and so on. It may be appropriate, however, to also keep track of other communications, such as newsletter announcements and even celebrations.

Change Management

Change management is the movement of an organization from its current state to some future and, it is hoped, more effective state (Pierce and Gardner 2002). Many books, articles, treatises, manuscripts, self-assessments, theories, and wise sayings have been written about change management. Perhaps the most important thing an EHR project manager can do about change is to recognize that it must be managed and to never forget the impact of any change on any individual, even when that individual may attest to being comfortable with change. It should also be remembered that change should never be made for the sake of change alone. Change must bring about value that accrues to the person required to make the change, the organization requiring it, and with respect to EHR, the ultimate beneficiary—the patient/consumer.

Many of the techniques and tools described in this chapter to build teams, manage conflict, and create effective meetings are components of change management. However, EHR

Table 4.10.   Change management strategies

Strategy	Description
Rational-Empirical	People are rational and will follow their self-interest—once it is revealed to them. Change is based on the communication of information and the proffering of incentives.
Normative-Reeducative	People are social beings and will adhere to cultural norms and values. Change is based on redefining and reinterpreting existing norms and values, and developing commitments to new ones.
Power-Coercive	People are basically compliant and will generally do what they are told or can be made to do. Change is based on the exercise of authority and the imposition of sanctions.
Environmental-Adaptive	People oppose loss and disruption but they adapt readily to new circumstances. Change is based on building a new organization and gradually transferring people from the old one to the new one.

Source: Bennis, Benne, and Chin 1969.

project managers also should recognize that change is quite unique to each organization. Warren G. Bennis is probably considered the father of change management. He describes four strategies that reflect how organizations approach change (Bennis, Benne, and Chin 1969). These are described in table 4.10.

Organizational change is significantly influenced by executive management's belief system. Although it is possible for an EHR project team to influence how change is managed in an organization, change management is often not effective when the assumed strategy is in conflict with the organization's actual strategy. A project manager should study other changes previously made in the organization to learn what the organization's overall change strategy has been, whether it has changed over time, and whether a new strategy is emerging, possibly due to new leadership or desired change brought about by executive management themselves.

Change management also requires consideration of the target population's size and professionalism, degree of resistance, and dependency on the organization; the stakes in making the change; the time frame for change; and the available expertise of the organization to effect change. If, indeed, the organization wants to change its change management strategy, ideally it needs to begin the process prior to initiating an EHR project and with smaller-scope projects to test and demonstrate their desire for change. Each change strategy has advantages and disadvantages associated with it; the strategy used should most closely reflect the needs and abilities of the organization.

Change Management Principles
Some principles that have been espoused about managing change can be summarized as follows:

- *Educating and communicating:* The more people know about the impending change, the more likely they are to become comfortable with it. Gain participation and involvement so that people not only know about what will be happening, but are actually a part of making change happen.

- *Supporting learning new skills and undertaking new tasks:* Some organizations provide computer skills building and then start to roll out e-mail and intranet services to get clinicians used to using a computer. Other things that can be done include structuring paper-based documentation to introduce templates, practice guidelines, and standard vocabulary.

- *Providing emotional support:* Demonstrating that the organization cares about its employees, medical staff, patients, and so on helps these individuals trust that when change comes, the organization will continue to aid and support them.

However, some tactics to managing change are less than successful. Following are examples of a few unsuccessful tactics:

- *Offering incentives to accept change:* Some organizations offer incentives because they know that some individuals believe they will lose something (such as time or stature) in the change. When an incentive can provide continuing value to all individuals, providing it can be effective. Unfortunately, however, incentives can be costly and can backfire in the form of expectations for compensation.

- *Using disincentives, manipulation, or coercion:* Unfortunately, it is not uncommon for some organizations to resort to these tactics when others fail or when they have prepared for the change less than they should have and are desperate for adoption. In some cases, these tactics can be unethical; at best, they can decrease long-term satisfaction, increase resentment, and destroy trust.

- *Ignoring the impact of change and establishing expectations that the change will occur over time no matter what:* Although not generating the dire consequences of disincentives, manipulation, or coercion, this tactic essentially abdicates the organization's responsibility and relies on peer pressure or group normative behavior to achieve the change. This tactic appears to be used more commonly than expected, perhaps as a result of lack of experience in managing change or a lack of awareness of the impact of change. It may result in change eventually, but at such expense to the organization in running parallel or hybrid systems that it never pushes forward to make other changes.

Reactions to Change

Project managers should encourage all managers in the organization to be change managers. Although a direct approach to managing change is important, everything done to communicate, build teams, engage users, and so on is part of the change management process. Supervisors and managers who do not support the change end up undermining it, either overtly or covertly.

Part of the role of the supervisor or manager in managing change is to recognize how each individual under his or her supervision is coping with change and addressing it with that individual appropriately. The range of reactions to change can be far greater than one anticipates. Dunham (2006) describes the following types of reactions to change:

- *Active support* is a situation where individuals indicate by word and deed that they are behind the change and are engaged and accomplishing key tasks in the project. Although it may not be expected that these individuals will need change management support, such support should not be disregarded because there can be a false sense of acceptance. Ensuring that these individuals have support and continue to be engaged is important. Acceptance is a somewhat passive form of support. In fact, it may be confused with acquiescence, lack of interest, or even passive opposition. These individuals may only need a bit more education or some other form of support to become comfortable and successful with the change.

- *Accept/modify* is a form of support where the individual states acceptance but wants to make changes continuously to plans, processes, screen designs, and so on. This individual is unwilling to state fear of change, but such ongoing modifications are often a way to return to the old and known ways. This is actually one of the most common problems in implementing an EHR. It offers so much opportunity for customization and tailoring that it is easy to overlook modifications as ways to return the system to old ways.

- *Acquiescence* is the state of mind where the individual accepts the inevitable but is not fully supportive. This individual may quickly turn into a more active form of resister or even leave taker if not managed appropriately.

- *Passive resistance* is the state where an individual truly is resistant to the change but will not admit it. Many clinicians find themselves in this position because of peer pressure. This type of individual is one of the most difficult to reach out to but probably represents a large majority. In many cases, it is necessary to assume that all but those who speak out directly for or against the change are passive resisters and work directly on education, engagement, support, coaching, counseling, and so on.

- *Active resistance* is the state where an individual assertively opposes the change. Such individuals are easier to deal with in some respects because you know where they stand. They sometimes can be turned around so successfully that they become champions for the change.

- *Leave takers* are individuals who will leave the organization to avoid accepting the change. In some cases, this may be for the best, although too many leave takers can disrupt the organization and fire up others who may not be quite ready to leave. In many cases, the latter individuals hope that their threats to leave will turn the organization away from making the change. These individuals may be more dangerous than the actual leave takers and should be managed directly, again through education, engagement, support, coaching, counseling, and so on.

Risk Management

In addition to change management, Doll (2005) suggests that good project managers manage risk to reduce uncertainty. As the healthcare industry knows from HIPAA, there are two components to risk: threats and vulnerabilities. **Risk management** utilizes an evaluation and response strategy to reduce the likelihood that a threat will exploit a vulnerability and jeopardize project success. The National Institute for Standards and Technology (NIST) identifies several response strategies to risks (Stoneburner, Goguen, and Feringa 2001):

- Eliminating the risk entirely if it is has a great potential for harming the project. For example, it may be necessary to remove a member of a team who is working at cross-purposes to the project, eliminate using certain devices if they prove to be ineffective, or drop a vendor when the solution is not working.

- Transferring the responsibility for the risk to a third party, such as outsourcing a function where the organization lacks expertise.

- Mitigating the risk reduces the probability or consequence of the risk. Mitigation is achieved through instituting various controls. For projects, these may include adding communication media, increasing project staffing, requiring certain approvals, and so on.

- Contingency planning to reduce the impact of a risk should always occur in EHR projects. This often includes a contingency budget but also may include back-up resources for programmers, additional support staff, and others.

- Taking no action is an appropriate response to risk when the risk is very small or will have minimal impact on the project. There is still the probability that it will not occur or will occur in an even milder form than anticipated. None of these actions would alter the project significantly.

Time, Cost, and Quality Management

Managing time, allocating budget, and achieving the project's deliverables are the key outcomes of managing a project. The next section on hard skills provides tools for managing time, cost, and quality; some of the soft skills associated with these outcomes include the following:

- *Discipline is an important part of managing time to plan.* Some organizations always start meetings late or run over. Instituting a plan to start and end on time and actually carrying it out requires perseverance.

- *Follow-up is essential to managing the budget.* Even then, however, if thorough planning for all costs has not been done in advance of the project, it is difficult to manage the budget. Anticipating elements of total cost of ownership, incorporating a contingency budget, and then managing to the budget can help overcome cost overruns.

- *Accomplishing tasks on time and within budget is important, but not if the desired outcomes are not achieved.* Building ongoing quality checks into the project plan where continuous feedback is checked is critical. Some of the most mundane elements of quality are often overlooked when there is a major project such as EHR. For example, something apparently as simple as a typo on a screen can be irritating to users at best and error generating at worst.

EHR Clinical and Cultural Transformation

Many EHR projects also have difficulty reaching appropriate completion or success because of the nature of the change the EHR brings about in the organization. This has been described as a clinical transformation or the systematic modernization of the healthcare industry on the basis of new and evolving clinical information systems. King et al. (2003) describe clinical transformation as consisting of the components listed in table 4.11.

Because the EHR represents a clinical transformation, the organization must recognize the need for a culture that supports such a transformation. This often requires a cultural transformation. *Hospitals and Health Networks* (*H&HN*) (2005) describes an organization with a culture that supports clinical transformation as one that is positive. Employees not only welcome change but actively look for ways to make improvements. In compiling a special supplement on cultural transformation, *H&HN* tapped the Baldrige National Quality Program, 2005 Health Care Criteria for Performance Excellence. The 11 core values for performance excellence are listed in table 4.12.

Table 4.11.   Components of clinical transformation

• Integration of enabling technology throughout the redesign process to maximize technology's impact
• Untethering of information to make it available at the time and place it is needed
• Clinical process improvement and standardization across the health system and sharing of knowledge across the system
• Evidence-based medicine and clinical care
• Sustained organizational and cultural change
• Transfer of knowledge and effective communication

Source: King et al. 2003, 40-41.

Table 4.12.   Core values for performance excellence

• Voluntary leadership
• Patient-focused excellence
• Organizational and personal learning
• Valuing staff and partners
• Agility
• Focus on the future
• Managing for innovation
• Management by fact
• Social responsibility and community health
• Focus on results and creating value
• Systems perspective

Source: *H&HN* 2005.

H&HN also identified barriers to cultural change, such as failure to set clear direction, lack of staff buy-in, fragmented communication, inadequate data collection and performance measurement process, failure to hold staff accountable for performance, lack of recognition and rewards program, satisfaction with the status quo, and insufficient leadership commitment and visibility.

Project managers would do well to study the core values and barriers to change as they approach the EHR clinical transformation.

Change in Health Information Management

The Joint Commission's Comprehensive Accreditation Manual for Hospitals (CAMH) includes a standard on Management of Information (IM) that is "designed to be equally compatible with paper-based systems, electronic systems, or hybrid systems." Departmental boundaries of the IT and HIM departments are not addressed but, rather, the functions, processes, and elements for performance with respect to the goal of supporting decision making to improve patient outcomes, improve healthcare documentation, ensure patient safety, and improve performance in patient care, treatment, and services, governance, management, and support processes (CAMH 2008).

The EHR will not only change the way clinicians document and use health information but will significantly change the nature of the IT and HIM departments.

Change in the IT Department

Change in the IT department will likely include significantly more outreach, user involvement, and focus on data and information. Implementing and maintaining technology is certainly a core function that will remain an important part of the IT function, but may be performed in a "department without walls" mode, often headed by a chief technology officer (CTO). IT staff can expect to physically and logically work much more closely with information system users. Technicians will team with informaticists who may be members of the medical, nursing, or allied health professions. Technicians will need a much better understanding of the data and information being processed rather than only the machinery that causes data collection and storage and screen design and report printing.

The IT department will be an active, but not sole, participant in EHR decision making. IT staff will be able to exercise their creativity and innovativeness through expanded adoption of information systems. Indeed, IT staff may require new skill sets in communications and healthcare operations.

Change in the HIM Department

The HIM department also can expect to find itself as a department without walls. A comprehensive, fully electronic EHR will ultimately mean no handling of paper charts, no filing of loose sheets, and no photocopying of records. Coding of diagnoses and procedures is being performed successfully online. With the use of standard medical vocabulary, coding eventually may become automated to the point where coding professionals will be monitoring data quality, managing vocabulary standards, and brokering data resources.

Transcription also has been affected by enhanced technology and ultimately may give way to voice and handwriting recognition and natural language processing, and certainly has already been significantly replaced by structured data entry. Transcription professionals may be managing data integrity and designing information presentation.

HIM professionals should take advantage of their new and expanding roles, and their opportunities to work with informaticists and, potentially, to earn informatics degrees. They are key members of the EHR project team. As liaisons between clinical users and IT staff, they ensure the privacy and security (including confidentiality, integrity, and availability) of health information, facilitate data use, and ensure that the legal health record can be represented from the EHR.

Changes for Informaticists

Several references have been made to the field of informatics and medical, nursing, and allied health informaticists. The American Medical Informatics Association (AMIA) defines medical informatics as a discipline having "to do with all aspects of understanding and promoting the effective organization, analysis, management, and use of information in health care" (AMIA 2004). Each of the medical, nursing, and health disciplines has developed its own special areas of emphasis and approaches to ensure the use of technology as an integral tool in helping to organize, analyze, manage, and use information. A number of universities offer master's programs in one or more of the informatics disciplines.

Conclusion

It should be clear from this chapter that many individuals contribute to envisioning, developing, and adopting an EHR. As a project, the processes required to achieve an EHR include requiring leadership commitment from executive management, through the project manager, to each individual project team member and ultimate EHR user. As a way of life in the future, the EHR demands changes that will realize improvements in all aspects of healthcare, from professional productivity through quality of care to patient/consumer satisfaction.

References and Resources

American Medical Informatics Association. 2004. What Is Medical Informatics? www.amia.org.

Bennis, W.G., K.D. Benne, and R. Chin, eds. 1969. *The Planning of Change.* New York: Holt, Rinehart and Winston.

Doll, B.A. 2005. Project management 101. *Journal of AHIMA.* 76(1):50.

Dunham, R.B. 2006 (Jan. 26). Managing organizational change. Presentation to MetaStar, Madison, WI.

Evans, C.C. 2006. Healthcare technology project ownership. *Journal of Healthcare Information Management* 20(1):34–38.

Frenette, R. 2003 (Oct.). IT project management 101. *ADVANCE for Health Information Executives* 7(10):75–78.

Garrity, C.E. 2002 (Aug.). Creating a balanced environment. *ADVANCE for Health Information Executives* 6(8):14.

Hammons, T., and J. Kralweski. 2005 (July 15). The adoption of electronic health records and associated information systems by medical group practices. Final report, AHRQ task order #5. Englewood, CO: Medical Group Management Association Center for Research.

Health IT Certification. Principles of HIT Project Management, V6.2, 2008.

Hospitals and Health Networks. 2005. Cultural transformation. Special supplement sponsored by the Baptist Health Care Leadership Institute. hhnmag.com/hhnmag/hospitalconnect/search/article. jsp?dcrpath=HHNMAG/PubsNewsArticle/data/backup/0504HHN__FEA_Gatefold&domain=HHNMAG.

Hughes, G. 2000. The value of project management expertise. *Journal of AHIMA* 71(10):72–73.

Isola, M., A. Polikaitis, and R.A. Laureto. 2006. Implementation of a project management office (PMO): Experiences from year 1. *Journal of Healthcare Information Management* 20(1):79–87.

Joint Commission. 2008. *Comprehensive Accreditation Manual for Hospitals: The Official Handbook.* Oakbrook Terrace, IL.

Joint Commission on Accreditation of Healthcare Organizations. 2006. Management of information. In *Comprehensive Accreditation Manual for Hospitals.* Oakbrook Terrace, IL.

King, L.A., et al. 2003. The digital hospital: Opportunities and challenges. *Journal of Healthcare Information Management* 17(1):37–45.

Knight, G. 2005 (June). Avoiding IT project management mistakes. *ADVANCE for Health Information Executives* 9(6):59–60.

Matson, E. 1996. The seven sins of deadly meetings. *Fast Company.* www.fastcompany.com/online/02/meetings.html.

McNamara, C. 1999. Basic guide to conducting effective meetings. The Management Assistance Program for Nonprofits. www.mapnp.org/library/misc/mtgmgmnt.htm.

Microsoft. 1999. *User's Guide for Microsoft Project 2000.* Redmond, WA: Microsoft Corporation.

Morris, S.A., et al. 2002. IT investment planning: The best hospitals. *Journal of Healthcare Information Management* 16(2):62–65.

Morrison, F. 2006. The standing operational implementation team-playing a vital role in successful project completion, implementation of operational initiatives, and process improvement. *Journal of Healthcare Information Management* 20(1):28–33.

Nickols, F. 2000. Change Management 101: A Primer. http://home.att.net/~nickols/change.htm.

Phillips, M.T., and E.S. Berner. 2004. Beating the system: Pitfalls of bar code medication administration. *Journal of Healthcare Information Management* 18(4):16–18.

Pickens, S., and J. Solak. 2005. Successful Healthcare Programs and Projects: Organization Portfolio Management Essentials, *Journal of Healthcare Information Management* 19(1):19–27.

Pierce, J.L., and D.G. Gardner, with R.B. Dunham (2002). Managing organizational change and development. Ch. 18 in *Management and Organizational Behavior: An Integrated Perspective*, pp. 627–654. Cincinnati, OH: South-Western College Publishing.

Project Management Institute. 2000. *A Guide to the Project Management Body of Knowledge (PMBOK Guide).* Newton Square, PA: PMI.

Radtke, Lisa. 2003 (Apr. 30). Tips and tools for facilitating meetings. *Wisconsin Health Information Management Association Conference Proceedings.* La Crosse, WI: WHIMA.

Rogers, E.M. 1995. *Diffusions of Innovations,* 5th ed. New York City: The Free Press.

Schade, S., and M. Gustafson. 2003. The evolution of balanced scorecard reporting systems. *ADVANCE for Health Information Executives* 7(9):65–72.

Schuman, S.P., moderator. 2004. Facilitator competencies. Electronic Discussion on Group Facilitation. Center for Policy Research, University of Albany, SUNY. www.albany.edu/cpr/gf.

Stack, J. 2002 (May). A crash course in project management survival. *ADVANCE for Health Information Executives* 6(5):49–53.

Stoneburner, G, A. Goguen, and A. Feringa. 2001. Risk management guide for information technology systems. National Institute for Standards and Technology special publication 800-30. Washington, DC: Department of Commerce.

Tuckman, B., and M. Jensen. 1977. Stages of small group development. *Group and Organizational Studies* 2:419–427. www.gmu.edu.

Tuckman, B. 1965. Developmental sequence in small groups. *Psychological Bulletin* 63:384–399.

Warner, H.R. 1995. Medical informatics: A real discipline? *Journal of the American Medical Informatics Association* 2(4):207–214.

Wyatt, J. 2004 (Feb.). Scorecards, dashboards, and KPIs keys to integrated performance measurement. *Healthcare Financial Management,* 76–80.

Chapter 5
EHR Goal Setting and
Impact on Quality of Care

An article in *H&HN*'s *Most Wired Magazine* observed that "Four years into the Department of Health and Human Services' 'decade of healthcare information technology,' little progress has been made in achieving the current president's goal of every American having a secure electronic health record (EHR) by 2014" (Towne 2008). This article also noted that "healthcare leaders are still arguing about the overall effectiveness of the EHR."

As everyone knows, statistics can be used to describe any viewpoint one cares to take. However, the referenced article makes an interesting point—although EHRs as a concept have been around long enough that their impact on quality of care should be able to be studied, the fact of the matter is that "complete" EHRs exist in only a few organizations—and even the definition of "complete" is elusive. In a June 2007 *Archives of Internal Medicine* report, it was stated that EHRs were used in 18 percent of all physician practices. Yet a *New England Journal of Medicine* report from June 2008 indicates that only 4 percent of physicians have an "extensive, fully functional" EHR. The American Hospital Association (AHA) estimates that 16 percent of hospitals use "fully operational" EHRs, whereas HIMSS Analytics (2007) indicates that not a single hospital reported achieving stage 7 on its EMR Adoption Model (that is, medical record fully electronic and sharable). Although these statistics may appear depressing, they could be viewed from the perspective that the industry is increasing its desire for more sophisticated systems and is pushing more complete utilization.

The bottom line really is that there is probably too small a sample of fully utilized, comprehensive EHRs to reach a valid conclusion about their effect on quality of care. Yet it is known that once down the path to EHR, few organizations want to turn back. There is definitely anecdotal evidence of productivity improvement, time savings, and reduced hassles, as well as patient safety and quality-of-care benefits.

A critical step, then, in both demonstrating and ensuring the value of EHR as promised by its proponents is to understand what benefits are feasible along the pathway to an EHR and to establish specific goals to achieve them. Even if benefits are difficult to quantify,

Key Terms

Adverse drug event	Evidence-based medicine	Meta-analysis
Anecdotal benefits	Fee-for-service environment	Productivity improvement
Baseline	Goal	Quantifiable benefits
Benefits realization study	Institutional review board	Quantitative benefits
Clinical trials	Managed care	Research methodology
Confounding variables		Return on investment
Cost–benefit analysis		SMART goals

goal setting begins the change management process and increases the chance for better adoption. This chapter:

- Enumerates improvements that can be realized along the migration path to an EHR

- Describes the importance of establishing quantifiable benefit expectations

- Provides examples to illustrate EHR benefits

Quantitative versus Qualitative Benefits

To discuss the benefits of EHRs in a fair and realistic manner, it may be appropriate to consider what the terms *quantitative* and *qualitative* mean with respect to benefits. Many chief executive officers (CEOs) ask for evidence of **quantitative benefits** before they are willing to make an investment in the EHR. They want to see a quantitative **return on investment** (ROI).

A good source for understanding the difference between quantitative and qualitative is from a **research methodology** perspective. An ROI analysis is actually quite similar to a research study in many respects. In her chapter on research methods in *Health Information Management: Concepts, Principles, and Practice*, Layman (2006) distinguishes between quantitative and qualitative research as described in table 5.1.

Given the description of quantitative and qualitative, one can suggest that a quantitative benefit is one that has a single truth; that is, by doing X, Y will surely happen. Unfortunately, outside something like a strictly controlled chemistry experiment in a laboratory, few things in life have a single truth or such a direct relationship. More frequently, multiple truths exist; that is, there are **confounding variables** that, within the context of research, would be said to confuse interpretation of the data. Not only could multiple factors contribute to the benefits of an EHR, which might be unrelated or not directly related to the EHR, even the act of analyzing processes to conduct an EHR fea-

Table 5.1.   Quantitative vs. qualitative research

Quantitative	Qualitative
Find the single truth.	Multiple truths exist simultaneously.
Apply the single truth across time and place.	Truths are bound to place and time (contextual).
Adopt a neutral, unbiased stance.	Neutrality is impossible because researchers choose their topics of investigation.
Identify a chronological sequence of events.	Influences interact with one another to color researchers' view of the past, present, and future.

Source: Layman 2006.

sibility study could result in improvements that probably should be—but will likely not be—attributed to an EHR.

Quantifiable vs. Anecdotal Benefits

Although it is clear that quantitative research is focused and limited to certain domains of study, CEOs and boards of directors will still say they want a quantitative ROI analysis to support adoption of the EHR. Considering the definitions of quantitative and qualitative research, all benefits of EHRs will be qualitative. Probably a better approach is to categorize EHR benefits as those that are quantifiable and those that are anecdotal.

Quantifiable benefits are tangible. They are described by a numeric representation, such as a percent of improvement, a number of full-time equivalent (FTE) staff reduction, or cost savings from not having to purchase paper record folders. Although CEOs typically want an ROI described in monetary terms, more are beginning to recognize the importance of having a benefits portfolio consisting of both cost savings and revenue enhancement as well as benefits relating to quality of care.

Anecdotal benefits are difficult to quantify in any manner and are described by specific examples of events that occurred or were avoided when the EHR was used. For example, describing the fact that a key nurse could not be recruited because the organization did not have an EHR is an anecdote that can be persuasive. Another example may be that an EHR improves care of diabetics by more closely monitoring their compliance with their treatment regimen. Anecdotal evidence of benefits can be strengthened in several ways. One way is to report anecdotes from similar organizations. An anecdote from an academic medical center will likely be looked on suspiciously in a community hospital. Another way to strengthen anecdotal evidence is through **meta-analysis**, which is integrating findings from many similar organizations that use similar systems. A pilot study is another way to support anecdotal benefits, although this is difficult to do with a project that is the scope of an EHR.

A distinction for providing evidence of benefits as quantifiable versus anecdotal is shown in table 5.2.

Table 5.2. Quantifiable vs. anecdotal evidence

Quantifiable/Tangible	Anecdotal/Intangible
Numeric representation (preferably in monetary terms)	Scenario-based case description
Requires establishment of metrics and baseline data for comparison	May reflect quantifiable data from other sources if organization is unwilling or unable to conduct its own study
Provides opportunity for course correction	Requires leadership faith in others' experiences; does not provide direct opportunity for course correction
Example: Today, organization spends Y dollars on transcription. EHR will reduce transcription by X percent, resulting in cost savings of Y − X dollars.	Example: EHR has contributed to attracting qualified nursing staff as evidenced by consistent comments in staff evaluations and applicant interviews.

Cost–Benefit Feasibility Study vs. Benefits Realization Study

Another issue with respect to quantifiable vs. anecdotal evidence of benefits is whether the evidence is to be used in a **cost–benefit analysis** or a **benefits realization study**. In general, these two forms of benefits studies have many similarities. Most important, both depend on clear vision, executive management support, and realistic expectations of benefits. But there also are key differences, including when they are performed, their primary purpose, and the level of detail. Table 5.3 distinguishes between these two types of studies.

Practical Issues in Benefits Studies

Very few healthcare organizations find any kind of benefits study to be easy. Indeed, few have quantified their existing processes, at least to the degree necessary to evaluate either potential benefits in a cost–benefit feasibility study or actual improvements for a benefits realization study.

Quantifying benefits is both an art and a science. Not everything can be studied in depth, but what is to be studied should be decided by not only how easy it is to study, but also how meaningful the study is to the organization. For example, it is easy and important to study lines and cost of transcription when looking to eliminate dictation and have clinicians enter data directly into the EHR. However, it is difficult to study how much time it saves a clinician in a day to use the EHR. If it appears that the project could be at risk for clinician complaints concerning productivity, a stopwatch time study could be done; but it probably will be of little value. If the study can be done so as not to interrupt workflow, which is one of the biggest problems, it is still likely to be discredited by those who were not included in the study. Such individuals may claim that their workflow is different or

Table 5.3. Cost–benefit feasibility study vs. benefits realization study

Characteristic	Cost–Benefit Feasibility	Benefits Realization
When performed	Before decision is made to undertake EHR initiative	Before decision is made to undertake EHR initiative *and* after EHR implementation
Purpose	To determine if an EHR initiative is appropriate for the organization at this time	To determine if anticipated benefits are realized
Additional value	May highlight "broken" processes to be fixed	• May highlight "broken" processes to be fixed • May contribute to system build • Will identify areas not meeting benefits for corrective action
What is measured	• All costs associated with acquisition of hardware and software, installation, implementation, and ongoing maintenance • Expected ROI from quantifiable benefits and anecdotal evidence (See further in chapter 11.)	Quantifiable changes associated with differences in processes, such as units of work, percent of improvement, and so on (See further in this chapter.)
Level of detail	• May be estimated and not detailed OR • Based on process assessment and detailed	Based on process assessment and detailed
Critical success factors	• Clear vision of EHR • Senior management support • Realistic expectations	• Clear vision of EHR • Senior management support • Realistic expectations • Valid metrics • Process assessment skills (See further in chapter 6.)

their work requires greater knowledge or expertise. Furthermore, it may actually take more time *per entry* to use an EHR, but save time in numerous other ways to ultimately produce an *overall* time savings. This is difficult to measure and even more difficult to persuade busy caregivers that such **productivity improvement** is true. More likely, other measures will be needed to help demonstrate this benefit.

Another practical matter is that to truly substantiate EHR benefits, a formal process needs to be established to ensure that the findings are valid and reliable. Some organizations undertake a formal study because it is part of the organization's broader research mission. For others, quantifying benefits is a way to achieve recognition. Still others find that the more benefits can be quantified, the more likely subsequent projects will be approved. This happens in part because the "record speaks for itself," but also because such studies can pinpoint problem areas early in the process where course correction can occur easily, contributing even further to benefits actually being achieved.

Many organizations also ask why it is necessary to study a process that is going to be changed. In general, the only answer may be to measure the difference. However, many EHR experts also advise against automating a process that is broken. If a process is suspected of being broken, a process analysis may be necessary to fix it prior to automation. Unfortunately, this is another thorny issue. Many organizations assume that automation will fix the broken process. So much of this has occurred in the past that many EHR systems were doomed to failure before they got started.

In preparing to describe the benefits of an EHR for an organization, there must be agreement that the resources needed to implement the EHR will be supplied. Some executives are so skeptical of EHR benefits that they hold back not only the appropriate level of funding but also their full support and encouragement. Lack of benefits sometimes can become a self-fulfilling prophecy. It is pointless to establish high expectations for benefits only to find that the "go" decision produces a scenario where the solution does not match the vision of the EHR on which the benefits were based. Disappointment then will be tremendous, and the projected benefits will be looked on with skepticism.

Whatever reasons apply for conducting a benefits study, the fact remains that the process is much like a research study. Benefits' expectations must be defined before the study begins, metrics must be designed, and then before-and-after or control-vs.-experimental samples must be taken and analyzed. The organization must be committed to carrying out such a study or must accept benefits on the faith that anecdotal evidence is real.

Goal Setting and Anticipating EHR Benefits

A **goal** is a specific, intended result of a strategy. But to be useful, goals must be **S**pecific, **M**easurable, **A**ttainable, **R**ealistic, and **T**imely (often referred to as SMART). The concept of **SMART goals** has been recognized for many years and no one can find a specific individual or entity to which to credit for the acronym. However, these traditional attributes, or ones that enhance their meaning further, are believed to be critical to achieving fast-paced results. (Enhancements for each acronym have been suggested: S for stretching, systematic, synergistic, and significant; M for meaningful, motivating, and magical; A for accountability, acumen, and agreed-upon; R for realistic, resonating, results-oriented, rewarding, rooted in facts, and remarkable; and T for tangible and thoughtful [Heathfield 2000].)

There are many reasons to set goals and anticipate EHR benefits. Certainly, determining whether there is a value proposition is important. Without anticipating there will be benefits, most organizations would not undertake the level of investment an EHR requires. However, in addition to identifying cost–benefit feasibility, the process, itself, of setting goals can have significant value. A recent research study (Amatayakul 2006) performed to identify best practices for EHR adoption found that organizations with well-established goals

Figure 5.1.   Importance of goal setting in EHR best practices study

Goals in Study Group	Existence of EHR	
	Present	**Absent**
Access to data/integration across care sites	3	4
"Paperless"	1	2
Part of corporate plan	0	0
Quality of care	1	1
Specific business objectives	2	3
None	0	6

From EHR Best Practices research study funded through Blandin Foundation, College of St. Scholastica, Margret Amatayakul, Researcher, December 2005.

for their EHR system were more likely to implement a comprehensive EHR. Figure 5.1 describes these findings. Although the sample size of the study was relatively small, not a single hospital or clinic that had a comprehensive EHR had no established goals for its EHR, whereas 38 percent of the hospitals and clinics without an EHR had no goals.

Goal setting, sometimes also referred to as benefits expectation setting, has several important values. Figure 5.2 summarizes the impact of goal setting.

Goal Setting and Education

When goal setting is performed during the planning stages for an EHR, it helps stakeholders understand what an EHR is, its scope and complexity, and what it means to actually achieve the desired benefits. A simple example is illustrative:

A small physician office considering an EHR brought in a consultant to assist with the selection process. When asked what they hoped to accomplish, the physicians noted cost savings among their anticipated benefits. This goal not being very specific, the consultant asked them to quantify what cost savings meant to them. The physicians said they understood that EHRs could reduce their transcription expense, maybe by 50 percent or 75 percent. This being a broad range, the consultant asked them what function they thought could be eliminated. The physicians suggested that note dictation could be eliminated, which they estimated accounted for about 75 percent of the office's transcription expense. When asked how the EHR would help reduce the expense of transcribing notes, the physicians literally had to stop and think a moment that they would no longer be dictating notes. When asked how they expected the notes to be entered into the EHR if not through dictation, the physicians were taken aback by the thought that they would have to "type" all the content themselves, fearing they would become transcriptionists. Finally, some product demos reassured them that templates with point-and-click data-entry options, drop-down menus, and perhaps even a structured patient self-assessment or personal health record would be available so that they would be doing very little typing. Furthermore, as the information was being entered, the template could be context-sensitive, recognizing, for instance, that the patient was diabetic, providing guidance on what information the physicians should not forget to collect. Even though a lot of typing would be eliminated through use of templates, the physicians were told they would have to review the vendor-provided templates to be sure they were what they wanted. Moreover, they would likely have to modify the templates to

Figure 5.2.   Impact of goal setting

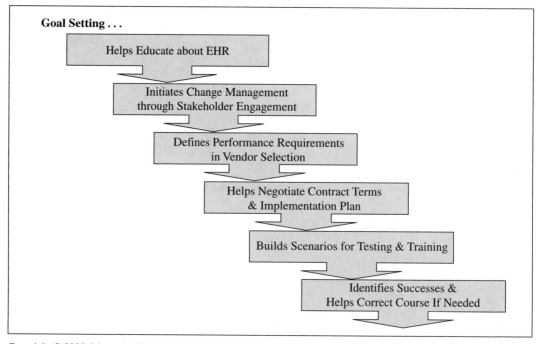

conform to their practice standards and certainly would have to achieve some level of standardization across the practice, in addition to keeping the templates up to date.

The entire process of establishing this goal explained a lot to these physicians. It was not that they had not seen some demos or had not discussed the benefits of EHR, but they had done so only from a 30,000 foot-level, so to speak. They had not yet internalized what the EHR would mean to them directly as they performed their work. Interestingly, the physicians in this practice went on to set several additional goals, finding that the exercise really forced them to understand how an EHR worked and helped them realize the changes it would bring about. They also felt better prepared to evaluate vendor offerings.

Goal Setting and Change Management

Going through a process of identifying goals for an EHR also can help potential users "buy into" the results, but the goals must be clear and complete. Generally, people who set their own goals are more inclined to commit to achieving them than if they are told what to do. However, clearly articulating the intent of the goals and paying attention to how they should be achieved also are critical elements of getting the goals adopted by all. An example from a hospital considering acquiring a point-of-care charting system is illustrative:

A large hospital about to embark on an electronic documentation system decided to start with nursing. As part of the planning, teams of nurses were created to review the various types of documentation they performed. The planners' purpose was to ensure that all the data currently collected could be accommodated through the electronic system, eliminated as unimportant, or identified as data to be collected by someone else or obtained from some other source. As one team of nurses started to review their patient admission documentation, they were surprised to find how many forms they used and how much time it took to complete them. In total, they identified 11 different forms and found that, on average, their completion took about 1.75 hours. The nurses then analyzed the data on each form and recognized that many of the forms contained duplicate data, some contained data from an information system elsewhere in the hospital, and some contained data that were not needed. The nurses estimated they could eliminate almost 1.25 hours by adopting a point-of-care charting system integrated with other systems in the hospital. The nurses then set as their goal the completion of admission documentation within 30 minutes. Interestingly, however, as they discussed their findings with their colleagues and as word spread about the time that would be saved, several nurses approached their union representative with concerns that the new system would cost them their jobs. Thus, although the planning and goal setting had been fine, the nurses had failed to state their goal in a way that articulated the true benefits of the new system, which would be to free up nursing time so that the nurses would be able to provide better information to patient families, support patients in following care instructions, take more care in administering medications to reduce errors, and so on.

Goal setting is important to the change management process. Those who set their own goals and understand what that means will be enlightened and will likely have a strong desire to see them accomplished. They can anticipate the change and be more accepting of it. However, in most healthcare organizations, not everyone can be involved in every planning and goal-setting process, so care must be taken to state goals in a manner that describes their actual benefit (for example, not just to reduce nursing time, but to make better use of it).

Goal Setting and Vendor Selection/Contract Negotiation

Although some components of an EHR will be implemented as part of a larger EHR project so that not every component is selected separately, where there is a need to select a product, goal setting can help both describe more fully what functions are desired and establish performance metrics the vendor should demonstrate. For instance, a clinic that reports HEDIS data to health plans may want to be able not only to collect the data in its EHR to avoid costly and error-prone abstraction, but also to evaluate the data it is submitting and perform its own analysis of them. If, for example, the clinic sets a goal of improving its childhood immunization rates by a certain percentage, it will want to evaluate products that can collect those data, embed clinical decision support to remind its providers to collect the data, and provide monthly or quarterly reports on its progress.

Goal Setting and Testing, Training, and Improved Adoption

With clear metrics and explicit descriptions of how the EHR will help achieve its specific goals, a healthcare organization has the ability to construct test scenarios and training tools to help focus its EHR implementation. For instance, a barcode medication administration record system is not just about scanning a patient's identification band and the medication being administered; rather, it is a complex system that, in addition to requiring connectivity with other information systems, requires considerable flexibility for use. If medications are normally distributed early in the morning, but a patient prefers to take them at night, the system must allow the nurse to make any adjustments in the schedule deemed acceptable. If medications are to be administered on a certain schedule, but the patient is in surgery at the scheduled time, the system should be sufficiently flexible to allow this variation without treating it as a medication administration error. If goal setting is focused on reducing medication administration errors, there must be accountability for such variations and these variations should be included in both system design and testing, and training. Any system that does not consider professional judgment will not be well adopted.

Benefits Description

However an organization uses its goal-setting process and benefits expectations development, there are some important considerations in describing goals and benefits. These are summarized in figure 5.3.

Benefits must relate directly to the organization or they will have little value. For example, if the provider has little **managed care**, identifying significant benefits associated with managed care contracting will have little influence. If the organization typically has not been involved in **clinical trials**, the ability to increase participation may or may not be of interest. EHRs for inpatient facilities are very different from those used in outpatient facilities and quite different from those used in physician offices, long-term care facilities, behavioral healthcare institutions, home health agencies, or any of the other places an EHR may be implemented.

A good way to decide how to determine the EHR benefits that would relate to an organization is to review the organization's current goals and objectives, or its strategic plan. What are its hot buttons (for example, to create a center of excellence or to enter a merger and acquisition mode)? What are its pain points (for example, patient satisfaction or high-cost/low-revenue areas)? Where does it identify what improvements are needed (for example, in utilization management or medication errors)? What issues is it facing (for example, staffing shortages, reduced reimbursement, a depressed economy)?

When the organization's goals and objectives are understood, it also is important to gain an understanding of its EHR vision. Again, it would be pointless to be describing the benefits of **evidence-based medicine** when the organization's strategy is limited to an EHR that only enhances access to health records through a document imaging project. However, if the organization's vision is limited by concerns for cost and benefits realization, it may be necessary to push the envelope a bit and describe benefits of a more comprehensive view of the EHR with the hope of creating a migration path toward a more robust system. Figure 5.4 summarizes the benefit outcomes that may be achieved as one moves along a migration path from a simple to a complex vision of the EHR.

Figure 5.3. Benefits description requirements

Benefits described for an EHR must:

- Relate to the type of organization
- Support the organization's strategic goals and objectives
- Reflect the vision of the EHR defined by the organization
- Be proposed within the context of their realization, whether by perception or formal study
- Be supported by resources and commitment of senior management

Figure 5.4.   Modeling outcomes from a simple to a complex vision of the EHR

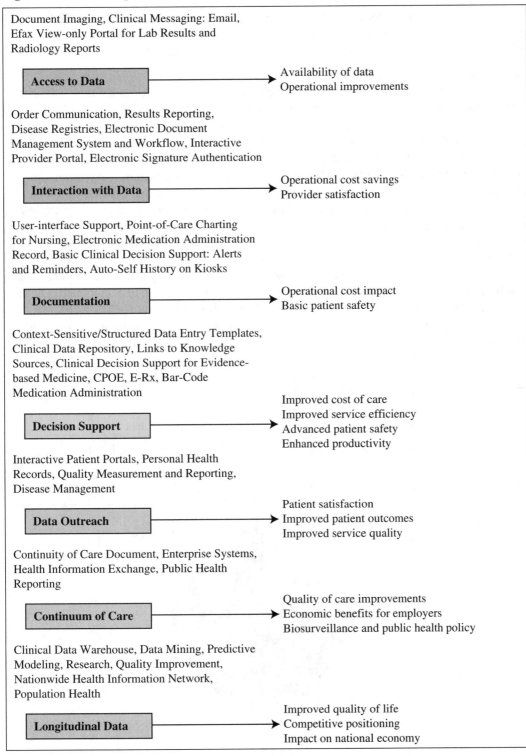

Economic Benefits

Economic benefits can be found relating to cost savings or cost avoidance, revenue increases or contribution to profit, and productivity improvements. Figure 5.5 identifies the different types of economic benefits. (These benefits are not necessarily accrued in these proportions.)

Cost Savings or Cost Avoidance

Cost savings result in the elimination of specific expenditures the organization now incurs. Most commonly, cost savings result from eliminating staff, usually through attrition and in operational areas rather than in direct patient care areas. Caution must be applied in evaluating staff elimination. Although some staff who leave may not have to be replaced as a result of an EHR, many staff are simply redeployed to other functions. Clerical staff are often redeployed to scan and index paper documents. Nurse productivity improvements through prescription refill/renewal automation in a physician office may be asked to take on patient recall functions (although this may generate an increased number of patients and thus impact revenue in that manner).

Other cost savings can result from reductions in liability insurance, forms reproduction, microfilming or other record archival processes, and paper chart storage. For example, at least one malpractice insurance carrier is offering between 2 percent and 5 percent discount on premiums to provider groups that get 75 percent of their providers using at least two of six functions in a CCHIT-certified EHR for at least one year (MMIC 2007).

Measuring cost savings is fairly straightforward, at least in relation to the other forms of quantifiable benefits. The organization's operational budget, in conjunction with the process redesign efforts, can provide most of the cost-saving information needed.

The term *cost avoidance* refers to any cost the organization presently does not or should not incur but will incur if specific steps are not taken. Examples of such costs include:

- Not having to expand the file area to house more paper charts

- Avoiding staff recruitment costs because the EHR has improved staff retention

Figure 5.5.   Types of economic benefits

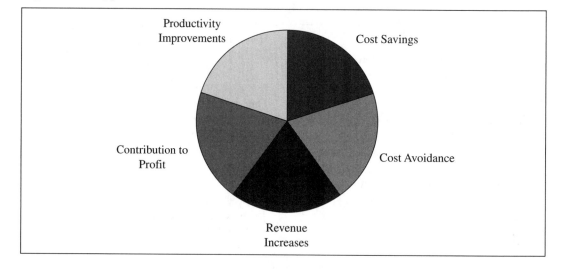

- Avoiding the cost of a specialty care referral when primary care physicians use rules-based decision support

- Avoiding the cost of repeat diagnostic studies when results are unavailable

- Not having to hire additional telephone receptionists as patient volume increases

- Avoiding more expensive medications through presentation of cost-effective alternatives

Several of these cost avoidance strategies are being seen as so important that key stakeholders in healthcare have been focused on their achievement. For example, one study associated with the formation of a health information exchange (HIE) found that 13.7 percent of all laboratory tests were potentially unnecessarily redundant and could save an average of $87.81 per test, or $31.8 billion annually across the entire country (Walker 2005). Several health plans, such as BlueCross BlueShield in a number of states and Aetna, are giving away e-Rx systems to physicians, valued at approximately $3,000 to $7,000 (including hardware, software, and network connectivity), in order to reduce the number, and hence cost, of brand-name drugs prescribed. Among the results of the program have been achievement of 59 percent of prescriptions written for a generic drug, 29 percent of prescriptions entered alerted a physician to a potential drug-drug interaction, and 2 percent of prescriptions entered alerted a physician to a potential drug-allergy interaction not previously reported by the patient (*Health Business Daily* 2007).

Cost avoidance is more difficult to identify than cost savings, but the organization usually has some experience with incurring costs it can avoid and measures of these can be taken. In a way, this becomes cost savings, although the categorization of benefits is essentially an artifact for purposes of discussion anyway. The experience of other institutions that have performed cost–benefit feasibility studies or benefits realization studies may be used as guides to estimate potential cost avoidance.

In considering cost avoidance, the organization must not include a cost that it will avoid if it has no plans to incur it; this inflates the benefits. For example, if the experience of other organizations demonstrates a reduction of two medication errors for every 100 prescriptions, but the organization's experience indicates a current error rate of only one medication error for every 100 prescriptions, this benefit should not be inflated beyond the organization's own experience. However, medication errors are a significant source of cost avoidance because they generally contribute to increased lengths of stay or avoidable office visits. When in doubt about a cost avoidance estimate, it is generally better to err on the conservative side and not include the estimate in the organization's benefits study.

Another example of an issue associated with cost avoidance is "false hope." For example, an EHR may be proposed when budget figures are analyzed for expanding warehousing for current and anticipated future volumes of paper charts. In the hope of avoiding this cost, the organization may consider an EHR that is paperless. However, current paper charts still exist and something must be done with them. Furthermore, there must be an absolute commitment on the part of the organization to avoid printing and to do away with paper charts completely at some point in the future. There may be some cost avoidance, but there will likely be some cost of archiving current charts or of scanning or abstracting them into the EHR and then destroying them. There can also be added cost if paper copies are printed, used in documentation, and have to be filed—not to mention the risk to patient safety if the paper annotation is not observed. In many cases, hospitals have found that some of the components of EHR have contributed to more paper having to be filed until such time as they declare the information system to be the official source of this information. The reason for the increased paper is that the systems often print out a full page for only one order, one result, or other component being documented. Some healthcare organizations also are finding significantly more duplication of record content. For example, a clinic migrating to the EHR, but not fully functional, found it was creating both a paper face sheet and an electronic face sheet that was being printed. Both had to be filed in the chart because different processes led to the same forms containing some different information.

Revenue Increases and Contributions to Profit

Revenue increases are achieved by using the EHR to attract more business or to ensure appropriate reimbursement for services—including participating in various incentive programs. For example, a clinic that can convert its file room to another suite of offices and examining rooms for a new physician is generating revenue through the new physician. Another example is that of increasing the number of annual physical examinations through an automated reminder system or booking aftercare at the time of discharge, which is likelier to secure the follow-up visit than if the patient were left to schedule the appointment at a later time. If days in accounts receivable can be reduced, the potential exists for increasing revenue through improved earnings on funds or paying down debt, which may avoid some cost. Emergency departments have found that patient workflow management systems have reduced the number of patients who left without being seen (increasing revenue) and the number of emergency department patients with lengths of stay exceeding 12 hours (providing financial benefit) (Jensen 2004).

Many ambulatory EHR systems link documentation directly to coding, and so improved coding can contribute to increased revenue. This includes improved documentation for evaluation and maintenance care coding, which also increases revenue and lessens the risk of reimbursement denials and penalties. Virtually all EHR systems link documentation to charge capture, which may hasten the ability to drop a bill or at least avoid lost charges. In a managed care environment, increased revenue may be achieved through documented cost savings and cost avoidance that will bring in a new contract or achieve a better contract with an existing client. Improved immunization rates and success with smoking cessation programs are examples of targets of managed care organizations that yield preferred pricing.

Revenue increases can be real, but understanding the organization's payer mix is essential in estimating revenue increases. In a managed care environment, more visits to the physician or longer lengths of stay (LOS) mean less rather than more revenue. Keeping people well and out of the care delivery system in a managed care environment contributes to both revenue increases (through better contracts) and profit (Rosenstein 1999). Alternatively, more visits and longer LOS have meant more revenue in a more **fee-for-service environment** and is one of the reasons for pay-for-performance incentives to keep people well, but not at the expense of lowered income for providers.

A number of revenue-enhancing incentives are being sponsored by Medicare and other payers. For example, under Medicare's Physician Quality Reporting Initiative (PQRI), eligible providers who meet the criteria for satisfactory submission of quality measures data for services furnished during the reporting period can earn an incentive payment of 1.5 percent of their total allowed charges for Physician Fee Schedule (PFS) covered professional services furnished during that same period. The 2008 PQRI consists of 119 quality measures, including two structural measures. One structural measure conveys whether a provider has and uses EHRs and the other e-Rx. To report the quality measures, CPT G codes or Category II codes must be supplied on the claim. To date, the measures are process-based rather than outcomes-based. For example, providers might report the level of the hemoglobin A1C for their patients (codes are available for reporting higher than 9, between 7 and 9, or lower than 7). Presumably, future such programs will consider actual outcomes, such as whether the patients' blood sugar was within certain acceptable boundaries (for example, 7 or less) or if it was improving (for example, moving from 9 to 8). It should also be observed that some incentives are actually sanctions. For example, the CMS Hospital Compare program provides full reimbursement to hospitals if they participate in quality reporting, but will discount the reimbursement if they do not.

The term *contribution to profit* refers to keeping more of what the healthcare organization earns (in comparison to revenue increases that cause the organization to earn more). As noted, any way to keep people well contributes to profit in a managed care environment. For example, tracking failed appointments and getting patients into a diabetes clinic so that they can be monitored should result in fewer complications and hospitalizations.

Productivity Improvements

Productivity improvements result primarily from time savings that may ultimately yield cost savings or other forms of benefits. For example, point-of-care charting improves productivity by reducing the amount of dictation, which contributes to cost savings in transcription time. Reduced time tracking diagnostic study results may improve physician productivity by freeing the physician to see an additional patient each day, which has the potential to increase revenue. The ability to provide access to patient information has been one of the primary incentives for the formation of HIE organizations.

Because most productivity improvements yield other forms of benefits, care should be taken not to consider one benefit twice. Furthermore, many productivity improvements may "only" contribute to clinical value (that is, they are more difficult to quantify, even though clinical improvements should be more highly valued). For example, relieving nurse time generally will not produce cost savings because the nurse must remain at work the entire shift. (Cost savings would only accrue if overtime could be reduced, part-time personnel could be eliminated, and so on.) However, if the nurse has more time to spend explaining instructions to patients and the result is better patient compliance with medications, the value is clinical. Although it is difficult to assign a monetary benefit to this type of value, which is often difficult to quantify in any way, it is real in that it contributes to not only clinical value, but also strategic value in patient satisfaction and quality of life for the care-giver.

Clinical Benefits

Obviously, many of the economic benefits also contribute to improved quality of care or what may be categorized as clinical benefits. Many clinical benefits can be readily quantified, but it is more difficult to assign monetary value to them. Contributing factors to clinical benefits include:

- Better access to clinical information
- Improved clinical decision making and disease management
- Enhanced documentation
- More tailored patient education
- More time to spend with patients
- Improved care
- Improved quality of life

Better Access to Clinical Information
Better access to clinical information not only contributes to care-giver productivity, but also contributes directly to better diagnosis and treatment. Information immediately accessible in the emergency department can ensure that patients' chronic conditions and current medications are readily available. Answering telephone inquiries and triaging patients in real time may prevent utilization issues as well as ensure that proper treatment is provided when necessary. Clinical information that is always available can provide a much more effective picture of a patient's health history. For example, in a busy inner-city outpatient department, the ability to have a single problem list that was always the first screen presented led to identification of an unusual syndrome in a patient that might otherwise have gone years without being recognized. Probably every user of an EHR has at least one such anecdote where availability of information led to faster or more accurate diagnosis and treatment.

Improved Clinical Decision Making and Disease Management
The mere act of making data available is a tremendous aid, but adding to that the ability to process the data, fire alerts, and reminders and to provide clinical guidance takes what has traditionally been a passive document and makes it a living tool. In fact, several physicians who have had EHRs for some time have suggested that the EHR may be the only practical way to apply practice guidelines while clinicians are delivering care to patients.

There have been many published reports of specific clinical improvements as a result of adding reminders at the point of care. These have included reminders to promote aspirin use in patients with coronary artery disease, flu shots for older patients, and ACE-inhibitor use in patients with congestive heart failure. Chronic disease staging, such as for diabetes and asthma, has been significantly improved through a more easily compiled longitudinal record of care. There has been **adverse drug event** (ADE) avoidance as well. For example, Kaiser Permanente of Ohio found that a reminder at the point of care reduced the number of hypertensive patients taking nonrecommended medications from 16 percent to 12 percent in 12 months.

Table 5.4.   Illustration of benefits from clinical interventions supported by the EHR

Measure	EHR Support	Result
Cervical cancer screening	Health maintenance alert triggers when female between ages 18 to 70 years has not had a Pap smear in last year	88% compliance with screening requirement
Screening for diabetic retinopathy	Best practice alert trigger if no dilated eye examination performed in last year	63% compliance with screening practice
Beta-blockers after myocardial infarction	Best practice alert trigger if patient has history of MI and not taking beta-blockers	95% compliance with screening practice
Pediatric well-child visits	Health maintenance alerts vary by age groups; based on frequency of requirements	86% compliance with screening requirements ages 3 to 6 years 63% compliance with screening requirements ages 12 to 21 years
Flu immunization rate	Influenza reminder program initiated through EHR database for at-risk population	53% rate of immunizations achieved

Source: Crowell, M., et al. 2000. The journey to a CPR in a large multi-specialty group practice. Sixth Annual Nicholas E. Davies Award Proceedings of the CPR Recognition Symposium, Computer-based Patient Record Institute, Inc. Healthcare Informatics Executive Management Series. Bethesda, Md.: HIMSS. Reprinted with permission.

Harvard Vanguard Medical Associates is a mixed-model health maintenance organization (HMO) with more than 25,000 physicians and more than 100 hospital affiliates in New England. For more than 20 years, the HMO has developed an EHR system that supports clinical interventions for targeted clinical procedures. Table 5.4 illustrates some of those interventions.

Enhanced Documentation

Although enhanced documentation may generally be regarded as an administrative issue, legibility, accuracy, and completeness all contribute significantly to quality of care. The idea behind computerized physician order entry (CPOE) systems is predicated on the notion that these three issues significantly contribute to medication errors. At issue with some CPOE systems, however, is that they address only legibility and may not add the clinical decision support necessary to provide value to the physician for using the system to ensure accuracy and completeness.

Most physicians see the entry of orders into a computer as a clerical function because it always has been. In the paper environment, the physician handwrites the order on an order sheet and someone else keys it into the computer system to be communicated to the various ancillary departments (laboratory, radiology, pharmacy, physical therapy, nutrition services, and so on) required to carry out the orders. This is computerized order communication, not CPOE as it is intended. Clearly, if the physician were to key the order into the system, it would be legible. If drop-down menus were used as aids to select medications, there would be less confusion among names of drugs that are similar so that the entry would be more accurate. However, if the system does not suggest that the dosage may be inappropriate, warn that the medication may be contraindicated due to allergy or another medication already being taken, provide alerts when drug orders and lab tests contradict each other, or prompt for additional information relative to route or frequency, it is no better than an automated aid for a clerical function.

CPOE systems supported by clinical decision tools also can contribute to better drug utilization, where more cost-effective options can be presented to the ordering physician or charges can be shown for various alternative medications. (This also applies to utilization of diagnostic studies, such as displaying the cost of studies, warning that an order for a lab test is inappropriate soon after a previous test, or identifying that an order repeats an order for a test where results already exist.) Moreover, such CPOE systems can contribute to enhanced documentation by prompting for attending physician sign-off on a therapeutic regimen or where indications for use of a certain drug need to be documented.

The benefits of CPOE and other components of EHRs are not new. Teich et al. (1996) have done extensive studies on the impact of clinical decision support on medication errors and adverse drug events. Table 5.5 provides a sample of some of the results identified at Brigham and Women's Hospital. An interesting feature of these findings is their attempt to describe monetary value as a result of the effects. This was done by estimating what an

Table 5.5.   Examples of medication errors reduced through CPOE

Intervention	Description	Means of Benefit	Potential #/Year	Effect	Savings $/Year
Ondansetron guidance	Changed default frequency for IV administration	Guided toward effective, but less-expensive dose	3,000 displays per year	92% switch to new dose	$500,000 in charges
Vancomycin guidance	Prompt to guide initial use of drug and to consider stopping after 3 days	Reduce overutilization; decrease spread of vancomycin-resistant *Enterococcus*	5,000 orders per year	Under study	Under study
Nephros/Gerios	Changes recommended dosing based on patient's renal function and age	Prevent adverse events due to failure to reduce drug dosing	106 adverse events per year	Not measured yet	$640,000 in costs*

*Estimated hospital cost savings based on prior analysis that shows that each adverse event costs $6,000 to the hospital. These costs are primarily due to extended length of stay and to additional testing and therapeutic measures needed because of the adverse event. This figure excludes cost and detrimental effect to the patient, as well as any liability the hospital may incur.

Teich, et al. 1996. Toward cost-effective quality care: the Brigham integrated computing system, Brigham and Women's Hospital. Second Annual Nicholas E. Davies Award Proceedings of the CPR Recognition Symposium, Schaumburg, Ill.: CPRI. Reprinted with permission from HIMSS.

average day of hospital care costs and how many more days a patient would have to use hospital services if the adverse drug event or medication error actually occurred. Not taken into consideration, however, were costs associated with hospital liability, which could be impressive. Also not included were costs associated with the detrimental effect to the patient. Although these would not accrue to the hospital, they do contribute an overall impact to the nation's economy (that is, they have a strategic impact).

A number of other hospitals, clinics, integrated delivery systems, and HMOs have contributed to the body of literature that supports quantifiable benefits from better access to clinical information, improved clinical decision making and disease management, and enhanced documentation. For example, LDS Hospital found that "cost impact studies of computerized adverse drug event monitoring showed some astounding results . . . in an 18-month period, only nine adverse drug events were reported using the conventional manual reporting mechanisms. During the same time interval, 731 adverse drug events were detected and verified by computer methods" (Grandia 1995). Queen's Medical Center reports that incorrect dosage, administration at the incorrect time, and incorrect route of administration were reduced by 78 percent since adopting its EHR (Davis et al. 1999). Evanston Northwestern Healthcare found that medication transcription errors reduced to zero, delayed administration of medications decreased by 70 percent, and omitted administration of medications decreased by 22 percent with the electronic medication administration record (EMAR) component of its EHR (Smith et al. 2004).

Not only does enhanced documentation through EHR systems contribute to these dramatic results, but other components of documentation also are enhanced. Documentation linked to charge capture and, specifically, codes for reimbursement have been mentioned previously. Another example is that patient-generated information can be incorporated into the record. Some providers are reluctant to put self-reported information in their records, fearing it may be too voluminous or inaccurate. However, an EHR with a patient interface can guide a patient through a self-history that captures only what is necessary for the visit and improves accuracy. The information then can be reviewed by the clinician and updated during the encounter. As a result, the encounter takes less time, the clinician may actually have more information to work with, and the patient is satisfied that all pertinent information has been relayed to the care-giver.

More Tailored Patient Education

Closely related to documentation is more tailored patient education. Although many providers keep a supply of a wide variety of instructional handouts available to give their patients, the EHR can not only generate the handout as needed, but also incorporate a patient's specific medications and other information that may be unique to his or her situation.

At Northwestern Memorial Hospital, an after-visit summary is printed for each patient. This not only includes patient instructions, but also an entire description of the details of the encounter, as suitable for the patient. Focus group studies were conducted in which this summary was found to have satisfied most of the patients' need for information surrounding an encounter (Tang et al. 1998).

More Time to Spend with Patients, Improved Care, and Improved Quality of Life

Many of the above benefits converge to impact workflow and hence contribute to more time to spend with patients, improved care, and improved quality of life for both patients and care-givers.

Wisconsin Hospital and Clinics found that because data did not have to be recollected at intake numerous times, nurse intake time was reduced from 35 to 20 minutes for initial office visits and from 35 to 15 minutes for return visits. Moreover, patients were considerably less frustrated by the fact that they no longer had to fill out forms with the same information for every part of the clinic visited (Dassenko and Slowinski 1995). Duke University Medical Center also found time saving at intake due to improved workflow (Renner 1996). In another study, Internet-based physician–patient communication systems were found to result in reduction in office visit spending. Not only could patients log on to request appointments, referrals, and prescription renewal and to obtain lab results, but they also were actually able to avoid a visit altogether in some cases by an e-consultation (Baker, et al. 2005).

Reduced transcription is a frequently cited benefit of EHRs. In addition to reducing the cost of transcription, clinicians who complete their documentation at the point of care find they have no need for dictation at the end of the day. This workflow change not only permits the clinicians to leave work on time, but also ensures more accurate documentation because recall is not a problem.

Many other workflow improvements have been found, such as the ability to coordinate with the business office, reduce chart pulls, improve making referrals, ensure drug recall ability, and find candidates for clinical trials. However, providers should be aware that much of the literature on workflow improvements resulting from EHRs comes from ambulatory settings. Fewer acute care settings have implemented a total EHR, but there are greater challenges with respect to workflow. For example, many clinicians report problems with data entry into an EHR rather than use of their traditional flow sheets in intensive care units (ICUs). Many ICUs utilize elaborate flow sheets that are often reproduced across multiple pages of a single long document. It may take a different orientation or a different type of monitor to accomplish the goal of this type of documentation. Physicians who conduct rounds also have identified that taking a group of trainees to a workstation at a nurses' station is not practical. Workstations on carts and handheld devices are starting to address some of these issues. One hospital decided to put a workstation and projector into the trainee conference room, where rounds were initiated. The trainees could review charts prior to the physical walk-through, thus reducing hallway congestion and contributing to patient confidentiality.

Other important considerations in workflow have to do not only with eliminating steps or placing workstations, but also with the look and feel of the information as it is presented on the screen itself. Different types of clinicians obviously need different views, and different individuals within a clinician type may have personal preferences. One physician may prefer to review patient results in graphic form; another may prefer a table. Even something as simple as whether tabs to different parts of the record are located on the top, bottom, or side of the screen may make a big difference in usability and hence adoption of an EHR. Color, too, is critical. Many men are color-blind, so males may find it difficult to be guided solely by color-coded text. It may be necessary to use icons in addition to color.

Finding benefits through workflow improvements can be "touchy" and requires both diplomacy and thorough analysis. Clinical workflows have existed for years and are ingrained in their users. Changing workflow is much like asking a left-handed person to write with the right hand. Unless forced to or compelled to through loss of the left hand, it is extremely difficult to persuade a "lefty" that doing something with the right hand is better. In addition to this state of mind, clinicians themselves are rarely able to see what workflow improvements may actually be worth adopting. Ideally, workflow changes should come about by the users themselves, but the old adage that "You can't see the forest for the trees" applies here. Therefore, process analysis and workflow studies will need to be conducted by someone who is an expert in process improvement. Moreover, this individual should be someone who is close enough to the clinical workflow to be considered reliable and yet far enough removed to be objective and able to pinpoint potential changes of value. Then, the clinician users must be convinced that they actually discovered the changes or at least validated them in some form of experiment.

Support for Quality Measurement, Reporting, and Improvement

As suggested at the beginning of this chapter, there is much debate over whether and how well EHRs are able to impact the IOM's quality aims of safe, effective, patient-centered, timely, efficient, and equitable care (IOM 2001). There are great expectations by the IOM, the federal government, and many others for health information technology (HIT) and EHRs to enable redesign of the healthcare system. It is clear from a sampling of the literature that a critical mass of EHRs and concerted study of quality benefits must be made.

An article in the *Archives of Internal Medicine* reflected on a retrospective, cross-sectional analysis of visits in the 2003 and 2004 National Ambulatory Medical Care Survey and found an association of EHR use with 17 ambulatory quality indicators. *Performance on quality indicators* was defined as the percentage of applicable visits in which patients received recommended care. The results revealed that for 14 of the 17 quality indicators, there was no significant difference in performance between visits with and without EHR use. For two quality indicators, practices using EHRs had significantly better performance; and for one quality indicator, visits to practices using EHRs had significantly worse quality. (Linder 2007) Of course, this article fails to observe that without EHRs, it was likely that retrieval of the study findings might have been impossible, or at best a costly abstracting process.

Alternatively, Hillestad et al (2005) found numerous potential health benefits and savings from EHRs, with a projected cost savings of $81 billion annually through healthcare efficiency and safety measures. Another study has documented significant quality improvements achieved by community health centers (CHCs) through the use of electronic patient registries (Landon 2007). In fact, this study has been cited as an example where healthcare quality has improved for those treated by CHCs with HIT but where limited federal funding of such centers may result in exacerbating health disparities among vulnerable populations (Shields 2007).

Benefits Realization Study

The benefits described here are numerous, impacting virtually every aspect of the care process and reflecting varying degrees of specificity. But as suggested earlier, a benefit is the result of change from the way something was done before using the EHR to how something is done after its implementation.

Some organizations are willing to take others' findings on faith that the benefits will accrue for them as well. Although few say they are willing to make this commitment of faith, most end up doing so because they do not want to conduct a rigorous benefits realization study. For such a study to be truly meaningful, it needs to be done properly because the study itself can be time-consuming and costly.

Understanding the potential scope of change in the specific organization is a critical part of benefits realization. It is not nearly as bad to project that benefits will not be as great at one organization as at another than it is to believe they will be as great and be disappointed. It also cannot be emphasized enough that benefits realization hones in on the need to ensure that the benefits are being met and to take corrective action, when necessary, to see that they are achieved.

The steps to a benefits realization study are listed in figure 5.6. The first step is to commit to a properly conducted study. The second step is to identify the benefits that are most likely

Figure 5.6.   Steps in a benefits realization study

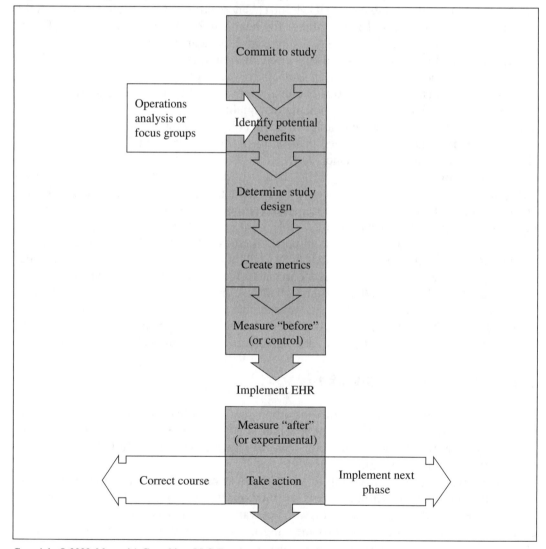

to accrue to the organization and be measured in the study. As noted earlier, these benefits are identified by reviewing the organization's goals and objectives, strategic plan, and vision for the EHR. When identifying benefits to measure in a benefits realization study, it is important to be realistic and reasonable. A solid set of a relatively small number of benefits is more powerful than a weak set of many benefits that will be tiresome to measure.

Determining a Study Design

A benefits realization study is not very different from a formal cost–benefit feasibility study. The primary difference is that a benefits realization study requires not only measuring "before" implementation and anticipating benefits, but also actually measuring "after" implementation. A **baseline** must be established to determine the degree of change. To attempt to be as quantitative as possible and eliminate as many confounding variables as can be identified, there are primarily two ways to structure the benefits realization study:

- A before-and-after study will measure processes before and after the EHR is implemented. Ideally, the time period in which the before measures are taken should be prior to any feasibility study or process analysis is undertaken because changes may occur as a result of these activities (although it is not uncommon to find that any attention paid to a process may result in a change in the process). However, the time period should not be so long before EHR implementation that other factors could make a difference, including changes in personnel, changes in clinical practices, user adoption of information technology elsewhere, and so on.

  The time period for taking the after measures should be sufficient for users to be comfortable using the system, but not so long that old habits are reinforced and the benefits of course correction are delayed. In the before-and-after situation, the same group of users should be involved. (Note: If a benefits realization study involves reviewing actual patient records rather than aggregate data only, it may be necessary to determine if this is considered a research study on human subjects, in which case it must be reviewed by an **institutional review board**.)

- A control and experimental study may be conducted to overcome the timing issues of the before-and-after study. EHR systems are frequently phased into a provider setting anyway, so there is generally an opportunity to identify a group of caregivers in one clinic versus another, one nursing unit versus another, or even one hospital of an integrated delivery network versus another. Although timing issues are not as great in this type of study, the variability of the users may be a factor. Even that the first implementation is compared to a "control" (the location waiting for implementation) vs. a later implementation when compared to a control could be a confounding variable.

The decision as to which type of study is constructed may have more to do with practical matters of when a decision is made to do the study and who is willing to participate. However the study is constructed, the confounding variables should be recognized and normalized to the extent possible. Obviously, the duration of the study is another factor in selecting the timing.

In addition to timing and duration of the benefits study, it is important to consider whether the population will be measured or whether a sample will be taken. Measuring the population (that is, all applicable situations) may be ideal and possible for some scenarios, but also may be difficult to achieve and impractical for many scenarios. The nature of the scenario, the number of occurrences of the event being measured, the importance of capturing each occurrence, and the validity and reliability of the sampling methodology are factors to consider. For example, if the goal is to measure ADEs, each of these is probably already being counted and studied in some manner. Including the population of ADEs in the benefits realization study is probably realistic and appropriate. Measuring patient satisfaction with a care-giver entering data into a workstation in the examining room may be something to study via sampling. In this case, however, the sampling process should follow the rules of sampling commonly found in research methodology texts or approved by a statistician.

Creating the Metrics

A critical step in the benefits realization study is that of creating the metrics used to measure the benefits. Many EHR vendors will offer metrics (and may offer, even eagerly, to conduct the study for the organization). Reviewing the literature and looking at vendors' approaches are useful ways to identify metrics that may apply to the benefits the organization is trying to achieve.

The most important thing about the metrics is that they truly measure what they are intended to measure. One organization wanted to achieve improvement in referrals. Although the organization could count how many referrals were made formally, it was concerned that many were missing. In addition, it wanted to understand why the referrals were made and how long it took for a patient to get to the referred physician. Although these are important issues, they represent a mix of easy and difficult items to measure. They also represent benefits that directly apply as well as some that may not be impacted by an EHR implementation and thus do not actually apply to the organization. Table 5.6 analyzes this scenario and proposes metrics for measuring applicable impacts.

It should be noted that in each case the same metric is used both before and after (or in the control group and experimental group if conducting the study as the EHR is phased in). If for some reason it is impossible to use the exact same metric, equivalent metrics should be found and everyone should agree to use them as equivalents.

When metrics are identified, it is important to obtain agreement on their applicability and the process by which they will be used. Ideally, the process of identifying the metrics to begin with included representatives who would be affected by the metrics. If so, obtaining agreement is part of the identification process. However, if it is unclear that all stakeholders are involved, it is essential to involve them at this point. When human behavior is being observed, it is important to explain not only that monitoring is going on, but also its purpose. Suggesting that a blind study may lessen the "risk" of change occurring during the "before" measuring process is really not fair, especially when it may impact the care process. It is just important to be cognizant of such an eventuality.

In addition to identifying and agreeing to what the metrics should be and how they will be applied, it is important to test the metrics. Testing should determine whether the metric is actually measuring what it is intended to measure and ensure that the measuring process is imposing no undue hardship or harm.

Table 5.6. Benefits realization metrics scenario

Benefit Statements	How EHR Can Help	Before-and-After Metric
Reduce number of referrals outside the organization.	EHR will present a list of internal physicians as first choice in making the referral.	Number of formal referrals. (Obtaining information about the "casual" referral, such as "You might consider seeing an ophthalmologist about that" is difficult, unless you want to interview patients as they leave.)
Ensure that referrals are made to appropriate level of care-giver (for example, do not refer a diabetic to an orthopedic surgeon for foot care when a podiatrist would do).	EHR will require referral justification as a drop-down menu and suggest alternatives.	Analyze each referral for appropriateness (Y/N). (This process may lead to pre-EHR improvement. It also can help identify the menu of reasons for referrals used to build the EHR.)
Always use formal referral process to document plan of care.	EHR will prompt the care-giver for disposition of patient before encounter is closed.	Number of records without documented plan of care. Number of records with documented plan of care, including and excluding referrals. Compare to number of known referrals. (This addresses more than referrals.)
Reduce time it takes for patient to be seen by referred physician.	EHR will coordinate with referral authorization process so that approval for referral is obtained prior to patient encounter ending.	Number of referral approvals prior to end of encounter. (The time it takes for a patient to be seen by a referred physician is only due in part to the referral authorization process. Other factors, such as patient compliance and referred physician schedule, are factors out of your control.)

After the metrics have been tested and any necessary adjustments made, they are implemented at both points in time or in both groups. Follow-up at regular intervals is important to ensure that the metrics continue to measure what is intended and that there are no problems. It also may be possible to take preliminary findings and determine whether sufficient information has been obtained so that the study can be stopped, if warranted.

Evaluating the Measurements

The final step in the benefits realization study is to analyze the results. In conducting "before" measurements, a baseline is obviously being formed. One analysis that should be conducted is whether there is a change within the period of the study. For example, if the goal of the EHR is to reduce outside referrals and the study's duration is 6 months, but the number of outside referrals steadily declines during that period, the act of monitoring this obviously has an impact even before the EHR is implemented. This is a behavior change that is good for the organization overall, even if potentially difficult to manage from a statistical analysis point of view. The question often arises whether the start, end, middle, or average (mean) measurement is the one to which benefits are keyed. Such an event should be anticipated during the creation of the metrics and a decision made at that time (which may vary by type of event). More dramatic results are obviously found if the start measurement is taken. It is not a good practice to be especially liberal when anticipating benefits. Thus, it could be argued that the end measurement is the only one directly impacted by implementation of the EHR. However, one also could argue that the study would not have been done except to begin the implementation of the EHR, which might speak to using the middle value or the mean value. Finally, it should be assessed whether the "good behavior" is likely to continue without the monitoring. If not, or if not with the same level of intensity, it is clear that the EHR will have a significant impact and the start measurement may well be applicable.

If such a phenomenon occurs in the control group when the study is constructed in that manner, the same reasoning should apply. However, the opportunity exists to determine whether the results are more dramatic in the experimental group (the one that has the EHR).

It also is possible to use the "before" or control measurements to gain insights into how an EHR should be designed to best improve on the outcomes of the process. In fact, this important benefit of such a study is often overlooked. Using a benefits realization study can be helpful in the system build process, as was illustrated in table 5.3.

As previously noted, the timing of the "after" or experimental group portion of the benefits realization study is important. Implementing the EHR will involve a learning curve, during which time all events could take much longer. If time is not a factor in the intended benefit, however, measurements could start as soon as practicable. Many of the decision rules contribute to evidence-based medicine, not to improving productivity, and should be initiated as soon as the EHR is implemented.

Some EHRs measure when a rule "fires," that is, when the data entered trigger an alert or reminder (for example, when a certain age criterion has been met, when the patient is on certain medications, or when the patient has not had a certain screening within a defined period of time). In other studies, the results of the rule being fired are measured. In this case, the alert or reminder occurs, but the system only tracks whether the alert is followed. For example, if there is a reminder for a mammogram, the benefit is measured only when the mammogram has been performed. Care should be taken to determine exactly what is to be measured because, again, there is the potential for behavior change to occur by virtue of knowing a rule may fire.

Before measuring the benefits, it is important to try to describe the level of improvement or degree of benefit desired. It also may be appropriate to anticipate a time period in which a goal will be achieved. Continuing with the referral example, if the goal is to reduce all external referrals except to those medically necessary, the process of measurement and evaluation must consider medical necessity and continue until such a goal is achieved. If this is taking a long time, factors that may be causing the goal not to be met must be considered. These may include those related to the EHR but also may be totally outside the scope of the EHR. For example, results showing that all medically necessary referrals are still not being made internally could mean that bringing certain specialists on board may be a consideration. However, if the volume of such referrals is small, it may not be appropriate to establish such a high goal as "all patients must be referred internally."

Correcting Processes

The goal of the benefits realization study should be to demonstrate that anticipated benefits are being met. If the study reveals they are not being met, adjustments in the study must be made or corrective action taken with respect to either the EHR and its use or other activities. The referral example used in this discussion is reflective of several types of problems. The study could have been constructed inappropriately (that is, expecting all referrals to be in-house). The EHR may not be supplying the support needed (perhaps a rule is not firing when needed, perhaps it is too easy to bypass the rule, perhaps the rule is wrong). Other factors may need to be addressed (such as availability of in-house caregivers to receive referrals).

It also has been noted that the "before" component of the benefits realization study can contribute to system build and, potentially, even the nature of the EHR system to be implemented.

Conclusion

Benefits found to be occurring as anticipated should be celebrated. Indeed, all milestones along the way to an EHR should be celebrated to keep up momentum. Sometimes there is a tendency to question why the study was done in the first place when the findings are positive. However, many factors make for successful implementation of an EHR. The care with which a benefits realization study is constructed, implemented, and used may actually be conveying a level of commitment and support that is not inherently obvious but is a powerful message that contributes to adoption of the system.

References and Resources

Aetna's E-Prescribing Pilot Causes Increases in Generic Drug Prescriptions and Formulary Compliance, 2007 (Nov. 5). *Health Business Daily*.

Amatayakul, M. 2006. Unpublished research study funded by the Blandin Foundation and sponsored by the College of St. Scholastica : Is an EHR for Everyone?

Amatayakul, M., and M. Cohen. 1999 (May). Participatory approach to cost/benefit analysis and achieving measurable CPR benefits. *TEPR Conference Proceedings*. Orlando, FL: Towards the Electronic Patient Record.

Aspden, P., et al., eds. 2004. *Patient Safety: Achieving a New Standard for Care*. Washington, DC: National Academies Press.

Baker L., et al., 2005. Effect of an Internet-based system for doctor–patient communication on healthcare spending. *Journal of the American Medical Informatics Association* 12(5):530–36.

Centers for Medicare and Medicaid Services, Hospital Compare. www.cms.hhs.gov/hospitalqualityinits/25_hospitalcompare.asp.

Centers for Medicare and Medicaid Services, Physician Quality Reporting Initiative. www.cms.hhs.gov/pqri.

Chaiken, B.P. 2003. Clinical ROI: Not just costs versus benefits. *Journal of Healthcare Information Management* 17(4):36–41.

Crowell, M., et al. 2000. The journey to a CPR in a large multi-specialty group practice. *Sixth Annual Nicholas E. Davies Award Proceedings of the CPR Recognition Symposium, Computer-based Patient Record Institute, Inc. Healthcare Informatics Executive Management Series*. Bethesda, MD: HIMSS.

Dassenko, D., and T. Slowinski. 1995. Using the CPR to benefit a business office. *Healthcare Financial Management* 49:68–73.

Davis, D.C., et al. 1999. Clinical performance improvement with an advanced clinical information system at the Queen's Medical Center. *Fifth Annual Nicholas E. Davies Award Proceedings of the CPR Recognition Symposium, Computer-based Patient Record Institute, Inc. Healthcare Informatics Executive Management Series*. Bethesda, MD: Healthcare Information Management and Systems Society.

Delio, M. 2003 (Jan.). Barcode tech drives nurses nuts. *Wired News*. www.wired.com/news/prnt/0,1294,57311,00.html.

DesRoches, Catherine M, et al. 2008. Electronic Health Records in Ambulatory Care—a National Survey of Physicians, *New England Journal of Medicine* 359(1):50–60.

Erstad, T.L. 2003. Analyzing computer-based patient records: A review of literature. *Journal of Healthcare Information Management* 17(4):51,57.

Grandia, L.D., et al. 1995. Building a computer-based patient record system in an evolving integrated health system. *First Annual Nicholas E. Davies Award Proceedings of the CPR Recognition Symposium*. Schaumburg, IL: CPRI.

Healthcare Information Management and Systems Society. 1995–2004. The Annual Nicholas E. Davies Award of Excellence. Available online from himss.org.

Healthfield, S.M. Beyond Traditional SMART Goals, About.com, 2000.

H&HN Team. 2005 (July). The 100 most wired: The quality connection. *Hospitals & Health Networks* 79(7):39–50.

Hillestad R., et al. 2005. Can Electronic Medical Record Systems Transform Health Care? Potential Health Benefits, Savings, and Costs, *Health Affairs*, 24(5): 1103–1117.

HIMSS Analytics. 2007. The EMR Adoption Model.

Committee on Quality of Health Care in America, Institute of Medicine. 2001. Crossing the Quality Chasm: A New Health System for the 21st Century, National Academy Press.

Jensen, J. 2004. United hospital increases capacity usage, efficiency with patient-flow management system. *Journal of Healthcare Information Management* 18(3):26–31.

Layman, E. 2006. Research methods. In *Health Information Management: Concepts, Principles, and Practice,* Second Edition, edited by K.M. La-Tour and S. Eichenwald. Chicago: AHIMA.

Landon, B.E., et al. 2007. Improving the Management of Chronic Disease at Community Health Centers, *New England Journal of Medicine.* 356(9): 921–934.

Linder, J.A., et al. 2007. Electronic Health Record Use and the Quality of Ambulatory Care in the United States, *Archives of Internal Medicine*, 167(13).

Midwest Medical Insurance Company (MMIC), Certified Electronic Medical Record Risk Management Premium Credit, October 25, 2007.

Morris, S., et al. 2002. IT investment planning: The best hospitals. *Journal of Healthcare Information Management* 16(2):62–65.

Renner, K. 1996. Electronic medical records in the outpatient setting. *Medical Group Management Journal* 43:52–74.

Rosenstein, A.H. 1999 (Feb.). Inpatient clinical decision-support systems: Determining the ROI. *Healthcare Financial Management,* pp. 51–55.

Shields A.E., et al. 2007. Adoption of health Information Technology in Community Health Centers: Results of a National Survey, Health Affairs, 26(5): 1373–1383.

Smith, T.W., et al. 2004 (Dec.). Transforming healthcare with a patient-centric electronic health record system. Evanston Northwestern Healthcare, Nicholas E. Davies Award of Excellence. Chicago: HIMSS.

Tang, P.C., et al. 1998. NetReach: Building a clinical infrastructure for the enterprise. *Fourth Annual Nicholas E. Davies Award Proceedings of the CPR Recognition Symposium, Computer-based Patient Record Institute, Inc. Healthcare Informatics Executive Management Series.* Bethesda, MD: Healthcare Information Management and Systems Society.

Teich, J.M., et al. 1996. Toward cost-effective quality care: The Brigham integrated computing system, Brigham and Women's Hospital. *Second Annual Nicholas E. Davies Award Proceedings of the CPR Recognition Symposium.* Schaumburg, IL: CPRI.

Towne, Jennifer. 2008 (June 11). The EHR's Impact on IOM's Aims. H&HN's *Most Wired.*

Walker, J. M., et al. 2008 (Feb. 28). EHR Safety: The Way Forward to Save and Effective Systems, *Journal of the American Medical Informatics Association.*

Walker, J., et al. 2005 (Jan.). The Value of Health Care Information Exchange and Interoperability, *Health Affairs.*

Chapter 6
Strategic Planning for the EHR Migration Path

Dwight D. Eisenhower is quoted as having said: "In preparing for battle I have always found that plans are useless, but planning is indispensable."

CIO magazine conducted a survey of CIOs and found that as many as 39 percent of respondents had no formal information technology (IT) strategy (Slater 2002). They contend that strategic planning is a frustrating, time-consuming endeavor, where plans are frequently threatened with obsolescence by technology changes and economic upheaval before the ink even dries. The process of planning can be time-consuming and distracts from, rather than contributes to, the real work of building and maintaining an adequate technology infrastructure. Alternatively, many suggest that it is indeed that environment that requires strategic planning. Project prioritization, risk analysis, understanding the likelihood of changes in the industry and technology, and setting appropriate expectations are key ingredients in managing the IT support for the changing and increasingly competitive environment of healthcare. Good planning helps achieve impressive outcomes with a minimum of frustration.

Because an electronic health record (EHR) is not a technology or an event but, rather, a journey toward goals for clinical transformation aided by technology, a migration path, strategic plan, or evolution along a set of generations, such as suggested by Gartner, a technology consulting firm, (Gillespie 2003) is very important. This chapter:

- Describes pathways toward the EHR

- Identifies ways to approach strategic EHR planning

- Links EHR planning to strategic organizational planning

- Discusses strategic planning for the EHR within specific healthcare settings and circumstances

Gartner Generations

Gartner proposes one of the most widely recognized descriptions of a pathway to an EHR. Despite that it was proposed in 2003, the generations and their level of functionality based

Key Terms

Analytical processing	Data warehouse	Implementation strategy
Best of breed	Dual-core	Legacy systems
Best of fit	Financing and acquisition strategy	Open architecture
Continuum of care	Functional strategy	Technical strategy
Data repository	Hospital information system	Transactional processing
Data strategy		

on the Gartner EHR generations illustrated in figure 6.1 are still valid today. (Each generation is described further below.) Although Gartner typically associates the description with a time line denoting availability of products or current industry progress in implementing an EHR, the illustration in figure 6.1 has avoided proposing a time line so that each organization can adopt its own. Any given organization may have started to plan some time ago or is just beginning to plan. It is hoped that organizations will recognize that any automation focused on clinical information is a start along the migration path. The generations provide a useful summary of the path that an EHR project might take for strategic planning purposes.

The Collector Generation

In the Collector generation, systems provide a site-specific, encounter-based solution to access clinical data. The industry also has described this functionality as clinical data display or results retrieval. In such an environment, there is no workflow support, no clinical decision support, and no knowledge management, and communications basically are uni-

Figure 6.1.   GartnerGroup generations of an EHR

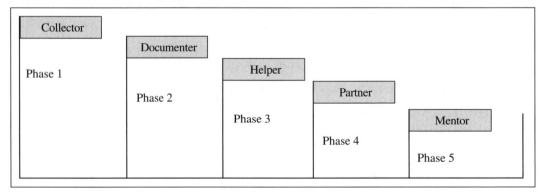

Source: Handler, 2001.

directional. For example, for order communications, nursing personnel are able to send an order to a departmental, or ancillary, system, but get no feedback on potential issues with the order or even an acknowledgment that the receiving system has received the order.

The Documenter Generation

Gartner describes the Documenter generation as the phase in which data capture occurs at the point of care. Simple documentation tools exist with minimal collection of discrete data. Graphic and tabular display for results management capability is included. Computerized physician order entry (CPOE) with drug–drug and drug–allergy alerts is provided in real or near real time. There is minimal access to knowledge sources and simple bidirectional communications. Electronic medication administration record systems might also qualify in this generation, as they are merely documents generated by a pharmacy information system without any associated closed-loop medication management processes.

It is interesting to note that this is only the second generation because many healthcare organizations are still very much in the early planning stages for even the most rudimentary CPOE system. Actually one major reason for the difficulty in getting CPOE systems adopted is that they lack the robust decision support capability that would return value to the provider using the system (Sternlieb 2004). In fact, many hospitals have implemented point-of-care charting systems before CPOE systems because of the lack of robust decision making in some of the current CPOE systems. The point-of-care charting systems, however, generally are not context-sensitive. That is, they provide a template to capture standardized data, but the template does not change to reflect the specific context of the data being entered.

The Helper Generation

The Helper generation includes more advanced EHR systems that cover episodes and encounters and use decision support to assist clinicians. Gartner qualifies that such a system must be able to function in ambulatory and acute care settings. The functions of documentation, data display, workflow, decision support, and knowledge management are beginning to be integrated; but communication across the ambulatory and acute care settings is still more complex than many products are designed to handle. When the systems are more integrated, they tend to be document-based rather than data-based. Although Gartner indicated in 2003 that it believes the industry is still in the Documenter generation, there has been enough emphasis on patient safety issues that many organizations that were in the Documenter generation in 2003 are likely in the Helper generation in 2008.

The Partner Generation

Gartner considers the Partner generation to be an advanced system that provides more complex decision support encompassing evidence-based medicine, and with comprehensive links to personal health records (PHRs). Some organizations with leading-edge EHR implementations have this level of EHR. Data from a survey conducted by the American Hospital Association in late 2006 reported that only 1 percent of hospitals offered a PHR, with 4 percent more in the planning stages.

When the Institute of Medicine (IOM) first conceived of the computer-based patient record (as it was then called), it was envisioned that information also would flow to and from patients. This was never widely recognized, and the concept of the PHR has grown up sometimes connected and sometimes disconnected from the EHR. Certainly the recent consumer empowerment initiatives from the federal government (ONC 2008; CMS 2007) and a number of health plans for value-driven healthcare make a PHR a much more important, integrating function of the EHR, despite that it remains a challenge for care delivery organizations to consider adopting.

The Mentor Generation

The Mentor generation is the most complex and sophisticated phase of EHR. In this phase, the system is fully integrated across the **continuum of care** and guides clinicians through highly advanced knowledge management, decision support, and predictive modeling. A key element of this generation is the notion of data flowing throughout the continuum of care and providing a feedback mechanism where information learned about treatment efficacy can be returned to the user in the form of evidence-based medicine.

Many organizations that are composed of multiple provider settings, typically called integrated delivery systems (IDSs) or integrated delivery networks (IDNs), do not even have an enterprisewide master person index, so in some respects the Mentor generation is quite futuristic. However, there also has been significant movement toward health information exchange (HIE), which would identify patients through an algorithmic matching process and locate their records through a record locator service. The HIE would be supported by a consent management process, potentially enabled by PHRs, and would utilize strong security services of authentication, access controls, and logging and auditing.

The path toward an EHR is long, winding, and variable. New technology, new legislation, and even new government initiatives such as the concept of the nationwide health information network (NHIN) continue to help change the course of the path.

The EHR Pathway

The Gartner set of EHR generations is one view of the path toward an EHR. Although much of the path toward an EHR forms a continuum of technological advancement, there are components that individual organizations may want to consider adopting at different times relative to their needs. In other words, each organization may be guided by the proposed generations in terms of what is commonly available or what has been typically deployed, but not necessarily what the organization itself plans to do.

Essentially, strategic planning for the EHR is deciding on the path, journey, or genealogy an organization wants to undertake to transition to an EHR. For as much as some might like to see a revolution where all aspects of the EHR are implemented at once, no one has yet been able to achieve anything but an evolution. Some organizations have gone far in certain areas, and many are just beginning down the path. Strategic planning will ensure a more orderly, logical, and, it is hoped, more cost-effective and efficient method to achieve the benefits the EHR provides.

Strategic Planning

In general, strategic planning determines where an organization is going over the next year or several years, how it is going to get there, and how it will know whether it got there (McNamara 1999b). The emphasis in strategic planning is not only the extended time period of the plan, but also the fact that the plan is high level and developed by executive management. Strategic planning establishes an overall purpose and set of goals to be accomplished. A strategic plan is not necessarily devoid of quantification, but it is not focused on task-level detail. It should specifically define the benefits to be achieved by its outcome. Moreover, there should be specific milestones to help executive management monitor the plan's progress.

For example, if one of the organization's strategic goals is to become a center of excellence in a specific medical specialty, the benefits of this initiative might be described by enhanced revenue stream and contribution to capital. The organization may expect a return on investment (ROI) of a specific payback period. Milestones would include opening a new wing by a certain date, recruiting a specified number of specialists, and achieving a percent of occupancy or utilization rate within an established period of time. Because the EHR should support strategic initiatives, each of these milestones should encompass components of the EHR. For example, the new wing should fully support wired and wireless access and the internal design should support point of care computing. Another supporting component might be that specialists be nationally recognized, able to attract patients from a regional geographic area, and support adoption of an EHR.

Even though the EHR can be identified as a strategic initiative in its own right, the more closely it can be linked to other strategic initiatives, the more likely it will be viewed as an integral part of them. However, because the EHR is such a resource-intensive activity and a significant change for an organization, it may still be appropriate to identify it as a strategic initiative as well as an integral part of other initiatives. Organizations that consider planning for an EHR only as a technology project often do not understand its scope and may later have difficulty gaining adoption or retaining funding levels. These organizations often view an EHR project as "only an IT project," rather than the clinical transformation it truly is. Adoption of EHR is indeed an activity that should tie to the organization's mission, goals and objectives, and other strategic initiatives. Numerous, more detailed plans associated with the EHR components will flow from the strategic plan.

Conducting Strategic Planning

Many healthcare organizations use a fairly standard approach to strategic planning. The components of a standard approach are listed in table 6.1. Typically, strategic planning is performed once a year or once every 2 or 3 years, often in a retreat environment with the entire executive management team involved. Sometimes additional resource people are included, depending on the issues faced by the organization. A facilitator may be used to overcome bias and other group process pressures as well as to prepare perspectives or to conduct comparative analyses in advance. At the conclusion of the strategic planning activity, a written plan is produced that summarizes the planning activity and records objectives, responsibilities, time lines, and so on. Executive management may plan regular meetings

Table 6.1.   Components of strategic planning activity

Strategic Planning Components	
Preparation	1. Who 2. When 3. Where 4. Why 5. How (See strategic planning models in Table 6.2.)
Strategic analysis	1. Environmental scan 2. Organization's strengths, weaknesses, opportunities, and threats (SWOT) 3. Organizational assessments
Strategic direction	1. Review and reaffirmation of mission, vision, and values (unless significant change in organization would create new statements) 2. Strategic goals 3. Strategic initiatives 4. Action plans and accountability
Process	1. Evaluate planning process and plan 2. Acknowledge completion and celebrate results

around reviewing the strategic plan, receiving reports, analyzing deviations from the plan, and generally monitoring progress.

Determining EHR Interest

However the actual strategic planning event occurs, much work goes into preparing for the event. Individuals who may contribute to preparing for an EHR discussion may include members of a general information systems (IS) steering committee, members of a special grassroots committee constructed to begin investigation of an EHR, or key individuals who have casually discussed the organization's readiness for an EHR.

Whatever group or individuals rise to the occasion or may be tasked by executive management to compile preparatory material, the first task is to gain an understanding of the interest for an EHR at the grassroots level. This must trickle up to executive management as evidence of readiness for an EHR. However, all the potential users of the EHR may need to be educated about it. Although physicians often are in a position of being a single point of failure for an EHR initiative, nurses, all other clinicians, administrative and financial staff, and other users must be educated, positive, and supportive (Hier 2002).

If strategic planning is being done in a hospital, physicians active in the medical informatics community may already be familiar with the concept and others may have adopted an EHR for their office practice. However, many physicians may have only heard stories and filtered this information with their own personal predilections. Even those physicians actively engaged in an EHR in some way may have personal biases and perceptions, especially because a hospital-based EHR is different from an office-based EHR. Hospitals also should note that acute care environments have different needs for EHRs than do ambulatory care environments. If the organization is a large physician group practice preparing for an EHR, many of the same planning principles apply. Physicians are not always able to persuade their colleagues that an EHR is an appropriate investment without the planning work described here. Smaller offices might study the same issues but perform their analysis in a less formalized manner.

Gauging User Readiness

There are several ways to gauge interest and readiness by potential users of the EHR. If the level of automation is already somewhat strong, listening to users describe what they would like to see "next" will offer much insight. Distributing literature about EHRs or encouraging representatives of various user types to attend professional meetings and trade shows where EHRs are described and demonstrated can provide value. Interest in reading or in attending the shows is one measure of interest in EHR alone.

Raising the issue in various forums and studying the response also will provide clues for readiness. Clearly, if people are talking about EHRs, asking the IT department, or commenting about their value to health information management (HIM) professionals, these are all good signs of interest. Finally, it may be appropriate to actually conduct a quick survey of interest.

Conducting a Survey

The survey tool displayed in figure 6.2 has been used successfully with more than 5,000 individuals in approximately 100 group practices to ascertain EHR readiness by physicians, nurses, and other personnel. It is constructed so that there is no pattern to similar answers. Respondents have to read each question to correctly provide an answer. The survey also includes questions where strong agreement is a positive indication of readiness and questions where strong agreement is a negative indicator. Figure 6.2 also illustrates results from actually conducting the survey. (Results also could be shown for different groups of respondents, for example, to determine whether there were differences in views between physicians and nurses.) In this example, the respondents were generally neutral with respect to cost, personal productivity, and depersonalization when using EHRs in the examining room. The only really negative indicator was that respondents did not believe their patients were expecting them to use an EHR. (This finding may vary by geographic location and population served. A negative response to this statement also suggests that there is potentially unfounded perception by clinicians, as many patients surveyed have had no objection to use of the EHR as long as physicians take steps to focus on the patient (Ventres et al. 2006). Perhaps the most favorable responses were that the respondents did not believe the EHR imposed unwanted discipline, believed the EHR contributed to increased office productivity, and understood that EHR implementation is a long-term commitment. No survey results should be taken at total face value.

Even though these results appeared to be quite positive, personal interviews and other indicators indicated that many potential users did not understand the full functionality of an EHR. This was probably why respondents did not view the EHR as contributing to their personal productivity (only their office productivity) or as imposing any unwanted discipline (although hopefully the EHR does not impose unwanted discipline, but will likely impose some discipline when decision support is applied). Clearly, the group of physicians and nurses who responded to this survey seemed interested but would need further education.

Figure 6.2.   EHR readiness assessment survey (with results)

Concerning EHRs	5 4 Strongly Agree	3 Neutral	2 1 Strongly Disagree
They contribute to increased office productivity	3.9		
They impose unwanted discipline			2.2
They are not as secure as paper records			2.7
They raise the quality of healthcare	3.5		
Our patients are expecting us to use them			2.4
Their cost is beyond our budget		3.0	
They will improve my personal productivity		3.2	
They are essential for keeping up to date	3.5		
Use in the examining room is depersonalizing.		3.1	
They are difficult to learn how to use			2.6
The effort to implement them is a long-term commitment	4.2		

Copyright © 2008, Margret\A Consulting, LLC. Reprinted with permission.

Constructing an EHR Briefing Paper

When executive management begins its discussions of an EHR, it also may need education. Even if management has discussed the EHR in the past, an update on its current industry status may be necessary. A well-constructed briefing paper can be useful. The briefing paper should:

- Outline a definition that is commonly accepted in the industry
- Illustrate the notion that the EHR is an infrastructure built over time
- Fairly outline costs and benefits
- Accurately reflect the current level of interest, understanding, and readiness of an EHR within the organization

It may be necessary to describe issues associated with current technology or the organization's IS vendor's capability to support an EHR if these issues are especially vexing for the organization. Finally, the briefing paper may outline typical steps to visioning and migration path development. However, the briefing paper should stick to facts and make recommendations only when requested. Incorporating speculation or desires from any one constituent group within the organization should be avoided.

Choosing a Strategic Planning Model

Various consultants or planning facilitators have their own set of terms to describe different types of strategic planning models. Just as there is no one standard set of terms to describe strategic planning models, there also is no one perfect planning model. Often organizations try different models for a period of time and then settle on one model or a hybrid. Models also can be integrated, using one form to creatively identify strategic issues and goals and another to determine how issues will be addressed and goals reached. Table 6.2 offers a set of strategic planning models from the Management Assistance Program for Nonprofits.

Strategic Planning Applied to the EHR

It cannot be emphasized enough that the EHR should emerge from strategic planning and support the organization's strategic initiatives. Although, ultimately, there will be specific plans associated with the various tasks that need to be conducted to establish an EHR infrastructure, the initial planning needs to be at the strategic level.

EHR Planning

The EHR as a strategic initiative does not imply that the EHR planning should be all top-down. Just as the EHR should not be considered solely as an IT project, so, too, should it not be simply an executive management initiative. There needs to be strong support at the grassroots level. In fact, executive management would be well advised to look for or cultivate such level of interest prior to committing to the EHR as a strategic initiative. Goal-setting and benefits expectations processes should be underway. All components of executive management, the user community, alignment with organizational mission, and technical capability must be part of the overall EHR plan.

Adoption of a Migration Path

Just as executive management adopts a vision of the organization as a whole, the organization's vision of the EHR must be articulated. The ultimate, long-range vision may be described, but because the EHR is more a path or genealogy, a migration path may be suitable to describe the journey. Some call this a transition strategy, but such language tends to imply a process to achieve use rather than a journey through phases of applications and their outcomes. A migration path suggests *what*; a transition strategy suggests *how*.

A migration path also suggests a more overall vision whereas a transition strategy should be used to move from one milestone to the next. Both are valuable tools and serve different functions. Figure 6.3 depicts a sample diagram of a migration path to describe the

Table 6.2.   Strategic planning models

"Basic" *Typically for small organizations or those with minimal planning experience*	1. Identify purpose. 2. Determine goals to accomplish mission. 3. Identify strategies or approaches to implement each goal. 4. Identify action plans to implement each strategy. 5. Monitor and update the plan.
Issue-Based *Suitable for experienced planners and large organizations updating current plans*	1. Update vision, mission, and values if necessary. 2. Conduct external and internal SWOT assessment. 3. Identify and prioritize major issues. 4. Design major strategies (or programs) to address issues. 5. Establish action plans. 6. Record in a strategic plan document. 7. Develop yearly operating plan. 8. Develop and authorize budget. 9. Conduct organization's operations. 10. Monitor, review, evaluate, and update strategic plan.
Alignment *Helpful for organizations experiencing a large number of internal inefficiencies*	1. Outline mission, programs, resources, and needed support. 2. Identify what is working and what needs adjustment. 3. Identify how adjustments should be made. 4. Include adjustments as strategies in plan.
Scenario *Appropriate for ensuring strategic thinking in the face of potential major change in direction*	1. Select several external forces (such as recently identified in news headlines) and imagine related changes that might influence the organization. 2. For each change in a force, discuss best-case, worst-case, and most likely case scenarios as a result of the change. 3. Suggest potential strategies in response to each of the three scenarios. 4. Identify common strategies among the scenarios. 5. Select the most likely changes to affect the organization and identify the common strategies to respond to the change.
Organic *This is a self-organizing approach as opposed to the typical linear plan that may be more suitable for certain cultures or when senior management changes*	1. Clarify organization's values using dialogue techniques. 2. Articulate group's vision for the organization, also using dialogue techniques. 3. Regularly dialogue about processes needed to arrive at vision. 4. Continually reinforce value of dialogue and patience. Focus on learning rather than method. 5. Agree on how to portray the results of this planning to key stakeholders.

Source: Adapted from McNamara 1999b.

Figure 6.3. Sample migration path toward the EHR

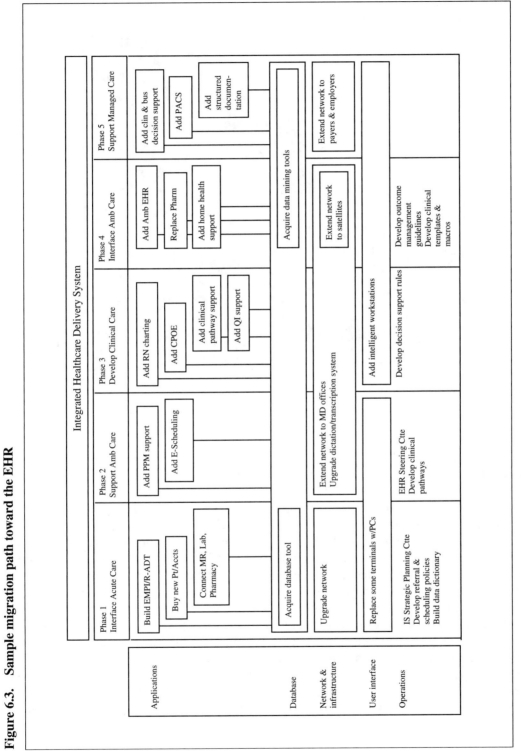

Figure 6.4.   Migration path described by building blocks

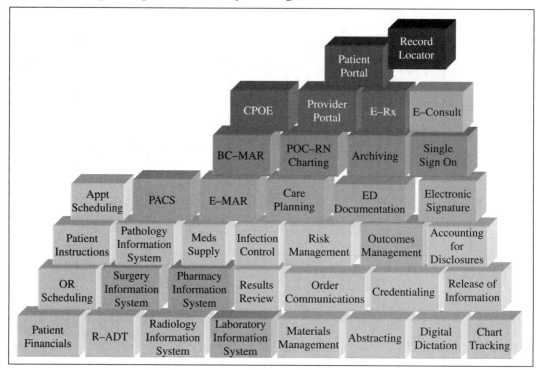

milestones toward the EHR. This example is drawn from a community-based IDN, with a hospital, owned physician practices, and a home health agency in a heavily managed care environment.

It is not necessary to construct a migration path using the particular format shown in figure 6.3. Different organizations may use a set of building blocks (figure 6.4), a step diagram (figure 6.5), a table, a narrative description, or other pictorials (figures 6.6 and 6.7). Several formats are illustrated not only to emphasize that format is not as important as content, but also to reflect that there is no one right path for all organizations. Each format, however, does have strengths and weaknesses for planning purposes.

A building block approach (figure 6.4) typically focuses exclusively on applications, where it would be ideal to include at other elements, such as operations and technology (such as when an EHR steering committee will be formed, when a medical director of information systems will be assigned, what interfaces are needed to connect applications, network upgrades, storage additions, and so on). This approach also does not definitely describe the time line, but only the sequence of implementations. Still, the building block approach emphasizes that the EHR is a system of components, a concept sometimes lost on stakeholders.

Figure 6.5.   Migration path described as a step diagram

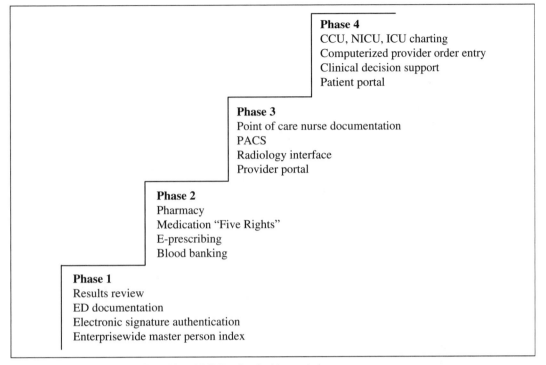

Phase 4
CCU, NICU, ICU charting
Computerized provider order entry
Clinical decision support
Patient portal

Phase 3
Point of care nurse documentation
PACS
Radiology interface
Provider portal

Phase 2
Pharmacy
Medication "Five Rights"
E-prescribing
Blood banking

Phase 1
Results review
ED documentation
Electronic signature authentication
Enterprisewide master person index

A step diagram (figure 6.5) is similar to the building block approach, although the time frame is a bit clearer and it is generally possible to include more elements, such as technical and operational aspects needed to support the applications. Although not included in this illustration, it would be easy to add the goal for each phase and even dates or other time line elements.

Figure 6.6 illustrates the applications, technology, and associated benefits, but provides no time line, and may be difficult to use when there are many more applications and technologies to include.

The flowchart in figure 6.7 uses color and line designations to illustrate current and proposed applications and some technology. It clearly illustrates the flow of information throughout systems, although without a time line it does not suggest the migration path as clearly. What applications will be implemented next? What supporting technology is needed?

Migration Path Construction

As illustrated in the variety of formats describe the EHR system, most organizations appreciate the need to gain an overview of the EHR and how it will be developed. A tool illustrating the various applications, supporting structures, and sequencing can provide such an overall picture and help establish milestones.

Figure 6.6.   Migration path as a picture

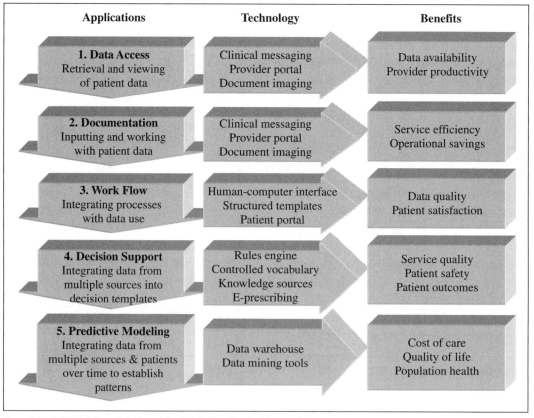

Copyright © 2008, Margret\A Consulting, LLC. Reprinted with permission.

As the migration path is planned, it also can highlight issues of appropriate sequencing and overcome a "stovepipe" mentality. For example, in one case, a hospital found itself planning a comprehensive electronic document management system for use by its HIM department. Another, separate document imaging system was being planned by its contracted emergency department physicians. Finally, an attempt also was being made to sell a third document imaging system to its radiology department, which had just acquired a PACS system and no longer had the pocket in the film jackets to store copies of the radiology order and report. Although there are differences in electronic document management systems based on workflow needs that may preclude one system being used for all three purposes, the acquisition of three systems of essentially the same type should be evaluated. It is hoped that a solution would emerge that would address at least two of the three needs, if not all.

A migration path also will help resolve issues of sequencing: Should a CPOE system be implemented in the hospital before or after a nursing documentation system? Should an e-prescribing system for the physicians be acquired before, simultaneously, or after a CPOE system? Should an electronic medication administration record system be imple-

Figure 6.7.   Migration path as a flowchart

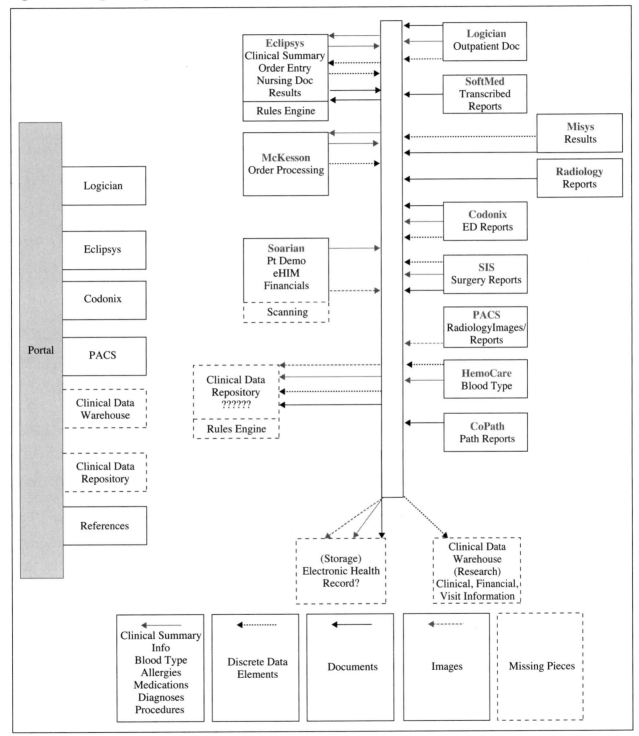

Used with permission, Children's Health System, Birmingham, AL.

Figure 6.8.   Migration path template

Timeline	Current	Phase I	Phase II	Phase n
Goals				
Applications: • Financial/ Administrative • Operational • Clinical				

Technology
• Database
• Network &
  Infrastructure
• Interoperability
• Human-computer
  interfaces
• Storage				

Operations • People • Policy • Process				

Copyright © 2008, Margret\A Consulting, LLC. Reprinted with permission.

mented prior to or after a new pharmacy information system? The answers to these questions depend on many factors, including the organization's infrastructure, goals, medical staff interest, and so on.

The construction of a migration path for the EHR might best include the following components, as illustrated in the template shown in figure 6.8:

- Time frame
- Goals
- Applications
- Technology
- Operations

Time Frame and Goals

The term *time frame* refers to the overall period of time in which the EHR is expected to be accomplished. Although planners prefer to plan for only 2 to 3 years, most healthcare organizations recognize that the planning horizon for an EHR is much longer than this. In fact, although some organizations have accomplished much in 5 years or so, many organizations take much longer. Indeed, it is for this reason that some organizations are hesitant to plan a migration path because they believe so much will change in 5 years or more. Although this is true, no one says such migration paths need to be cast in concrete. They can easily be modified over time. However, realistically portraying a time frame helps establish sequence and provides an appreciation for the scope of the endeavor and hence its cost implications.

It may be appropriate to start with phases and then add actual dates later. The phases can be described across the top of the migration path. Most organizations like to describe the current state of their information systems, using the first column in the migration path to do so. However, in the example in figure 6.3, the IDN did not include such a benchmark.

It is generally desirable to have a place to record the primary goal or goals for each phase. Although goal setting should be very explicit, the detail can be provided in an attachment. In figure 6.3, the IDN associated an overarching goal with each phase.

Applications

Applications are identified next in the migration path. Applications are the most commonly described component of a migration path. Some organizations try to simplify their migration path by listing only the applications related to clinical information. Others prefer to include all applications because there may be a need to pass information among any and all applications.

If all applications are listed, it is a good idea to group them, perhaps by financial/administrative, operational, and clinical applications. In an IDN, some effort also may be given to grouping the applications by type or organization, such as hospital, clinic, and so on.

It should be noted that the applications are described by their function and generally not by vendor name. This is not simply an artifact of this discussion occurring in a reference book, but the fact that not all stakeholders may know what a particular product is when identified only by vendor name. If the organization wants to illustrate that it has a "best-of-breed" situation, the vendor name can be listed in parentheses after the functional description (for example, radiology information system [GE], laboratory information system [Cerner], pharmacy information system [McKesson], R-ADT [Siemens], medication supply [Pyxis], and so on).

Acquisition Strategy

The term **best of breed** refers to the fact that several different vendors are used to supply the various applications in the organization, because each vendor is believed to provide the best application in its class. The result of a best-of-breed IT strategy may mean that the organization has a challenge in getting the various systems to exchange data and requires interfaces to do so.

The opposite of best of breed is **best of fit**. In this situation, virtually (though not absolutely) all applications are provided by a single vendor. This frequently makes it easier to add new applications from that vendor, but potentially even more difficult to add products from other vendors. Many organizations find that their best-of-fit financial/administrative and operational system vendor is not as strong in EHR as they would desire. Alternatively, best-of-breed organizations find it very difficult and costly to sustain this approach.

Table 6.3.   IT acquisition strategy

Best of Fit	Dual Core	Best of Breed
One primary vendor	Two primary vendors: • Financial/Administrative • Operational or Clinical	Many vendors
Generally found in small hospitals or corporate organizations seeking standardization	Both moving to this strategy	Generally found in large, stand-alone or academic medical centers
Generally simpler to implement and maintain	Viewed as either a consolidation strategy or a means to achieve a comprehensive EHR	Generally more difficult to implement and maintain due to interface requirements for exchange of data

Copyright © 2008, Margret\A Consulting, LLC. Reprinted with permission.

As a result of the disadvantages of being at one extreme or the other, many organizations are migrating to a "**dual-core**" strategy, where one primary vendor supports financial/administrative applications and possibly the operational applications and another primary vendor supports the operational and clinical applications or just the clinical applications.

These IT acquisition strategies are illustrated in table 6.3.

Technology

In the past, technology was fairly consistent based on IT strategies and vendor recommendations. As organizations look to EHR systems and different technologies become available, technology to support EHR applications becomes more of a decision factor. Technology issues especially include database structures, network and infrastructure, interoperability strategies, human–computer interfaces (input/output devices), and storage.

Database Structure

Database structures relate to how data are processed. Databases may be optimized for **transactional processing**, such as in the everyday tasks performed by an EHR. This is characteristic of a **data repository**. Databases may also be optimized for **analytical processing**, such as evaluating population health data or performing predictive modeling. This is characteristic of a **data warehouse**. In addition to these broad categories, issues of whether to purchase an incumbent vendor's database or acquire a third party can be particularly important. A vendor's database may or may not be very robust; be able to handle discrete data as well as images; be easy to retrieve data from; and be useable for data mining. Buying one's own database means a tremendous amount of development work, not only to structure the database, but generally also to develop the presentation applications that permit data entry into the database and retrieve data from the database.

Network and Infrastructure Capability

Network and infrastructure capability is obviously a major requirement for an EHR. Many times, decisions about new network structures such as wireless, more remote access, and Web-based architectures are made at the time an EHR is considered. These can play an important role in ease of use, response time, and reliability of the system as well as the ubiquity of the EHR functionality. Telecommunications capability may well need to be enhanced.

Interoperability

Interoperability strategies especially relate to the IT strategy, the openness of the vendor's systems and how well they comply with industry standards, and the need to exchange data. Most organizations are recognizing a significantly greater degree of need and interest in exchanging data across the continuum of care.

Human–Computer Interfaces

Human–computer interfaces, or user input/output (I/O) devices, are singled out as a highly critical element for user adoption. Although this may be considered part of the general technology infrastructure, generally there are critical decisions to be made that directly impact users. Choices can also significantly impact the cost of the systems.

Storage

Storage also is becoming a much bigger issue than ever before. Stored data must be more readily accessible when organizations become paperless. The volume of data becomes much larger as entire chart contents now must be archived as opposed to operational data that are not needed for a very long time, because the paper chart is the legal record of care. In addition, the data to be stored are physically of much greater size. EHR systems need to store discrete data, images of documents, and, frequently, voice files and pictures, which are huge. How these data are stored is literally becoming a separate management function.

Operations

The final category of information captured in a migration path addresses the operational elements that need to support EHR planning, selection, implementation, adoption, and benefits realization. Operational elements address the people, policies, and processes need to effect an EHR. Some examples of operational elements include project management, clinical informatician support, clinical data preparation, and policies on rule use and how they will be described, used, or not used. Plotting these elements on the migration path not only helps identify the potential impact of any change to one area on all other areas but also serves as a high-level plan.

Critical Success Factors for EHR Planning

Different organizations will construct different models of a migration path or may choose to use different tools to plan their EHR. However the broad view of the EHR is presented, the critical success factors of planning the EHR include:

- Creating the vision
- Identifying the planning horizon
- Gaining agreement

- Developing a financing and acquisition strategy
- Developing functional, data, and technical strategies
- Carrying out a vendor selection process
- Planning the implementation
- Conducting benefits realization

Creating the vision, identifying the planning horizon, and gaining agreement have been emphasized throughout the initial chapters of this book. Each of the other factors is introduced in this chapter, with in-depth discussion provided in the remaining chapters.

Financing and Acquisition Strategy

The **financing and acquisition strategy** refers to how the EHR is paid for and acquired. This includes whether the organization designs and builds its own system or acquires one from a vendor. It also addresses financing options such as purchase, lease, or various partnering/codevelopment options. Some vendors offer a discount when organizations are willing to implement a prototype of a new version of an EHR and assist in its further refinement. Some vendors also have linked up with pharmaceutical companies, hardware vendors, and other suppliers to provide reduced prices in exchange for using their products or obtaining data. Major employers in the area may be a source of funding if they are interested in negotiating reduced costs of care. Finally, private foundation or government grants or contracts are potential sources of funds. Although some of these options may provide significant benefits, they should be approached with a full understanding of what the organization must do to obtain the funding support.

A strategy refers to a high-level planning activity. Thus, the policies surrounding vendor selection would be included in the financing and acquisition strategy, although the actual steps in vendor selection would not be considered at this point. For example, some organizations prefer the best-of-fit approach, only considering purchasing from the vendor that has supplied products to them in the past. Other organizations may consider a best-of-breed approach, because they want the best system for each application and are willing to address integration issues. The dual core strategy, which combines these strategies, is becoming more common. This often arises when the organization has a best-of-fit strategy for its core components and then opts for a different vendor to supply its clinical components, as long as they can be interfaced with the core vendor's products.

Other policies considered in the financing and acquisition strategy include the purchasing requirements that stipulate the stability of the vendor business, the number of other installations it must have, the size and type of clients, and so forth. Some organizations are more willing to assume risk than others. The financing and acquisition strategy must reflect the degree of risk-taking a healthcare organization is willing to accept.

Although financing and acquisition strategies should be addressed early in strategic planning, they generally are not carried out until after functional, data, and technical strategies have been identified. Hence, financing with ROI is discussed in chapter 11 and EHR selection is discussed in chapter 12.

Functional Strategy

The **functional strategy** describes how the EHR system performs with respect to its users and in relationship to its boundaries with other systems. There are essentially two levels of functional strategy. The first is that which supports the overall migration path. Executive management approves this functional strategy.

A more detailed level of functional strategy defines the specific, detailed functions to be performed and generally serves as a set of functional specifications for vendor selection. This level of functional detail may require a process assessment to be performed. A process assessment entails a detailed review of operations, workflow, and outcomes to both identify process improvements needed prior to EHR implementation and establish the functional requirements necessary to support improvements in processes through an EHR. Process assessment is discussed fully in chapter 7.

Functional assessment entails studying the various groups of processes and translating that discussion into a statement of functional needs that can be taken to a vendor or IS designer for development. Functional needs assessment is discussed fully in chapter 8.

One way to distinguish processes from functions is to consider that functionality is what is "bought" in an EHR; processes must be built into the functions of an EHR. Processes are unique to the organization; functions are provided by a vendor.

Data Strategy

The **data strategy** refers to the overall manner in which the organization plans to use data standards and build its data infrastructure. Although most EHRs are built on a data repository, not all are. A few EHRs have been constructed through a tightly integrated set of systems and applications. Whatever the data infrastructure is going to be, however, strategic-level decisions must be made about the infrastructure, adoption of standards, and the degree to which narrative vs. structured data will flow throughout the migration path. Data infrastructure is discussed in chapter 9.

Technical Strategy

The **technical strategy** describes what IT will support the EHR and how it will be structured. The technical strategy at the highest level describes, for example, whether the EHR will run in a client/server environment, use Web-enabled technology, include a wireless network, and so on. At a minimum, the technical strategy should identify the hardware, operating system, programming languages, and database structures that will be used. Specific technical standards to be used should be identified (for example, all intraorganizational communications must adhere to Health Level Seven [HL7]).

Finally, the technical strategy should be flexible enough to allow for the rapid pace of technological change and, as far as possible, should be built on **open architecture** so as not to limit choice. (The term *open architecture* refers to the fact that elements of different information systems work together through the use of standards that are not proprietary.) Technology infrastructure is discussed in chapter 10.

Although functional, data, and technical strategies may seem beyond the scope of an executive management strategic planning session, certain philosophical issues do need to be understood and addressed at that level. For example, one organization developed a comprehensive vision of the EHR and gained acceptance for it from the user community, only to find that its primary **hospital information system** (HIS) vendor could not currently support such a system. Many healthcare organizations have many application systems from many different vendors and could potentially add a new EHR vendor to the mix; others have highly consolidated systems. Healthcare organizations have invested a huge amount of money over time to gain a tightly integrated information structure predominantly from a single vendor, even though it may not be cutting edge. (These older systems are often referred to as **legacy systems** [Keener 2000]). The organization then must decide whether it will replace its legacy system, attempt to interface with the system, persuade the vendor to move toward a more sophisticated vision of an EHR, or withdraw from its original goal for the time being.

Implementation Strategy

The **implementation strategy** describes the sequence in which an organization undertakes discrete project tasks such as infrastructure building, new application system implementation, and organizational change. These tasks are prioritized based on clinical and strategic need. Issues of dependency and precedence also are considered in developing an implementation strategy. For example, some organizations believe that all elements of the technical infrastructure should be built at once and the applications phased in over time. Although this approach may seem ideal, the rapidly changing pace of IT and system upgrades may mean installing new technology on an old platform.

Another strategy is a phased approach, where pieces of infrastructure are implemented in accordance with a given application requirement. Although this offers distinct advantages, some organizations find that it results in a piecemeal approach in which no application is fully implemented.

Each organization must weigh the risks associated with each implementation approach and select the one with which it is most comfortable.

The implementation strategy also addresses the philosophy of how rapidly users are trained and expected to be fully operational using new applications. A slower-paced implementation, where all system functionality is fully tested and users fully trained, and a more rapid implementation, where some system issues are addressed while users are still learning, both offer benefits. Yet another approach is to fully implement a system and require users to learn various parts of the applications on their own.

Another aspect of the implementation strategy is cutover. Will everyone be required to use the new system at a certain date, or will people be allowed to phase in their use over time? Providers have different philosophies about this and also change their philosophies based on economic factors.

Finally, a good implementation strategy includes benefits realization as a key component in ongoing operations and maintenance. Chapter 5 established the basic construct of a benefits realization study. Chapter 11 relates the benefits realization study to ROI and chapters 12 and 13 include vendor selection issues as well as specific installation and continual enhancement issues.

Strategic Planning in Different Healthcare Settings

Although the basic concept of a migration path and strategic planning does not vary with the type of provider setting, the actual path itself and the nature of the specific strategies do vary among settings.

Acute vs. Ambulatory Settings

The differences between acute care and ambulatory care are the most striking differences among various types of provider settings. However, there also are differences at the application level within a given setting. For example, many hospitals implementing CPOE find that the discharge medication order is actually a prescription the patient carries to a retail pharmacy. The electronic flow of information for inpatient orders (CPOE) and discharge prescriptions (e-prescribing [e-Rx]) is quite different. These differences are illustrated in table 6.4.

When an IDS begins planning for an enterprisewide EHR, the differences between acute care and ambulatory care become so important that they may not be overcome by a single system. A few vendors are approaching an integrated EHR environment to overcome these differences and make it easier for users to operate within the continuum of care (Vegoda 2002). Still, workflow differences are such that accommodations must be made and there are likely still to be significant—and needed—differences within settings in an IDS.

Table 6.4. CPOE (in acute care) vs. e-Rx (in ambulatory care) Characteristic

	CPOE	e-Rx
Workflow	Tightly coordinated	Tightly coordinated
Communication	Formal	Formal
Primary user	Provider	Provider
Secondary user	Clinical pharmacist	Retail pharmacist
Data content	Structured	Structured
Data volume	Low density	Low density
Primary data source	EHR	Practice management system
Secondary data source	Pharmacy	Health plan/PBM and drug knowledge databases
Information flow	Location-centric	Geographically dispersed
Data input	Stationary	Mobile
Data transmission	Closed	Open

Other Forms of Care Delivery Settings

For the most part, differences in other provider settings, such as long-term care, home health, diagnostic facilities, and others are more a matter of scale.

Typically, a long-term care facility is highly regulated and has a standard data set that is easily automated, but the facility remains similar to the acute care environment from the perspective of workflow, communication, primary user, information flow, and IS decision making. Long-term care facilities typically have significantly lower budgets, but their decision-making demands are less, so their IS can be simpler. Strategic planning for an EHR in a long-term care facility should still focus on benefits, but the remaining strategy components are typically more straightforward. Many long-term care facilities are part of a corporate structure and derive their IS from the corporation. However, a given long-term care facility within a corporation may be ripe for a pilot test of an EHR.

Home care environments are more of a hybrid between the acute and ambulatory settings. Again, their data needs are simpler than in either of these environments, so their decision support is not as dramatic as in either the acute or ambulatory environments. However, their communication demands and user interface requirements may be greater. Home health agencies may be looking at portable devices and their security as well as the ability to transmit from multiple locations with vastly different capabilities. Home care processes include a number of both operational and clinical issues.

Diagnostic facilities may be similar to most other ambulatory care settings, although they are typically more focused and thus may be simpler in their data and decision-making requirements.

Academic vs. Community Organizations

In addition to differences in EHRs as required by the setting in which care is delivered, there are differences between academic and community types of organizations. Although both may typically have acute and ambulatory care components, and thus pose the same challenges of integrating information across the continuum of care, the organizational structures, uses of data, and users of data may be significantly different as to warrant attention when planning an EHR. Academic medical centers actually vary considerably. Some are quite centralized, with a central IT department, a faculty practice plan, and even a hospital. Alternatively, academic medical centers can be highly decentralized, where each faculty member literally maintains a separate office and IS. Some universities own hospitals; others are affiliated with a hospital only by virtue of the faculty medical staff.

In addition to the administration–physician construct unique to all of healthcare, the academic medical center adds the dimensions of teaching and research. Political issues can be intensified in an academic medical center. On the other hand, because of their strong interest in research, an academic medical center may be ripe for more formal study of new technology, benefits realization studies, and so on. They typically have more experience obtaining grants and contracts, and may be willing to extend that experience to the EHR.

Managed Care vs. Fee-for-Service Reimbursement

The method of reimbursement often has an impact on the goals of the EHR. A managed care organization may be a true health maintenance organization (HMO) with both payer and provider functions. Some HMOs include both acute and ambulatory care, although many provide just ambulatory care. More important, however, the types of decision support, the ability to impose change, and the interaction with patients may be quite different between a HMO environment and a fee-for-service environment. However, many fewer strictly fee-for-service environments now have some elements of managed care.

For-Profit vs. Nonprofit Ownership

Finally, the nature of ownership can impact strategic planning for an EHR. A for-profit environment may be looking at a much broader deployment of an EHR. Although it also may look for the lowest common denominator among its organizations for implementing an EHR, the for-profit environment has the most to gain by economies of scale and data-mining capabilities. Nonprofit organizations typically are more focused on a variety of benefit types and hence a broader array of functionality.

Although there are differences among the types of provider organizations with respect to an EHR, one should avoid stereotyping because each individual organization is as unique as any other. By the same token, each organization also shares the basic goal of high-quality patient care and, in that respect, will be looking for a core set of values and benefits from an EHR.

Conclusion

In a healthcare organization, the tipping point for an EHR is when strategic planning recognizes the supporting role the EHR places in every planning component. Such a position requires the combined efforts of all stakeholders: executive management, users, technology experts, and support staff.

In fact, most organizations with exemplary implementations of EHRs indicate that whereas lack of physician support is the single point of failure, executive management support is the most critical success factor. If the EHR is not a passion of the CEO, chances for success are far less than if the CEO is a strong supporter (Baldwin 2003). This passion is felt throughout the organization.

All users are critical to the success of an EHR and must be involved in the earliest planning stages. However, the missing link is often the physician community and it is for this reason that so much emphasis is placed on physician adoption. Entire CPOE systems have failed simply because physician needs were not addressed.

Strategic planning in which a clearly defined migration path is established sets the stage for the more focused planning and detailed tactical plans necessary to carry out the organization's vision of the EHR. A migration path also should be sufficiently flexible to permit new factors to be addressed. Whether these factors are new technology, change in organizational structure, regulations, or other, the migration path must be flexible enough to accommodate—and stable enough to withstand—the various external and internal influences.

References and Resources

American Hospital Association. 2007. Continued Progress: Use of Information Technology. http://www.aha.org/aha/content/2007/pdf/070227-continuedprogress.pdf.

Andrews, Robert. 1993. *The Columbia Dictionary of Quotations*. New York: Columbia University Press.

Baldwin, F.D. 2003 (May). CPRs in the winner's circle. *Healthcare Informatics,* 33–36. www.healthcare-informatics.com/issues/2003/05_03/cover.htm.

Centers for Medicare and Medicaid Services. 2008. http://www.MyMedicare.gov.

Department of Health and Human Services. 2008 (June 3). Office of the National Coordinator for Health Information Technology. The ONC-Coordinated Federal Health IT Strategic Plan: 2008–2012. http://www.hhs.gov/healthit/resources/HITStrategicPlan.pdf.

Frenette, R. 2003. IT project management 101. *ADVANCE for Health Information Executives* 7(10):75–78.

Gillespie, G. 2003 (July). Enterprisewide implementations: Helpful tips for CIOs who take on the universe. *Health Data Management,* 29–38. www. healthdatamanagement.com/html/current/PastIssueStory.cfm?ArticleId=8692&issuedate=2003-07-01.

Gladwell, M. 2000. *The Tipping Point: How Little Things Can Make a Big Difference*. New York: Back Bay Books/Little, Brown and Company.

Handler, T. 2001 (Feb. 12). CPR generations: An update. Gartner Research Note Research Note Number TG-17-6518. Stamford, CT: Gartner Inc.

Hier, D.B. 2002 (Oct.). Physician buy-in for an EMR. *Healthcare Informatics*, 37–39.

Jones, C.M. 2003. An overview of knowledge management. *ADVANCE for Health Information Executives* 7(5):53–55.

Keener, R.E. 2000 (Aug.). Upgrade or replace: CIOs on their HIS legacy systems. *Health Management Technology*, 16–18. www.healthmgttech.com/archives/h0800upgrade.htm.

McNamara, C. 1999a. *Basic Overview of Various Strategic Planning Models*. St. Paul, MN: The Management Assistance Program for Nonprofits.

McNamara, C. 1999b. *Strategic Planning: Basic Guidelines for Successful Planning Process*. St. Paul, MN: The Management Assistance Program for Nonprofits.

Ringle, M., and D. Updegrove. 1998. Is strategic planning for technology an oxymoron? *CAUSE/EFFECT* 21(1):18–23.

Rishel, W, V. Riehl, and C. Blanton. 2007 (May 31). Summary of the NHIN Prototype Architecture Contracts: A Report for the Office of the National Coordinator for Health IT. Gartner, Inc. http://www.hhs.gov/healthit/healthnetwork/resources/summary_report_on_nhin_Prototype_architectures.pdf.

Slater, D. 2002. Mistakes: strategic planning don'ts (and dos) *CIO Magazine* (June 1).

Sternlieb, J.M. 2004. Physician perspective: Perks and pains—the trials of information technology (IT) implementation initiatives. *Journal of Healthcare Information Management* 19(1):13–14.

Vegoda, P. 2002. IHE: Integrating the healthcare enterprise. *Journal of Healthcare Information Management* 16(1):22–24.

Ventres, W., S. Kooienga, and R. Marlin. 2006. EHRs in the exam room: Tips on patient-centered care. *Family Practice Management* 13(3):45–47.

Chapter 7
Healthcare Process Assessment

When vision, goals, and a strategic plan have been determined for the EHR initiative, planning for changes in workflow and processes must be initiated. Many organizations have discovered that not putting enough attention on workflow and process improvement in the EHR planning stages can have serious negative impacts—from not fully understanding what functional requirements are needed for an EHR to loss of productivity during go-live, costly rework of the implementation, and potential unintended consequences of poorly designed EHRs. Process assessment may go by many different names, but the result is a clear understanding of current workflows and processes and how an EHR will impact them. This chapter:

- Identifies the importance and scope of process assessment
- Describes the purpose and timing of the process assessment effort
- Identifies the steps in process assessment
- Describes process assessment tools
- Provides tips on ensuring solid process improvement through managing team empowerment, group facilitation and adopting process improvement techniques

Importance and Scope of Process Assessment

Understanding how current work is performed and the sequence of steps involved in order to make improvements is the general purpose of what this book terms **process assessment**.

Terminology and Methodologies

Such process assessment is not new—neither in general nor to healthcare. It has been a longstanding technique, adopted in multiple different settings, with many different approaches,

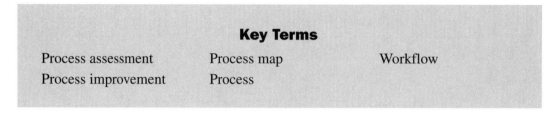

and sometimes with similar approaches going by different names. For example, some would suggest that process assessment is only the act of studying a **process**, which is the manner in which work to be completed to achieve a particular result is performed. These same experts would argue, then, that process assessments must be documented, perhaps in a process map (the documentation process being referred to as process mapping). A **process map** is the depiction of the process that is being assessed. Finally, process assessment must be coupled with **process improvement**, or the analysis of the current process to determine ways to make it more efficient and effective. Process improvement may also be referred to as process redesign or process reengineering. A variety of statistical and analytical methods may aid the improvement identification. Still other techniques may be needed to implement the improvement. When process assessment is performed to describe a desired process, or set functionality, for instance for the EHR, use case modeling may be used to define a scenario that is the ideal state incorporating process improvement. Still other experts would observe that no process stands alone, but is naturally a part of a **workflow**, which is the sequence of steps and hand-offs taken within a process. They would couple workflow and process mapping together.

The different approaches to identifying and implementing improvements may include Lean, Six Sigma, TQM, ISO9000, Kaizen, and others. These methodologies have similarities and differences, and are often combined to achieve the most value of each. For example, Lean is a methodology that is used to accelerate the velocity and reduce the cost of any process by removing waste (George 2008). Six Sigma is most closely associated with defects and quality. These might be combined with the Kaizen philosophy of continuous improvement throughout all aspects of life into a Lean Kaizen methodology complemented with Six Sigma.

Process Assessment Purpose

What should become apparent in considering the number of techniques and methodologies is that there has been a continual quest for improvement in work; and that over time, many have attempted to find better ways to make such improvements. However, it should also be observed that almost all of the formal methodologies that have emerged are grounded in manufacturing, sales, and other non-healthcare fields; and frequently focused on "man" and "materials" rather than the data-information-knowledge continuum. So, while much can be learned from these techniques, they may not necessarily apply directly without some modification to implementing health information technology (HIT) in general and EHR in particular. As a result, the process assessment techniques described herein combine many of the principles of continual quality improvement, but are focused on the information payload that is the EHR. In fact, a good mantra to keep in mind is:

> EHR is not about automating charts ("material") and you can't automate people ("man"), but about automating data collection and using information to generate knowledge that improves the care delivery process, empowers consumers, and transforms the health services industry. (Amatayakul 2008)

Put another way by Dr. David Smith of Riverton Family Health Center in Utah:

> "The single area that requires the highest level of attention during the planning and deployment of an electronic medical record is practice workflow."

Process Assessment Case Studies

"A man's errors are his portals of discovery." —James Joyce

A practice administrator on the East coast explains what happened when they did not attend to process assessment: "Since we didn't map out most of our EHR workflows before we went live, we had to figure out a lot of them as we went along." As a result, documentation for some EHR workflows, like reports from so-called noninterfaced labs that came back on paper vs. electronically had to be figured out via trial and error in the middle of office visits. This created long waits for patients and bottlenecks that lasted for weeks." In addition, in this practice's quest to figure out how to enter results for in-house labs, some nursing staff at the site entered the data in one part of the EHR, the so-called workflow module, whereas others entered data directly into individual patient EHR visit notes, creating more confusion and delays for physicians looking for lab results (Houck 2006). It can be noted that most EHRs will automatically populate or fill in results that are entered into one part of the record into other sections, but variations do exist, and without studying both current and changed workflows, it may not be clear exactly how any given EHR works.

Workflow and process improvements are not confined to the ambulatory setting, although the ambulatory setting is often less likely to recognize the need for or be willing to take the time to perform a concerted process assessment. A good example of a redesigned process is related by Guite and others (2006), where the nursing admission process was studied in depth prior to EHR implementation. Challenges faced by the nurses included considerable duplication of documentation, complex rules for coordinating care, and pressure to accelerate patient discharge. The result of convening stakeholders from the admissions department, nurses, and other departments that would potentially be a part of the future process, was an electronic admission referral process (EARP) that simplified the work of nursing and led to more appropriate referrals to the ancillary departments. It was found that more than 25 percent of the patients could have information imported from a previous encounter and that eliminating duplicate documentation also improved patient satisfaction. More accurate and complete admission information also is used to monitor and support a variety of quality efforts, including CMS core measures.

Figure 7.1.   The right way to implement an EHR is not necessarily the new way, my way, your way, or the old way—but likely a combination that achieves the five rights for EHR.

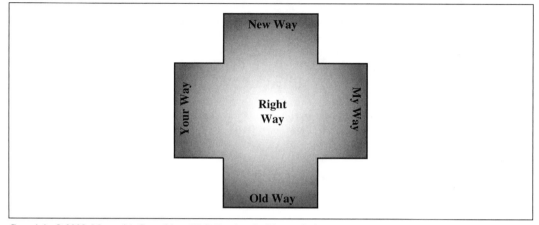

Copyright © 2008, Margret\A Consulting, LLC. Reprinted with permission.

As there are concerns that clinicians are not taking full advantage of EHRs and that inefficient and ineffective processes are often not corrected prior to implementing EHRs, there is great need to ensure that processes and workflow changes brought about by an EHR are understood and adopted. However, it is also essential to understand where an EHR's processes and workflows do not fit a given situation and to not force clinicians to change how they work only to fit a computerized system. Instead, process assessment is needed to make the *right* changes (see figure 7.1) for the *right* EHR (see table 7.1).

Three examples of lack of attention to process assessment have become classic in the industry:

> One is the experience at Cedars-Sinai Medical Center in Los Angeles, when a physician "revolt" required them to remove part of their CPOE system. While no one intends to set themselves up as an example, the Cedars-Sinai experience has provided significant lessons learned for the industry. They have attributed much of their CPOE implementation problem to inadequate education and physician involvement, lack of consideration for human factors, inadequate study of workflow, "functionality issues" in the software, weak pilot testing (in OB only), and a too aggressive rollout (two weeks per floor) (Polaschek, et al 2003).

Another experience was reported in *Pediatrics*, the journal of the American Academy of Pediatrics (Han 2005), with the headline "Unexpected Increased Mortality After Implementation of a Commercially Sold Computerized Physician Order Entry System." In this case, a CPOE system typically used primarily in general hospitals (with a large percentage of patients being adults) had not had incorporated control points for pediatric cases, which often require dose adjustments and have many more precautions than for adults. The Academy offers an opportunity for readers of its journal to post comments on its Web site, under a heading "Post-publication Peer Review (P3R)." Don Levick, MD, MBA, President Medical Staff Physician Liaison Information Services at Lehigh Valley Hospital posted this telling comment:

Table 7.1. Five Rights for EHR

> • *Right clinical data*: The EHR enables complete and accurate data capture in the manner that is most meaningful for all users and uses—be it structured, standardized, and encoded data; narrative information; or clinical images
>
> • *Right presentation*: The EHR provides a human–computer interface that enables the most efficient and effective means of capturing (such as via context-sensitive templates or self-administered questionnaires) and displaying data (facts, findings, observations, plans, rationales, and conclusions recorded by clinicians, consumers, and others about patient care), information (narrative and graphical displays), and knowledge (alerts and reminders)
>
> • *Right decision*: The EHR supplies clinical decision support that is context-sensitive, tailored to the user, and based on scientific evidence, which is kept current at all times, and which provides a means to document legitimate reasons when professional judgment calls for overriding the proposed support
>
> • *Right work processes*: The EHR supports processes and workflows that are most efficient and effective for all users and uses
>
> • *Right outcomes*: The EHR supports value-driven healthcare, with the right quality and cost results

Copyright © 2008, Margret\A Consulting, LLC. Reprinted with permission.

> The issue with CPOE is usually not in the software, but in the *process change* that is required to successfully implement such a complex system. These challenges were well documented in the article . . . But *rather than conclude that work process and infrastructure issues must be completely understood, investigated, and resolved prior to implementation*, the authors conclude that hospitals should monitor mortality rates after CPOE implementation.

One other similar study was reported in *JAMA*, entitled "Role of CPOE Systems in *Facilitating* Medication Errors" (Koppel et al 2005). In this article, 22 discrete ways in which medication errors were facilitated by a CPOE system were described. The system has reportedly been replaced with a newer product. Koppel is quoted as observing that it still has "oodles of problems," although despite this believes that CPOE deployments can offer "extraordinary advantages" in reducing many mistakes as long as the hospital provides "vigilance and self-examination" to ensure proper functioning (McGee 2005).

Unfortunately, all too often EHRs are expected to improve performance "magically" (Towne 2008). Instead, EHR implementation requires careful attention to detail, engagement of all stakeholders, and careful design of processes and workflows with accompanying training, change management, and reinforcement of new behaviors. For example, in one study of electronic reminders for diabetes and coronary artery disease, 71 percent of physicians were found to prefer clinical decision support in an electronic format over a paper-based system, although lack of stakeholder engagement, proper training, reinforcement resulted in only one-third of the physicians reporting on a follow-up survey noticing the electronic reminders and taking action on the recommendations (Sequist et al. 2005).

Purpose and Timing of Process Assessment

Although there is an increasing recognition that EHR is not about technology or product but about process, process assessment, if performed at all, is often postponed until the EHR implementation stage. This timing is unfortunate because process assessment begun early

Table 7.2.   Multiple Benefits of Process Assessment Performed Over Time

When	What	Why
Planning	Current process mapping	Initiates change management by highlighting processes that need improvement
Assessment	Process improvement	Addresses process that need to be improved prior to EHR implementation so bad processes are not carried forward into the EHR Acclimates users to potential changes, such as standardized templates and order sets
Selection	Use case scenarios	Describes the desired functionality for process improvements Enables cost–benefit analysis to determine potential return on investment
System build	Proposed process mapping	Enables the EHR to be configured in a way that will help achieve process improvements for right outcomes
Testing	Use case models	Ensures integrated system testing, not just unit testing of each system part
Training	Improved process map	Serves as training tool and documented procedure for ongoing reference
Benefits realization	Process assessment	Utilizing all components of the previous steps validates that new processes are working, helps celebrate success, and identifies course correction where necessary

in the EHR project can offer a number of benefits. Table 7.2 lists the key benefits associated with each time an aspect of process assessment should be performed.

Conducting process assessment in the early planning stages of EHR not only prepares the organization for the technological change, but it also often helps identify process changes that can take place immediately, achieving an early payback for the work effort. An early process assessment also helps ease change into an organization in which resistance to change is a major impediment. Process assessment also can help determine the EHR project's feasibility and assess its potential results in order to obtain management/clinical leadership approval. It should identify where changes in processes are needed, as well as what modifications need to be made to the system itself to reflect organizational processes that need to remain intact. Identification of potential process improvements with the EHR also helps change management. Finally, early process assessment can help produce projected cost savings. When an organization requires a thorough cost–benefit justification for an EHR project, what and how processes will be redesigned must be understood in order to identify potential cost savings. When an organization intends to do a comprehensive benefits realization study after EHR implementation, the analysis phase of process assessment can produce data for the baseline and the final, improved process documentation helps focus the study on the impact of the EHR.

Table 7.3.   Steps in Process Assessment for EHR

1. Identify processes to be assessed; that is., those that will be impacted by the EHR being acquired.
2. Create process assessment teams of individuals who perform the process now and those who will be impacted in the future.
3. Select process assessment tools suitable to the process assessment purpose, and learn how to use the tools.
4. Map the process as actually performed. Avoid identifying opportunities for improvement now, or critical controls built into current processes may be overlooked.
5. Validate maps to ensure they reflect current processes, all variations, and the information payload.
6. Collect all forms and reports that are part of the process to be automated.
7. Obtain baseline data to define expectations for change and for use in benchmarking for benefits realization studies.
8. Identify potential problems and determine their root cause (not just symptoms).
9. Identify changes that would address root cause of problems: Some may be addressed now; others will require EHR.
10. Identify other desired improvements from use of an EHR.
11. Document proposed changes by creating a proposed map.
12. Use new processes to create use case scenarios to identify EHR functional specifications, and later to build out the EHR application to achieve improvements. (This may require a second "improved" with EHR map.)
13. Test new workflows and processes.
14. Train all on new workflows and processes.
15. Incorporate changes in workflows and processes into policy and procedure.
16. Conduct benefits realization and celebrate successful change/correct course as necessary.

Steps in Process Assessment

Although the purpose of the process assessment may vary with the timing of its performance, the steps in performing process assessment are very similar at whatever time they occur. Table 7.3 provides the steps typically performed in process assessment, noting variations depending on timing and purpose.

Processes to be Assessed

The first step is to identify processes to be assessed. Although all processes in an organization could benefit from process assessment, if the focus is on implementing an EHR, then the processes to be assessed at this time will relate to those impacted by an EHR. For hospitals, the processes to be assessed should follow its EHR migration path, as not every process needs to be assessed for any given component implemented. However, if the hospital plans a comprehensive EHR rollout, then a comprehensive set of processes will be assessed. Table 7.4 identifies potential processes for hospitals and clinics that would be assessed during an EHR project. This may be modified for any specific organization and its migration path.

Process Assessment Teams

Although a single management team, consultant, or vendor can provide leadership, education, direction, and assistance, teams composed of the people who will actually implement the redesigned processes and use the EHR are much more successful. Teams should be

Table 7.4.   Processes to be Assessed for an EHR Project

Hospitals	Clinics
• Admission/discharge/transfer • Patient assessment • Medications reconciliation • H&P/differential diagnosis • Care planning • Provider order entry • Procedures • Medication administration • Patient monitoring • Patient care charting • Care coordination • Charge capture/coding • Reporting	• Scheduling and registration/check-in and check-out • Patient intake • Results review • H&P/encounter notes • Care plan/guidelines • Medication management: medication list maintenance/ prescribing/ refills/ compliance • Order entry • E/M coding • Charge capture • Patient instructions

responsible for the actual workflow and process mapping, analysis, redesign, and feasibility testing. For EHR process assessment teams to be effective, their membership should be interdepartmental and interdisciplinary. The EHR will cut across all departments and have multiple potential users. Teams also should solicit the input of all users in their respective areas and keep them abreast of progress made. Including individuals at the lowest feasible levels of the organization heightens the staff's sense of ownership of, and responsibility for, the assessment. Finally, teams should be rewarded for most accurately mapping workflows and processes as they are actually performed—not how a policy or procedure says they should be performed. If actual processes are not mapped, workarounds, delays, and other factors that contribute to today's issues will not be identified so they can be overcome. In addition, any controls points that have been added that must carry forward to the EHR may not be identified. Mapping current processes should find all the "warts." As a result, this is not the time to lay blame on staff for the problems that have arisen in the current processes.

Process Assessment Training

People within the organization are selected to participate on process assessment teams because they are intimately familiar with current processes. However, the organization cannot assume they know how to do process assessment, fully understand the features and functions of an EHR, or even know how to function as a team. Thus, orientation and training in these areas are essential.

Orientation to an EHR system must be comprehensive, with a fair amount of coaching. A single product demonstration will not suffice. It is best when preliminary reading materials followed by seminars and including distribution of actual demonstrations or Web sites with demonstrations are provided. As processes are analyzed and redesign work begins, at least one expert in EHR systems should be available to answer questions, coach, and work with the teams to help them understand what is feasible.

Process Mapping Validation

Once a current process has been mapped, it is important to validate that it is complete and accurate, and that it reflects information flow—bearing in mind that the EHR does not automate either the chart or people, but rather the collection and processing of data into useful information. This is often challenging because it is easy to see where the chart and people are at all times, but it can be difficult to understand what data are being processed mentally. It is for this reason that the persons actually performing the processes—including nurses and physicians—should map their own processes.

It can be helpful for an unbiased observer (who may be a consultant or simply someone in the organization not engaged in performing the process) to ask key questions about the maps. This will help ensure the process has been thoroughly described. Table 7.5 provides a set of questions that may be helpful in validating the completeness and accuracy of current process maps.

Process Changes

Once it is time to begin analyzing the current workflows and processes, it is necessary to focus on what changes are appropriate, and when they can be implemented. Following are some of its key elements of evaluating processes for improvement:

- *Free team members to make appropriate changes.* Too often, management is taught to control processes rather than to change them. Changes proposed by nonmanagement staff are often looked on as situations out of control. The process assessment teams must understand that they are free to make appropriate changes. The result

Table 7.5.   Key Questions to Validate Current Process Maps

• Is the scope of the process appropriate for EHR mapping?
• Are these all the tasks performed in this process?
• Does the map focus on information flow or only the chart or the person? Are all sources of input and uses of information identified?
• Are clinical decision-making tasks performed mentally included?
• Are some tasks performed only occasionally? Are they included? What triggers their performance?
• Are there tasks performed differently *by* different people or *for* different people? If so, are the variations included or more than one map made?
• Are some tasks performed outside of this process, but impact its boundary?
• Are there some tasks identified that really are not a part of this process, and could be dropped or placed at the boundary?
• What tasks are critical? That is, if not performed, the process is meaningless; or must be included in any new HIT adopted? Highlight these.
• Are there tasks not performed today that would improve efficiency, patient safety, and outcomes?
• Were all associated forms, reports, job descriptions, policies, and procedures collected?
• Did you collect baseline data if desired? Do you have benchmark data for comparison? Do you have plans to acquire such?

may still not be a change in the process, but a modification of the technology, and the decision then will have been made within the appropriate context. For example, when evaluating the process of nursing documentation, the technology may accommodate point-of-care charting. This is a significant change from charting at the nursing station. Neither is right or wrong, and nursing personnel should be open to understanding the ramifications of each. They may initially think point-of-care charting is too intrusive for their patients and decide to keep charting at the nursing station. However, it is possible that this will not alter the process sufficiently to improve documentation or productivity. An alternative then may be identified, such as charting at kiosks placed strategically throughout the nursing unit.

- *Solve problems rather than symptoms.* The hardest part of any problem-solving situation is defining the exact problem. Symptoms are often obvious, but to find the root of the problem, it is imperative to dig deep. This is analogous to pulling a weed out of a garden. If the root is left in the soil, the weed will grow back. Similarly, if only the symptoms of a problem are solved, the problem will most likely recur. A healthcare example that is currently a major issue relates to patient safety and medication errors. Many assume that computer physician order entry (CPOE) is the solution. However, a study of the flow of the entire process and quantifying where errors are occurring at each step may reveal that errors are occurring primarily around formulary access, pharmacy processes, or medication administration. Each environment may be different.

- *Stay focused on the ultimate goal.* Speeding up or compounding ineffectiveness is another common result of automation. The goal of the EHR project should not just be to "go paperless" but, rather, to improve the organization's use of health information to achieve its strategic initiatives. Although achieving a paperless environment is ultimately appropriate, focusing exclusively on going paperless can put blinders on process redesign efforts. Teams also should understand that islands of information systems have long characterized healthcare computing. This is due in part to the nature of systems development over time, how organizations have functioned, the often-insular nature of various medical specialties, and sometimes backlogs in information technology (IT) departments that have led to acquisition of departmental systems. For whatever reason, each of these information systems has had its own database. An EHR environment must be able to tap all these databases. Current technology has approached this problem by creating a central repository of information to which everyone has specified access. Even newer technology achieves the ability to share data across disparate databases through application of browser-based technology. Because departments typically are reluctant to give up the perceived power associated with having their own database, the benefits of sharing data must be made clear. Departments should be advised that sharing data enhances everyone's access and that data translated into information is the achievement of real power for the organization as a whole.

- *Focus on the primary customer.* The first step in an EHR project may be to determine who the EHR's customers are. There are actually several. Ultimately, the most important customer may be the patient or the individual about whom the EHR provides information. In fact, limiting the term EHR to a focus on "record" may be a misnomer because of the much broader scope of the information that can be processed in an EHR system. Many view the clinician users as primary customers, and indeed they probably are the users most affected by the process changes brought about by EHR implementation.

- *Study existing systems only enough to understand them without limiting break-through thinking.* Sometimes processes can be studied at such a level of detail that the overall impact on the organization becomes unclear. Just as an initial reaction to an event or intuition about something is often the best guide, so, too, should teams rely on their experience and expertise to know when a process is right or when a redesign makes sense.

- *Look at the big picture.* The scope of the EHR project is to improve results throughout the organization. Process changes will necessarily affect many, from the physician (who learns the value of clinical decision support as part of the medication-ordering process) to the coder in the HIM department (whose job may change to reviewing coding quality), the materials manager (who achieves an automated inventory), and even the CEO (who has the ability to produce executive reports at the desktop). Process teams must solicit all these areas for input and ensure that all affected areas are covered in any assessment. The goal of EHR process assessment should not be simply to change processes for the sake of change but, rather, to improve outcomes.

Process Assessment Tools

A variety of process mapping tools are available. Table 7.6 identifies some of the process mapping tools and their advantages and disadvantages.

Process Diagramming Tools

Process mapping can be kept at a simple level, where even just sticky notes are used to record tasks. They can be placed on a big sheet of paper or a wall to illustrate the flow and then analyzed for improvement. One advantage of using this form of process mapping is that users can be process mapping as they are performing their work tasks. Given a stack of sticky notes that fit into a pocket, users can make a record of each task as they perform their work. This usually means they spend less time formalizing the overall diagram and get quite an accurate representation of what is actually happening. Alternatively, the result of a simple sticky note mapping is not an easily transferable document, and there is some loss of mapping integrity because the various symbols or other aids available in the tools are often not incorporated. Still, this could be a good way to start the mapping process or to ensure a map's accuracy.

Process diagrams are among the most commonly used tool, although more often used in a manufacturing rather than information flow project. Table 7.7 provides the traditional flow process chart symbols, their interpretation, and examples of how they might be used to map information flows.

Figure 7.2 provides an example of a swim lane process map for the referral management process in a clinic. This map utilizes the same symbols as the process diagram, but depicts flow across department boundaries. Swim lanes can be can be vertical, as illustrated in Figure 7.2, or horizontal, as illustrated in table 7.6, which also illustrates a swim lane

Table 7.6.   Process mapping and system flowchart tools

Tool	Illustration	Advantages	Disadvantages
Process Diagram		Using standard symbols, process diagrams can map both the tasks and their sequence of current or improved processes easily.	Process diagrams do not lend themselves to extensive annotation, so may be difficult to translate into EHR system requirements.
Swim Lane Chart		Swim lane charts add the dimension of clearly identifying the different roles people play in a process. They may simply use boxes, colored boxes, or the process diagram symbols.	Because the focus of EHR process mapping should be on the information flow, the swim lane chart can put too much emphasis on the person or chart.
Flow Process Chart		This chart uses symbols from the process diagram to characterize narrative descriptions of tasks. These charts add the ability to record time a task takes and quantity of work performed.	The flow process chart is an older tool and often focuses on person or chart rather than information flow. They are more difficult to use in illustrating branching logic or decision points, which are often illustrated by indention of the narrative.
System Flow Chart		System flow charts are universally recognized. Although they use a different set of symbols than the process diagram or flow process chart, they are still standardized. These are ideal charts for illustrating decision points.	As most charts, the amount of narrative that can be accommodated in a system flowchart is limited. Many overcome this by keying narrative descriptions to the symbols where necessary.

chart created only with colored boxes as opposed to process diagramming symbols (this was also generated using a computer program).

When attempting to map processes performed by clinicians, especially physicians, use of charting symbols may seem too technical. Flow process charts can be a way to incorporate the narrative a physician may be willing to document for a clinical process with the symbols that may be applied to a chart form later, if desired. Figure 7.3 is a blown-up version of the flow process chart included in table 7.6.

Table 7.7.   Flow process chart symbols

Symbol	Process	Example
◯	Operation make-ready	Sorting
●	Operation do	Coding
⇨	Transportation	Faxing
▽	Storage	Permanent file
☐	Inspection	Proofreading
D	Delay	Awaiting signature

Figure 7.2.   Sample swim lane process map

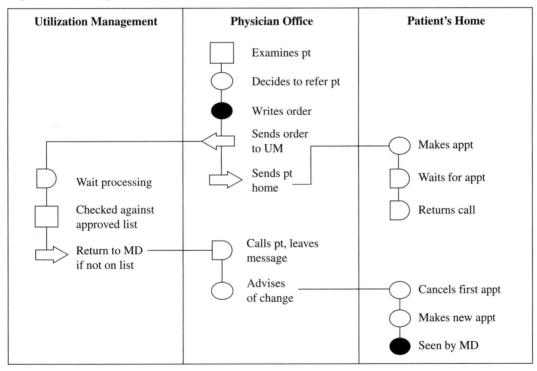

Figure 7.3.   Flow process chart

Flow Process Chart

Process:
☐ Present   ☐ Proposed
☐ Person   ☐ Material

	Operation	Transportation	Inspection	Delay	Storage	Distance in feet	Quantity	Time
Analysis (✓): Why is it done this way? / Why is it done by this person? / Why is it done at this time? / Why is it done at this location? / Why is it done—is it necessary? **Details of Present/Proposed Process:**								
1.	○	⇧	☐	D	▽			
2.	○	⇧	☐	D	▽			
3.	○	⇧	☐	D	▽			
4.	○	⇧	☐	D	▽			
5.	○	⇧	☐	D	▽			
6.	○	⇧	☐	D	▽			
7.	○	⇧	☐	D	▽			
8.	○	⇧	☐	D	▽			
9.	○	⇧	☐	D	▽			
10.	○	⇧	☐	D	▽			
Totals:	○	⇧	☐	D	▽			

Performed by:

Date:

Notes

Summary:	Present		Proposed	
	No.	Time	No.	Time
Operations				
Transportations				
Inspections				
Delays				
Storages				
Totals:				

System Flowcharts

System flowcharts are those most often used for workflow and process mapping associated with adopting information technology. They are familiar to most people who would perform this work, and are relatively easy to explain to others. The basic system flowchart symbols are provided in table 7.8. Of special note in EHR process mapping is the decision

Table 7.8.   Basic flowchart symbols

Basic Symbols	Purpose
	Terminator—designates where a process begins and ends
	Process—performance of an operation
	Decision—directs flow to two or more branches depending on the alternatives available. If there are more than three options a circle with multiple branches may be used instead. If there are many options, a decision table may be referenced (see figure 7.4).
	On-page and off-page connectors—designates when the flowchart extends to another location on a page or to one or more pages
Special Symbols	**Purpose**
	Manual operation—indicates where a manual operation must occur in a largely electronic workflow
	Document/s—indicates where a paper-based form or document is used, potentially an external document to be scanned
	Magnetic storage/direct access storage—often used to designate a database as well as storage
	Display—terminal or workstation monitor Manual input—keyboard

Figure 7.4.   Sample decision table

Conditions	Condition Alternatives								
	Printer does not print	Y	Y	Y	Y	N	N	N	N
	Red light is flashing	Y	Y	N	N	Y	Y	N	N
	Printer is unrecognized	Y	N	Y	N	Y	N	Y	N
Actions	Action Entries								
	Check power cable			X					
	Check printer-computer cable	X		X					
	Ensure printer software is installed	X		X		X		X	
	Check/replace ink	X	X			X	X		
	Check for paper jam		X		X				

Copyright © 2008, Margret\A Consulting, LLC. Reprinted with permission.

symbol. Sometimes the decision making attempted to be mapped is so complex that it is difficult to draw in a system flowchart. A decision table may be needed to illustrate all the decision points. A sample is shown in Figure 7.4. Sample before-and-after system flow-charts are illustrated in figure 7.5.

It is important to note that in implementing its EHR, NorthShore University Health-System (formerly Evanston Northwestern Healthcare [ENH]) developed 500 high-level workflow charts similar to those illustrated for medication administration. These eventually developed into 2,000 detailed workflow charts (Smith 2005).

As the NorthShore University HealthSystem teams proceeded with the redesign of the workflows, they simultaneously gathered all paper documentation tools and order sets. Working with the clinicians, the teams analyzed and classified the data elements to enable them to redesign the clinical information gathering by units. They then worked with IS staff to build the documentation in their system so that users would enter data into the system only once. From there, it could be shared, retrieved, and reused by any clinician in the care and outcomes management of the patient across the continuum of care (Smith 2005).

Use Case

Use cases are another tool that may be used to describe workflows and processes. Although use cases can easily be used in process assessment at all stages in the EHR project, they typically have been more closely aligned with defining functional requirements. This is because they generally relate a scenario that focuses more on the desired state rather than current state. Use cases are described fully in chapter 8.

Document Analysis

Such a document analysis can be conducted using vendor-supplied worksheets or a set of spreadsheets, such as illustrated in figures 7.6 and 7.7. In the first spreadsheet, every document is analyzed. In the second, a database is created of all data elements appearing in all the documents.

Figure 7.5.   Sample before and after workflow charts

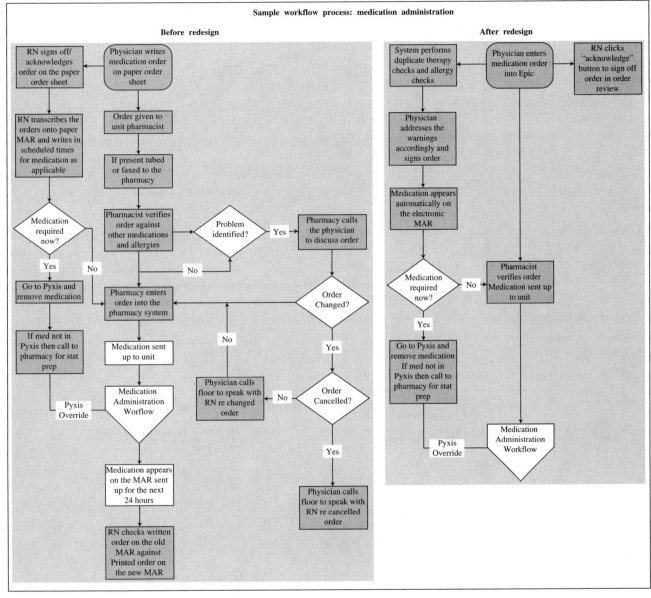

Used with permission: NorthShore University HealthSystem

Figure 7.6.   Document analysis: Document review

EHR Forms Inventory

Form #	Form Title	Current Version	Data Elements	Entry Responsibility	Frequency of Use	Validation Responsibility	Frequency of Validation	Purpose	Disposition: Medical Record Communication Reference	Omissions	Analysis
C2	Chart Note	12/1999	Med Rec No.	Reception	98%	None		Identification	Medical Record		
			Pt Name	Reception	100%	MD	?	Identification			
			Date of Visit	?	97%	MA and MD	?	Documentation			
			Temperature	MA	98%	None		Care Plan		Signature of MA	
			Pulse	MA	98%	None		Care Plan			
			Respiration Rate	MA	97%	None		Care Plan			
			Blood Pressure	MA	85%	MD	75%	Care Plan			Often repeated by MD
			Reason for Visit	MD	98%	None		Care Plan			Asked by MA but not documented
			HPI	MD	98%	None		Care Plan			Parts asked by MA but not documented
			Findings	MD	98%	None		Care Plan			
			Procedures	MD	63%	Coder	Audit	Documentation			
			Plan	MD	98%	Coder	Audit	Documentation			Includes Drug Name and Dose if prescription
			Diagnosis	MD	97%	Coder	Audit	Care Plan Documentation			
			Signature of MD	MD	98%	Coder	Audit	Documentation			
			Date of Signature of MD	MD	78%	Coder	Audit	Documentation			
	Prescription	6/2002	Pt Name	MD	100%	Pharmacist	?	Prescription	Communication	Med Rec No.	Would be helpful for reference & refills
			Pt Address	MD	75%	Pharmacist	?	Prescription			
			Pt Phone No.	MD	75%	Pharmacist	?	Prescription			
			Diagnosis	MD	63%	Pharmacist	?				
			Drug Name	MD	100%	Pharmacist	?	Prescription		Allergy	Generates 12 calls per week
			Dose	MD	100%	Pharmacist	?	Prescription		Contraindications	
			Refills permitted	MD	97%	Pharmacist	?				Would be helpful to have in MR for reference & refills
			Generic permitted	MD	96%	Pharmacist	?				Would be helpful to have in MR for reference & refills
			SIG	MD	98%	Pharmacist	?	Prescription			
			Signature of MD	MD	100%	Pharmacist	?	Prescription			
			Date of Signature of MD	MD	97%	Pharmacist	?	Prescription			

Figure 7.7.   Document analysis: Data element database

EHR Forms Database

Current Data Elements	Current Definition (& Reference)	Occurs in Chart Note Y/N	Occurs in Prescription Y/N	Required for:	Data Origination Screen #	Primary Source: Entry ID Reference Pt Portal	Validation Required by	Required in Rule #	Lexicon
Allergy to Drugs		N		MR	103	MA	MD	4.32	
Allergy to Food		N		MR	103	MA		4.32	
Blood Pressure		Y			201	MD			LOINC
Date of Signature of MD		Y	Y						
Date of Visit		Y				Reception			
Diagnosis	Narrative & ICD Code	Y	Y			MD			ICD
Dose		Y	Y	Rx					
Drug Name	Narrative	Y	Y	Rx				4.32	RxNorm
Findings		Y							
Generic permitted		N	Y						
HPI		Y				Pt Portal	MD		Medicin
Med Rec No.		Y	N						
Plan		Y							
Procedures	Narrative & CPT Code	Y		Bill					CPT
Pt Address			Y						
Pt Name		Y	Y						
Pt Phone No.			Y						
Pulse		Y							
Reason for Visit		Y							
Refile permitted		N	Y						
Respiration Rate		Y							
SIG	State Bd of Pharmacy		Y						
Signature of MD		Y	Y						
Temperature		Y							

Figure 7.8.   Sample comparison of processes across sites

Name Box	A	B	C	D	E	F	G
1	Medication Refill Process Mapping						
2		Site 1	Site 2	Site 3	Site 4	Site 5	Site 6
3	Contact Person						
4	1. Refill request faxed/called from pharmacy to clinic	X	X	X	X	X	X
5	2. Fax retrieved by medical records staff	X	X	X	5% of refils are faxe	X	X
6	3. If request called into clinic, Registrars will leave a message (in IDEAL) to have medical records pull the chart	If request is called into clinic, Registrar will contact Pharmacy to have refill faxed request faxed to clinic	If called, phone room leaves a message for medical records to pull chart	X	If called, message left with either Registrars or Triage. If Triage, RN will create a message (via IDEAL) for MR to pull chart	X	If request called into clinic, call is directed to the CMA, who handles all refill requests
7	4. Medical Records pulls the chart and delivers it to the Medical Assistant's inbox	X	MR pulls the chart and places it in the prescribing provider's "in-box"	MR pulls the chart and places it in the triage "in-box" for review	MR pulls the chart and delivers it to the "in basket" at Peds nursing station	MR pulls the chart and delivers it to the "in basket" at nursing station	If the request is for an antibiotic, narcotic, sedative, or migraine medication, the CMA requests the chart from MR. For all "routine medications, patient info. is looked up in IDEAL

Healthcare organizations also have found that mapping processes across (nursing) units, clinic sites, or other organizational units helps standardize processes. This makes it easier for staff to float among the units as necessary and provides for enhanced adherence to clinical practice guidelines. The process maps themselves can be compared for this purpose or a spreadsheet can be created to illustrate differences, such as shown in figure 7.8.

Baseline Data Collection

Another aspect of process assessment is baseline data collection. This is the process by which the volume of work, time to complete steps, and number of errors or near-misses are identified. Baseline data collection helps identify opportunities for improvement, set goals and expectations for what can be accomplished with the EHR, and for benchmarking how well the EHR is performing.

Some organizations find the process of baseline data collection tedious and time consuming, especially when they have "faith" that the EHR is needed and will achieve intended results. Just as was suggested that setting goals and expectations is important (in chapter 5), being able to objectively assess the results of EHR implementation is critical to forward progress. However, it is true that baseline data collection must be performed in a manner that is useful, and not simply an exercise that may detract from patient care or be viewed as disciplinary.

Considerations for baseline data collection include determining what data will be collected, how frequently data will be collected (for example, all data or only a sample), how it will be collected (for example, manually, as a by-product of another task, or automated), how it will be summarized (for example, individualized or aggregated), and how it will ultimately be used.

When baseline data are then used in benchmarking, there are also important steps to take to ensure that apples to apples comparisons are being made. In fact, a reason often given for not doing benchmarking is that it is difficult to make valid comparisons. A classic example in a hospital is medication errors. In almost every case of implementing an electronic or bar code medication administration record (EMAR/BC-MAR) system, the number of medication errors increases—not because the system contributes to making errors but because capturing baseline data for medication errors is very difficult. With better reporting capability the number appears to increase when the actual number may actually have decreased. The definition of medication error also needs to be considered. For example, many BC-MAR systems have tight windows of time for administering medications without calling out an error state, so that what might not have been considered an error in the manual environment may now be considered an error by the system. Hence, it is important to make sure benchmarking is performed by knowledgeable individuals, that those who are performing the processes have contributed to their design—including the benchmarking study, and that all benchmarking studies are followed up with appropriate celebration and course correction.

Process Improvement

The final steps in process assessment relate to process improvement. While recognizing the types of changes that may be feasible now and appropriate for the future are important, process improvement is not solely about change, but also about empowering people to transform their practices to achieve best outcomes.

Team Empowerment

A process assessment is a comprehensive undertaking with many people and even different types of teams coming together at different points within the EHR initiative. There are obviously going to be checks and balances within an EHR project so that no one group can be a significant outlier. Each set of people and teams, however, should be given not only responsibility for the work of process assessment, but also appropriate authority to carry out the work and responsibility for seeing to it that redesigned processes are carried out. If a process assessment team believes that its recommendations will not be carried out, it will not succeed.

Process assessment teams may be composed of individuals who have not previously participated in the type of team required for process assessment. Team building was extensively discussed in chapter 4. With respect to process assessment teams, it is important to recognize that people tend to differ according to their preference for working at a certain level of detail, making decisions, acting as overseers or finishers, and so on. The most desirable process assessment team brings together different types of people who can contribute in their unique way to the common good.

After the group is formed, it needs a leader. The leader's role is not to direct the group to a specific conclusion but, rather, to facilitate the proceedings, keep the group on track, and encourage everyone to participate.

Group Facilitation

Specific techniques are used to facilitate the type of thinking required to assess processes (Kubeck 1995, 254–57). These include:

- *Brainstorming:* In this technique, as many ideas for the redesign of a process as possible are suggested without any critique. In fact, the most unusual, wild, or crazy ideas are usually the ones that spark creativity among group members. When all the ideas are on the table, the group returns to each one to seek clarification or enhancement. Still, no criticism of any idea is permitted. As clarification is provided, new ideas may be identified. Over the course of this process, people may withdraw ideas that are clearly out of scope or unworkable. Usually, one idea emerges that is the most creative and yet the most manageable.

- *Double reversal:* This is a type of brainstorming technique that helps overcome the lack of ideas. In this technique, members of the group are asked to describe the worst way a process could be redesigned. Team members then sort through the ideas generated to determine whether any of them could, if reversed, improve or even totally redesign the system.

- *Nominal group process:* This technique is similar to brainstorming, except that ideas are generated outside the group and then brought to it for consideration. Group members first discuss the meaning and implications of the ideas and then rank-order them in order to reach consensus on one.

- *Probing:* Probing is often used when individuals find it difficult to break out of their paradigms. In probing, a facilitator uses various questioning techniques. Probing questions such as "What do you mean by that?" elicit greater detail about an idea just mentioned. A similar type of questioning technique is to ask a series of why questions to uncover personal concerns, political realities, and cultural issues. Mirroring questions are used to prevent misunderstanding and are basically restatements of what has been said. Mirroring also tends to elicit further description without appearing to be accusatory, which other probing questions can sometimes appear to be. Many people believe that the best type of question for eliciting detail is an open-ended question. Although open-ended questions are critical in brainstorming, sometimes a series of close-ended questions with yes or no answers or questions that provide only specific facts can be equally effective. A trained facilitator knows when to use each type of question to maximize results in a minimum period of time. Figure 7.9 describes facilitator competencies.

Figure 7.9.   Facilitator competencies

> **A facilitator . . .**
>
> - Is effective in distinguishing process from content
> - Carefully manages the scope of the project
> - Uses time and space intentionally
> - Is skillful in evoking participation and creativity
> - Is practiced in honoring the group and affirming its wisdom
> - Is capable of maintaining objectivity
> - Is skilled in reading the underlying dynamics of the group
>
> - Orchestrates the event drama
> - Releases blocks to the process
> - Is adroit in adapting to the changing situation
> - Assumes responsibility for the group journey
> - Can produce powerful documentation
> - Demonstrates professionalism, self-confidence, and authenticity
> - Maintains personal integrity

Source: Schuman 2004. Reprinted with permission from the Institute of Cultural Affairs, ICA-USA: Chicago, IL.

Process Improvement Techniques

As the process assessment team starts to analyze workflows and processes for improvement—whether now or with an EHR—there are some specific things to look for that may signal areas for improvement. These are identified in Box 7.1:

Box 7.1.   Opportunities for Improvement

> - Bottlenecks
> - Sources of delay
> - Rework due to errors
> - Role ambiguity
> - Unnecessary duplications
>
> - Long cycle time
> - Lack of adherence to standards
> - Lack of information
> - Lack of quality controls

Copyright © 2008, Margret\A Consulting, LLC. Reprinted with permission.

Caution should be applied in process assessment not to strip away processes that mitigate risk. For example, what may appear to be duplicate or unnecessary may be needed redundancy to ensure quality. In healthcare, licensure requirements also contribute greatly to who may perform what task, so apparent role ambiguity may be the result of such credentialing. Cycle time may also be driven by outcomes. These and other examples are important for clinicians to evaluate as part of risk analysis and proper due diligence on any changes process improvement techniques may suggest.

Effecting Change

Change management is the process by which an organization gets to its future state: the vision (Lorenzi and Riley, 1995, 150). Much has been said about the need for change

Figure 7.10.   Facilitator techniques

- Balanced Scorecard

- Benchmarking

- Best Practices

- Business Process Reengineering

- Continuous Quality Improvement (CQI)

- Cultural Change

- ISO9000

- Knowledge Management

- Learning Organization

- Management-by-Objectives

- Outcome-Based Evaluation

- Program Evaluation

- Quality Circles

- Statistical Process Control

- Strategic Planning

- Total Quality Management (TQM)

management to facilitate adoption of the EHR, and many techniques have been used to help empower those in process assessment teams to think "outside the box." Figure 7.10 lists some of the techniques commonly deployed to effect the changes identified and validated as necessary through process assessment. In using such tools, team members will take ownership of the change, which increases the likelihood that the change will be successful.

However, change management has many other components. The role of education has been discussed extensively. Providing feedback is another critical element. Process assessment team members may initially fear proposing changes that could result in the elimination of their jobs or the jobs of their subordinates. There are many ways to implement EHR systems and achieve cost savings without laying off employees. EHR implementation is a long-term process, and attrition will be a significant factor in achieving cost savings through staffing changes. The long-term process also allows for staff retraining so that they can take on new jobs within the organization or be more marketable outside. However, management must be open, honest, and responsive to these issues or creative process assessment will not occur and the level of benefit achieved through an EHR will not support the investment.

Role of HIM and IT Professionals in Process Assessment

HIM and IT professionals have a vested interest in the EHR and in process assessment. They both play valuable roles in process assessment. Both HIM and IT professionals are trained in the techniques described earlier. However, other members of process assessment teams may be unfamiliar with these techniques. Thus, it may be appropriate to apply some just-in-time training on the various techniques rather than bombard everyone with all they have to learn up front. If process assessment is not their primary job and they are expected to apply the various techniques over time, it is best to provide training as required.

A word also should be noted about the appropriate role of the HIM and IT professional in process assessment. The purpose of process assessment is to make the organization's processes compatible with the EHR and to ensure that EHR systems do not replicate but, instead, improve current processes. Because HIM and IT professionals know how to use the tools, an obvious role for these professionals is that of trainer or facilitator.

However, facilitators are supposed to remain neutral and unbiased. If the HIM or IT professional has strong ideas about what an EHR should be and how it should function, the facilitator role would be the wrong choice. The facilitator role leaves the individual in the role out of the decision-making process and without influence. However, each situation is different. It may be possible to provide training but leave the actual facilitation to someone else. In another situation, the position of trainer may be considered outside the primary decision making, in which case the HIM or IT professional may prefer to be a member of the assessment team.

Conclusion

The EHR affects an organization and its members like no other system. Although it necessarily imposes change to achieve its improvement objectives, how process assessment is undertaken can have a significant impact on its success.

It is critical to understand that the scope of assessment for an EHR project extends beyond a department or a single function. Similarly, it is unwise to view an EHR project as changing the organization's fundamental mission.

Redesigning processes to accommodate the EHR initiative should be undertaken by the users themselves to achieve the most realistic designs and commitment to the final result. Process assessment techniques are as much about focusing on change and empowering people as they are about the specific tools that help identify and document appropriate changes. Moreover, conducting a process assessment effort in a healthcare environment is challenging because it changes the nature of the teams commonly found there. Team participation, however, combines good idea generation with an appreciation for working with others.

References and Resources

Briggs, B. 2003 (Oct.). Medical records, IT lines blurring. *Health Data Management*, 80–84. www. healthdatamanagement.com/html/current/PastIssueStory.cfm?ArticleId=9062&issuedate=2003-10-01.

Cassidy, A., and K. Guggenberger. 2001. *A Practical Guide to Information Systems Process Improvement*. Boca Raton, FL: CRC Press LLC.

George, M. 2008, Integrating Lean and Six Sigma. www.isixsigma.com/library/content/ask-02.asp.

Graham, B.B. 2004. *Detail Process Charting*. Hoboken, NY: John Wiley & Sons.

Guite, J. et al. 2006. Nursing admissions process redesigned to leverage EHR. *Journal of Healthcare Information Management*. 20(2):55–64.

Han, Y.Y., et al. 2005 (Dec.). Unexpected increased mortality after implementation of a commercially sold computerized physician order entry system. *Pediatrics* 116(6):1506–1512.

Harmon, P. 2003. *Business Process Change: A Manager's Guide to Improving, Redesigning, and Automating Processes*. San Francisco: Morgan Kaufmann Publishers.

Houck, S. 2006. (August). Migrating workflows from paper to your EHR. California Academy of Family Physicians. http://www.familydocs.org/news-media/practice-management-news/august-2006.php.

Koppel et al. 2005. Role of computerized physician order entry systems in facilitating medication errors. *Journal of the American Medical Association*. 293(10):1197-203.

Kubeck, L.C. 1995. *Techniques for Business Process Assessment: Tying It All Together*. New York: John Wiley & Sons.

Lorenzi, N.M., and R.T. Riley. 1995. *Organizational Aspects of Health Informatics: Managing Technological Change*. New York: Springer-Verlag.

McGee, M.K. 2005. (March 9). Computerized systems can cause new medical mistakes, study says. *Information Week*. http://www.informationweek.com/news/management/showArticle.jhtml?articleID=159400302.

Nickols, F. 2000. Change Management 101: A Primer. www.home.att.net/~nickols/change.htm.

Polaschek, J., et al. 2003. (November 10). Lessons from the front line—The good, bad, and ugly: The Cedars-Sinai CPOE experience. Proceedings of the American Medical Informatics Association.

Schuman, S.P., moderator. 2004. Facilitator Competencies, Electronic Discussion on Group Facilitation. Center for Policy Research, SUNY Albany. Available online from albany.edu/cpr/gf.

Sequist, T.D., et al. 2005. A randomized trial of electronic clinical reminders to improve quality of care for diabetes and coronary artery disease. *Journal of the American Medical Informatics Association* 12(4):431–437.

Sharp, A., and P. McDermott. 2001. *Workflow Modeling: Tools for Process Improvement and Application Development*. Norwood, MA: Artech House, Inc.

Smith, D, and Newell, L.M. 2002. A physician's perspective: Deploying the EMR. *Journal of Healthcare Information Management*. 16(2):71–9.

Smith, T., et al. 2005 (Dec.). Transforming healthcare with a patient-centric electronic health record system. Evanston Northwestern Healthcare, Nicholas E. Davies Award of Excellence. Chicago: HIMSS.

Thiagi Inc. 1999. Secrets of Successful Facilitators. Online Workshops by Thiagi. www.thiagi.com/article-secrets.html.

Towne, J. 2008. (June 11). The EHR's impact on IOM's aims. H&HN's Most Wired Magazine. http://www.hhnmostwired.com/hhnmostwired_app/jsp/articledisplay.jsp?dcrpath=HHNMOSTWIRED/Article/data/Spring2008/080611MW_Online_Towne&domain=HHNMOSTWIRED.

Van der Aalst, W., and K. van Hee. 2004. *Workflow Management: Models, Methods, and Systems*, Cambridge, MA: MIT Press.

Chapter 8
Functional Needs Assessment

The following quote introduces the Institute of Medicine (IOM) report, *Key Capabilities of an Electronic Health Record System,* commissioned by the Department of Health and Human Services (HHS) in spring 2003:

> Knowing is not enough; we must apply.
> Willing is not enough; we must do.
> —Goethe

The functions of the electronic health record (EHR) are what we "apply" in order to "do." A functional needs assessment describes the key capabilities or application requirements for achieving the benefits of the EHR as the organization has envisioned it. Where process assessment looked at very specific tasks, functional needs assessment describes the overall purposes the EHR must achieve. This chapter:

- Describes the scope and purpose of a functional needs assessment for the EHR

- Offers models for understanding EHR users and uses, and the functionality required to achieve the benefits of the EHR and to support its beneficiaries

- Explains how to conduct a functional needs assessment

Scope and Purpose of a Functional Needs Assessment

There are many different views of what constitutes an EHR system and a migration path over which EHRs proceed to be developed, with corresponding levels of benefits to be achieved. Thus, any given organization must identify the functional needs required to achieve the desired benefits of the EHR it envisions.

Information Infrastructure

The full scope of functional needs, data requirements, and technical capabilities may be considered the overall **information infrastructure**. Figure 8.1 displays a schematic of what an information infrastructure looks like.

Meeting the information needs of users is the objective of every information system. Although the EHR effects a clinical transformation, when considered in relation to the core business of the healthcare organization, the EHR must receive data from, and supply data to, virtually every financial/administrative, operational, and clinical system, both within and outside the enterprise. Following is an example:

> A primary care physician covering emergency services meets with a patient presenting with chest pain. Using a clinical pathway, the physician is directed to conduct certain types of clinical assessments based on symptoms and signs observed and in response to specific interventions. After the assessment results are entered, an administrative protocol may determine that the physician is not credentialed to perform further interventions and that a referral to a specialist, such as a cardiologist, must be made. The administrative system may advise which cardiologist is on call or, if the patient is found to be stable and the referral is for follow-up care, the financial system, which manages the payer rules, may provide the patient with a list of specialists in the health plan's network to contact.

What makes the EHR such a complex system to implement is not only the interrelationships of all the applications, but also the integration of all the other components of the information infrastructure. The EHR requires all applications to work together. In addition to being a technical challenge, this is a policy, organizational, financial, and political challenge.

Borrowing from the classic **data-processing model**, applications are the *output* of the overall information infrastructure. To get the desired output, the right *input* must be provided; hence, functionality rests on an information infrastructure. The information infrastructure supports the system's input capabilities. Achieving output from input is the *processing* component that includes analytical tools and technology. An input–processing–output process is not truly a system without the users and uses of information. These are the beneficiaries and benefits of the system. Some of these are internal organizational users and uses; others are external to the organization.

For an organization to ensure that it has the necessary infrastructure to support the desired EHR benefits, a logical process must be undertaken to identify the full scope of the information infrastructure needed to achieve an EHR. This begins with the **functional needs assessment** (described in this chapter), moves to a data infrastructure assessment (described in chapter 9), and completes the cycle with a technology infrastructure

Figure 8.1.   Information infrastructure schematic

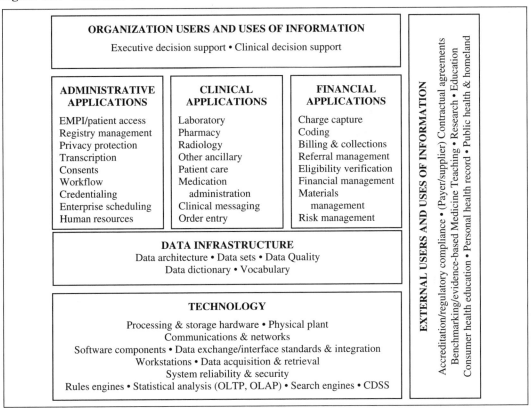

assessment (described in chapter 10). The end result of these assessments is a statement of requirement specifications that can be used to benchmark current capabilities, identify gaps, evaluate vendor offerings, and, ultimately, construct the EHR system.

Models for Understanding Functional Requirements

A functional needs assessment process should begin with identifying the organization's internal and external information needs.

In its Comprehensive Accreditation Manual for Hospitals (CAMH), The Joint Commission recognizes that an organization's "provision of care, treatment, and services is a complex endeavor that is highly dependent on information" (CAMH 2008). As such, in its management of information standard for accreditation, The Joint Commission requires organizations to "treat information as an important resource to be managed effectively and efficiently." It goes on to indicate that managing information is an active, planned activity and that the process of identifying information needs must be performed well to achieve "the goal of the information management function [which] is to support decision making to improve patient outcomes, improve healthcare documentation, assure patient safety, and improve performance in patient care, treatment, and services, governance, management, and support processes" (CAMH 2008). The Joint Commission standards are designed to be equally compatible with paper-based systems, electronic systems, or hybrid systems. The Joint Commission further recognizes that "the quality of care, treatment, and services is affected by the many transitions in information management that are currently in progress in health care, such as the transition from handwriting and traditional paper-based documentation to electronic information management, as well as the transition from free text to structured and interactive text"(CAMH 2008).

The Joint Commission requires that hospitals "base their information management processes on an assessment of internal and external information needs." They should identify "the flow of information throughout a hospital, including information storage and feedback mechanisms," and identify "the data and information needed: within and among departments, services, or programs; within and among the staff, the administration, and the governance for supporting relationships with outside services and contractors; with licensing, accrediting, and regulatory bodies; with purchasers, payers, and employers; for supporting information needs between the hospital and the patients; and for participating in research and databases" (CAMH 2008).

Identification of Uses and Users

When the outputs of an information system are understood, inputs should reflect both uses and users of the system. The IOM report, *Key Capabilities of an Electronic Health Record System,* identifies primary and secondary uses of an EHR system (IOM 2003). These are identified in table 8.1.

IOM has been a consistent proponent of EHRs. In its report, *The Computer-based Patient Record: An Essential Technology for Health Care*, published in 1991 and revised in 1997, it identified numerous representative individual and institutional users of patient records. Broad categories of these users included those listed in table 8.2.

Functional Requirements Models

Once outputs and inputs have been identified, the process part of the data-processing model needs to be considered. Such a model outlines the functions that are performed with the input to produce the output. There are several sources of functional requirements models. Although they may contain different levels of detail, structured in somewhat different manners, and have

Table 8.1.   Primary and secondary uses of an EHR system

Primary Uses	Secondary Uses
Patient Care Delivery	Education
Patient Care Management	Regulation
Patient Care Support Processes	Research
Financial and Other Administrative Processes	Public Health and Homeland Security
Patient Self-Management	Policy Support

Source: Reprinted with permission from *Key Capabilities of an Electronic Health Record System: Letter Report* © 2003 by the National Academy of Sciences, courtesy of the National Academies Press, Washington, D.C.

Table 8.2. Categories of users of an EHR system

Individual Users	Institutional Users
Providers	Health care delivery facilities, such as ambulatory surgery centers, donor banks, nursing homes
Consumers	Management and review of care organizations
Support personnel	Reimbursement of care organizations, such as business health care coalitions, employers, and insurers
Patient care reimbursement personnel	Researchers
Others, including accreditors, lawyers, researchers, journalists	Educators Accreditation and licensure bodies Policymakers

Source: Reprinted with permission from *The Computer-based Patient Record: An Essential Technology for Health Care,* Revised Edition, pp. 76–77, © 1997 by the National Academy of Sciences, courtesy of the National Academies Press, Washington, D.C.

somewhat different purposes, the models—thankfully—build upon each other. The IOM contributed its model to Health Level Seven (HL7), which in turn is being used by CCHIT.

Institute of Medicine

When the IOM produced its first report on EHRs in 1991, it identified a set of user requirements for patient records and record systems. These were confirmed as continuing to be valid in the 1997 revised IOM report and continue to be reaffirmed through 11 years of work by Andrew and Bruegel (2005). The original IOM user requirements for patient records and record systems are reproduced in table 8.3. These user requirements were validated in the creation of the revised edition

With renewed interest in EHRs occurring as a result of patient safety concerns, the federal government asked IOM to provide further guidance on the key capabilities of an EHR system. In *Key Capabilities of an Electronic Health Record System,* IOM identified that an EHR system includes (IOM 2003, 1):

- "Longitudinal collection of electronic health information for and about persons, where health information is defined as information pertaining to the health of an individual or health care provided to an individual

- Immediate electronic access to person- and population-level information by authorized, and only authorized, users

- Provision of knowledge and decision-support that enhance the quality, safety, and efficiency of patient care

- Support of efficient processes for health care delivery"

IOM envisioned the critical building blocks of an EHR system to be the EHRs maintained by providers and by individuals (also called personal health records [PHRs]). It also updated its list of core functionalities, which are identified in table 8.4.

Table 8.3. Original IOM user requirements for patient records and record systems

Requirements Categories	Examples
Record Content	Uniform core data elements Standardized coding systems and formats Common data dictionary Information on outcomes of care and functional status
Record Format	"Front-page" problem list Ability to "flip through the record" Integrated among disciplines and sites of care
System Performance	Rapid retrieval 24-hour access Available at convenient places Easy data input
Intelligence	Decision support Clinician reminders "Alarm" systems capable of being customized
Linkages	Linkages with other information systems (for example, radiology, laboratory) Transferability of information among specialties and sites Linkages with relevant scientific literature Linkages with other institutional databases and registries Linkages with records of family members Electronic transfer of billing information
Reporting Capabilities	"Derived documents" (for example, insurance forms) Easily customized output and other user interfaces Standard clinical reports (e.g., discharge summaries) Customized and ad hoc reports (for example, specific evaluation queries) Trend reports and graphics
Control and Access	Easy access for patients and their advocates Safeguards against violation of confidentiality
Training and Implementation	Minimal training required for system use Graduated implementation possible

Source: Reprinted with permission from *The Computer-based Patient Record: An Essential Technology for Health Care*, p. 80, © 1991 by the National Academy of Sciences, courtesy of the National Academies Press, Washington, D.C.

Table 8.4.   2003 IOM core functionalities for an EHR system

Core Functionalities	Examples
Health Information and Data	Key data using standardized code sets where available Narrative (clinical and patient) information Patient acuity/severity of illness/risk adjustment Capture of identifiers
Results Management	Results reporting Results notification Multiple views of data/presentation Multimedia support
Order Entry/Management	Computerized provider order entry
Decision Support	Access to knowledge sources Drug alerts Other rule-based alerts (e.g., significant lab trends, lab test because of drug) Reminders for preventive services Clinical guidelines and pathways Chronic disease management Clinician work list Incorporation of patient and/or family preferences Diagnostic decision support Use of epidemiologic data Automated real-time surveillance
Electronic Communication and Connectivity	Provider–provider Team coordination Patient–provider Medical devices Trading partners (external) Integrated medical record within and across settings
Patient Support	Patient education Family and informal caregiver education Data entered by patient, family, and/or informal care-giver
Administrative Processes	Scheduling management Eligibility determination
Reporting and Population Health Management	Patient safety and quality reporting Public health reporting Deidentifying data Disease registries

Source: Reprinted with permission from *Key Capabilities of an Electronic Health Record System: Letter Report,* p. 7 and extractions from pp. 13–19, © 2003 by the National Academy of Sciences, courtesy of the National Academies Press, Washington, D.C.

The 2003 IOM letter report also provides a grid of more detailed capabilities by time frame (specified as 2004–5, 2006–7, and 2008–10) and site of care (hospitals, ambulatory care, nursing homes, and care in the community [personal health record]).

Health Level Seven (HL7)

In addition to publishing its guidance on EHR functionality, IOM's 2003 work contributed to HL7 work, which was the **standards development organization** targeted by HHS to develop a standard for an EHR system functional model.

The HL7 EHR System Functional Model was balloted as a final ANSI-approved standard in spring 2007. It is provided in appendix B and is based on the framework illustrated in figure 8.2

In a press release, HL7 noted that the intent of the standard is to provide all stakeholders involved in describing EHR system behavior with a baseline understanding of the functions. It noted that some of the functions are visionary and very few vendors will have the ability to incorporate all of them right away. HL7 further noted that some of the functions are more important to one care setting than to another. Subsequently, HL7 has developed guidance to enable the creation and registration of functional profiles that provide a standardized description and common understanding of functions sought or available for special situations, such as an intensive care unit, cardiology practice, or even primary care delivery in another country. The first such profile to be registered related to emergency

Figure 8.2.   HL7 EHR-system Functional model

Direct Care	DC.1	Care Management
	DC.2	Clinical Decision Support
	DC.3	Operations Management and Communication
Supportive	S.1	Clincal Support
	S.2	Measurement, Analysis, Research, and Reports
	S.3	Administrative and Financial
Information Infrastructure	IN.1	Security
	IN.2	Health Record Information and Management
	IN.3	Registry and Directory Services
	IN.4	Standard Terminologies and Terminology Services
	IN.5	Standards-based Interoperability
	IN.6	Business Rules Management
	IN.7	Workflow Management

Source: Health Level Seven 2007. Copyright © 2007 by Health Level Seven, Inc.

medicine. The second profile released describes the legal EHR. At the time this book was updated, a third profile on vital records was being developed.

Finally, HL7 has recognized the importance interoperability plays both across disparate applications within a care delivery organization as well as within a health information exchange. It developed an EHR Interoperability Model with EHR Data Exchange Criteria as a Draft Standard for Trial Use (DSTU) in February 2007. (A DSTU is one that will be evaluated by the industry for a 2-year period, after which it will be refined and reballoted with the goal of achieving a final ANSI-approved status.)

Certification Commission on Health Information Technology

In spring 2004, President Bush called for widespread deployment of health information technology (HIT). Subsequently, HHS established the Office of the National Coordinator for Health Information Technology (ONC) and the American Health Information Community (AHIC). In July 2004, ONC issued the Framework for Strategic Action, which included in its broad goals the "private sector certification of HIT products" (Thompson and Brailer 2004). In response, AHIMA, HIMSS, and the National Alliance for Health Information Technology (The Alliance) funded and launched the Certification Commission on Health Information Technology (CCHIT). Its purpose was "to accelerate the adoption of robust, interoperable HIT throughout the U.S. healthcare system, by creating an efficient, credible, sustainable mechanism for the certification of HIT products" (CCHIT 2005). Since then, several other organizations have joined the effort and CCHIT has been awarded a HHS contract to develop and assess EHR and network certification criteria and inspection processes. The role of CCHIT within the HIT strategic landscape is illustrated in figure 8.3.

CCHIT's scope of work includes product certification for EHRs in ambulatory care settings, which it started in fall 2006, product certification for EHRs in inpatient care settings which it started in fall 2007, and assess certification of infrastructure or network components (such as regional health information organizations) through which EHRs operate by fall 2008.

For the ambulatory care EHR product certification, CCHIT has identified functionality, interoperability, and security criteria. These are largely drawn from HL7's EHR System Functional Model, various other healthcare interoperability standards development organizations, and HIPAA and other security standards. Several hundred criteria were identified, and use cases created as test scenarios. A crosswalk between the criteria and the scenarios has been developed to guide vendors and consumers concerning the time frame over which various criteria will be required in products for them to be certified. Figure 8.4 illustrates a sample of the crosswalk. Each year, CCHIT updates the criteria. As a result criteria changes; hence, for example, in 2006, ambulatory EHRs were not required to have e-Rx, although by 2007 they were.

Inpatient criteria for CCHIT certification focus primarily on EHR foundational components (including patient and provider demographics, allergy information, medication list functionality, results retrieval, and order communications) necessary to support CPOE and medication administration functionality. Other functions supporting other applications will be evaluated in the certification process in subsequent years.

Although only the most nationally recognized and broadest-in-scope EHR functional models have been described here, there are numerous other sets of functionality lists. Drury conducted a comparison of five such lists as evidence of their proliferation (2006). The

Figure 8.3.   Role of CCHIT within the Health IT Strategic Landscape

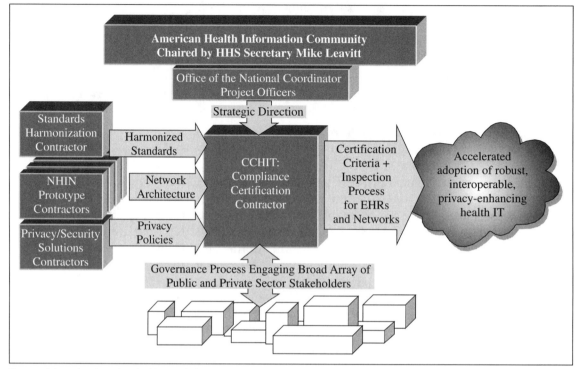

Source: Adapted and reprinted with permission from Certification Commission for Healthcare Information Technology (CCHIT^SM), © 2006.

Centers for Medicare and Medicaid Services (CMS) Doctors Office Quality-Information Technology (DOQ-IT) initiative conducted by the **quality improvement organizations** (QIOs) in each state also has identified an EHR Selection Tools and Resources list, which lists a number of different resources for identifying ambulatory EHR functions (Lumetra, 2005). There are many purposes for this review, comparison, and discussion of standards for EHR functionality models, including:

- The level of activity reflects the general level of interest on the part of the healthcare delivery system to move more rapidly to adoption of an EHR.

- The degree of commonality in both statements of purpose and functionality, after terminology is normalized, demonstrates that there is a relatively stable and comprehensive set of features and functions that have consistently been recognized as comprising the EHR.

- The multiple versions with different terminology and time frames reflect that the task is complex, and if the development and acquisition of an EHR is to be achieved by the "masses," there must be a standard that supports greater "mass production" and lower cost of ownership. Although systems must be customizable to accommodate

Figure 8.4. Example of CCHIT inpatient EHR criteria

Inpatient Certification Criteria
Final 08 Criteria
July 16, 2008

© 2008 The Certification Commission for Healthcare Information Technology

08 Criteria #	Source WG	Certification Track	Category	Category Description	Criteria	Compliance			Discussion/Comments	Source or References	Test Script Reference
						2008 Certification	Roadmap 2009	Roadmap 2010 and Beyond	Compliance Key: P = Previous Criteria M = Modified for Year N = New for Year O = Provisional		
IP 08.19	IP	IP	8. General Ordering Requirements	Create and communicate orders that are complete and actionable.	The system shall provide the ability to associate an order of any type (including medication order) with a related clinical problem(s) and/or diagnosis code(s) and description.	N				DC 1.7.3 DC 2.4.1 CCHIT Amb Criteria	IP 2.03
IP 08.20	IP	IP	8. General Ordering Requirements	Create and communicate orders that are complete and actionable.	The system shall provide the ability to allow the entry of orders to be activated at a future date and time including admission orders, discharge orders, and post-op orders.	N				CCHIT Amb Criteria	IP 3.14
IP 08.21	IP	IP	8. General Ordering Requirements	Create and communicate orders that are complete and actionable.	The system shall have the ability to clearly define one time medication orders within a single encounter that do not include a designated start date, stop date or time to be administered (i.e. unscheduled). Medication needs to remain visible as an active order.			N	For example, a vaccine ordered to be given at the time of discharge but the patient has been hospitalized for 44 days with a current discharge date.		
IP 08.22	IP	IP	8. General Ordering Requirements	Create and communicate orders that are complete and actionable.	The system shall provide the ability to print orders for all order types.	M					IP 3.34
IP 08.23	IP	IP	8. General Ordering Requirements	Create and communicate orders that are complete and actionable.	The system shall have the ability to select individual groups of orders for printing.			N	Example: i.e., active, discontinued, nutrition activity, radiology, lab, blood bank, etc. often printed in preparation for a down time.		

(continued)

Figure 8.4.   (Continued)

ID	IP	Section	Objective	Requirement	Status	Notes	Reference 1	Reference 2
IP 08.24	IP	8. General Ordering Requirements	Create and communicate orders that are complete and actionable..	The system shall provide the ability to enter conditional orders that can be activated when certain criteria and conditions are met.	N	For example, draw blood culture when temperature > 39.0 centigrade		IP 1.056, 2.08
IP 08.25	IP	8. General Ordering Requirements		The system shall alert the user when parameters for conditional orders are met and the order becomes active.	N	For example, draw blood culture when temperature > 39.0 centigrade		
IP 08.26	IP	8. General Ordering Requirements	Create and communicate orders that are complete and actionable..	The system shall provide the ability for a clinician to save frequently used and institutionally approved orderables of order sets as "favorites" or "preferences" to facilitate retrieval and ordering.	N		DC.1.7.1	IP 2.19
IP 08.27	IP	8. General Ordering Requirements	Create and communicate orders that are complete and actionable..	The system shall provide the ability to access orders for a patient by different views.	P	For example, Active, Discontinued, All, Date, Ordering Clinician, and Type.		IP 1.079
IP 08.28	IP	8. General Ordering Requirements	Create and communicate orders that are complete and actionable..	The system shall have the ability to allow the hospital to specify orders that always require co-signatures.	N	For example, V188 DNR or chemotherapy orders.	CCHIT Amb Criteria	
IP 08.29	IP	8. General Ordering Requirements	Create and communicate orders that are complete and actionable..	The system shall provide the ability for cosigned orders to retain and display the identities of both the ordering and cosigning providers.	N	This criterion will be required for inpatient in 2880 and has been proposed for Foundation in 2009.	CCHIT Amb Criteria	IP 3.11

variations, there also must be interoperability of system components and comparability of data to achieve longitudinal information for the care of patients across their lifetime and continuum of care.

Functional Needs Assessment Process

One may wonder if functional requirements models exist and even product certification is underway, why a given organization should replicate the process of defining its own requirements. Each organization needs to define its functional requirements for a number of reasons, including:

- *Every organization starts from a different vantage point.* Some organizations may have minimal automation, others may have highly specialized automation, and still others may have moderate automation across the entire organization. Some may operate on older platforms that do not support some of the newer functionalities. Defining requirements relative to the technical infrastructure present is essential.

- *Every organization has different needs.* What one organization may consider an essential requirement, another may consider only "desirable." As the CCHIT criteria evolve, more and more functions will be certified, which means that not all functionality is included now.

- *Every vendor offers a somewhat different approach.* Although many of the products are offered by vendors, they are not always offered in a single product or even through a single vendor. Organizations need to decide whether they want to (1) focus on a single vendor and accept that vendor's offerings (whatever they may be), (2) work with a core set of vendors that can achieve a broader set of functionalities, or (3) get best-of-breed for all the functions and attempt to integrate them.

- *Other elements of product selection must be considered.* The CCHIT emphasizes that company history and viability, staffing, number and type of clients, nature of implementation and training provided, level and quality of support and, of course, cost, are all factors that must be considered.

Any given organization's functional needs assessment, therefore, needs to utilize functional requirements models as resources, but those models also must reflect the organization's capabilities and needs.

Identifying Functional Requirements

A functional needs assessment often begins with a survey of users. Although this is important, users need to be sufficiently educated about EHR functionality. Without fully understanding the depth and breadth of functionality, users may be able to identify only limited requirements initially. But after some functionality is implemented, they may begin to see the potential and recognize that EHRs are capable of providing much more. If a full set of functionality is not planned for in advance, however, the wrong choice of vendor can be made or, potentially, the migration path may be piecemeal and result in disparate components that do not support one another. Because healthcare users typically are highly specialized and therefore focused on a specific activity, they often do not see the big picture or understand how an action in one area impacts another area.

Despite the shortcomings of surveying users and alternative means that aid functionality description, the process of engaging users is critical to successful EHR selection and implementation. The survey process initiates an educational effort and engages users from the start. As users more fully understand the EHR's functional capabilities, they can contribute much more to the planning effort.

Surveying Users

Several approaches can be taken to survey users. A good way to start is with a core set of users who have been exposed to EHR systems through personal interest or use of them in other settings. A group facilitation technique may be used to ensure that the process of surveying users provides value to the organization. The nominal group process works especially well if users are anticipated to be opinionated. For example, an individual who has used one product extensively may be favorable to the vendor and push hard for the organization to adopt the vendor's product regardless of the functionality. On the other hand, a user who has a bad experience with a product may introduce bias against the vendor of that product. The process of surveying users on EHR functionality should be vendor neutral.

After core users have identified a set of functionalities, it is possible to construct a questionnaire in which others are asked to rank the importance of the set to them and identify any missing functions they believe are important or desirable. Again, an "educated consumer" is needed to be able to discriminate among functionalities. If most of the questionnaires come back with every function checked as critical, the questionnaire may have only served as a token process to engage users. At best, users will think they have contributed to the process. Unfortunately, many may recognize the shortcomings of the process and feel they have not been provided the opportunity for true input. Additionally, if the core group is not representative of the full user community, the questionnaire might be viewed as a way for certain individuals to steamroll a process. Another negative effect of such a questionnaire is that potential users may have the mistaken impression that because they checked off everything, the system will ultimately provide everything.

It may be appropriate to use the set of functional requirement statements included in such a questionnaire as the starting point for focus group discussions. After experienced and inexperienced users have provided a sufficient volume of input, it may be effective to return to the questionnaire format as validation and refinement of all the input received. If it is possible to construct the questionnaire in a manner that asks potential users to identify what they could live without, or over what time frame they would envision implementation, the questionnaire may be more time consuming to complete but result in more valuable information.

Use Cases

Another approach to defining functional requirements is the use case technique, which is often easier for clinicians to provide. A use case is essentially a scenario that describes a system's behavior as it responds to a request that originates from outside of that system.

Box 8.1.   General sections of a use case

- Use Case Name
- Version
- Goal
- Summary
- Actors
- Preconditions
- Triggers

- Basic Course of Events
- Alternative Paths
- Postconditions
- Business Rules
- Notes
- Author and Date

Use cases describe the interaction between a primary actor, or initiator of the interaction, such a nurse, and the system itself, such as providing a notification that a patient is due medication. Use cases may be described at different levels of complexity and do not require a standard template or structure for documentation, although such are available for use if desired. When engaging clinicians in use case development, it is easy to simply ask them to think about some patient care events that are typical, unusually complex, and unusually easy. They may choose to write these down, perhaps in a list, much like the flow process chart described in chapter 7 or relate them to a systems analyst who may take notes and put them into a flow chart format.

In formally documenting a use case, much as any other process mapping or systems flowcharts, it is desirable to use a standard format for ease of subsequent use. The typical sections of a use case are listed in box 8.1.

Once the use cases are developed, each of the conditions, triggers, events, alternative paths, and business rules can be analyzed to determine what functions must be in the EHR for their support.

The American Health Information Community (AHIC) established by HHS Secretary Leavitt has been very involved in creating use cases for the nationwide health information network (NHIN), which have then been used by the Healthcare Information Technology Standards Panel (HITSP) to develop interoperability specifications. Figure 8.5 provides an example of a use case from the Harmonized Use Case for Electronic Health Records (Laboratory Result Reporting) released by the Office of the National Coordinator for Health Information Technology in March 2006.

This use case diagram is embedded within a 30-page document where preconditions are qualified—including that the scenario depicted in this use case is one in which a clinician is receiving laboratory results via the NHIN. This is distinctly different than if the clinician were only receiving lab results from an internal laboratory information system (IS). There are also business rules associated with this scenario that are explained in the narrative. For example, CLIA regulations require that the ordering clinician must receive laboratory results before anyone else may have access to them. Within the diagram itself, the top row of symbols depicts the actors, while the remaining boxes and flow lines depict the basic course of events. Note that there are no alternative paths in this particular use case example, but that it is designated Flow Scenario 1. Other scenarios in the set of use cases depict alternatives.

Figure 8.5.   Example Use Case

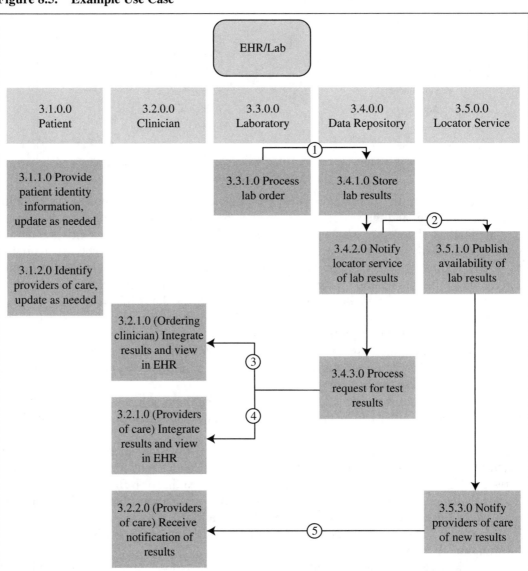

Flow Scenario 1
Ordering clinician receives results integrated into the EHR; providers of care receive text results or notification of test results

1. Lab sends test results to the data repository.
2. Data repository sends to the locator service the location of the results in the repository.
3. Data repository sends the test results to ordering clinician's EHR system (local or remote) or other clinical data system.
4. Data repository sends the test results to the providers of care who can accept the results in an EHR system (local or remote).
5. Locator service notifies the providers of care who don't have an EHR system that can accept lab results.

Source: AHIC Harmonized Use for Electronic Health Records (Laboratory Result Reporting), http://www.hhs.gov/healthit/usecases/documents/EHRLabUseCase.pdf

This use case illustrates how simple it can be for any user to develop a scenario, yet how powerful the result can be for those compiling functional requirements. For instance, in the case of the EHR/Laboratory Results in the NHIN, functional requirements would include (listed in order of their description in the use case):

- Patient identity matching

- Consent management

- Record locator service

- Laboratory results repository

- Notification of results availability to ordering clinician with EHR

- Notification of results availability to ordering clinician without EHR

- Verification of ordering clinician receipt date

- Process request for and provide laboratory results to providers of care with EHR

- Notification of new laboratory results availability

Verifying User Requirements

In addition to interviewing users and engaging them in developing scenarios, or use cases, other sources of information can be collected that can contribute to functional specification. Some of these steps are discussed in the following sections.

Inventory Current Functional Capabilities

Inventorying the functional capabilities of systems already in place not only helps potential users to see the scope of current capabilities, but also establishes a baseline on which to understand what essential functional capability may be missing that is needed in support of other, more robust capabilities. Another dimension may be to survey actual use of current functional capabilities. This may help describe the degree of change management and education/training needed for an EHR.

Conduct an Applications Inventory

EHR functions depend on the availability of source systems to supply data. Another approach to specifying functional requirements is to identify all the applications that currently exist and how they may be related to one another (or not). Figure 8.6 shows a sample tool frequently maintained by information technology (IT) departments to describe information systems (IS) interfaces. This is a good way to start an applications inventory. Any systems that are not interfaced or any applications that are an integral part of a larger system should be added to the list. Systems that are not interfaced but might exchange data with an EHR may include, for example, operating room scheduling systems or emergency department systems. Applications that are an integral part of a hospital IS might include patient access, patient care charting, charge capture, and so on.

Figure 8.6.   Sample tool to describe IS interfaces

Information System Interfaces												
System	Interfaced with	User Dept.	Data	PHI	Support	Type	Frequency	Std	I/O	Medium	Transmission	Comments

Copyright © 2008, Margret\A Consulting, LLC. Reprinted with permission.

Source systems generally perform three major categories of functions:

- *Administrative functions* for the departments they serve that are independent of the EHR; for example, inventory management, staff scheduling, quality control, accounting, and billing services

- *Ancillary care functions* that are specific to the application, such as specimen management in a laboratory system, dosage management in a pharmacy system, and nurse scheduling in a nursing system

- *Feeder functions* in which source systems send data to, and receive data from, the EHR system, often by means of order communications and results retrieval components (for example, a pharmacy system would need to send prescription information to, and receive prescription information from, the EHR system)

Healthcare organizations often lack all the source systems required to meet certain desired functional requirements of EHR systems. It is useful to conduct an applications inventory in which the sources and uses of data are identified so that this information can be applied to the organization's migration path because it may be necessary to install one source system before another. For example, a laboratory IS must exist before an order communication system that sends orders to a laboratory can be implemented.

Perform a Physical Review of Reports

For required reports, the organization should assess whether all fields are complete and whether the information reported is current, accurate, and complete. Users also should be asked whether there are any desirable reporting activities in which they do not participate because they do not have sufficient or easily accessible data. If so, copies of these reports should be obtained and analysis of them included in the needs assessment.

Perform an Ad Hoc Analysis of Information Requirements

An ad hoc analysis of information requirements is performed to capture the most difficult of information needs, such as those that occur on a nonroutine, informal reporting basis. For instance, a physician treating a patient may suddenly decide that certain specialized knowledge would be helpful to arrive at a diagnosis. Although the EHR system is not constructed to routinely capture all the data needed to fulfill such requirements, as many of these types of needs as possible should be identified as well as an ad hoc manner in which to fulfill them. In this scenario, it may be appropriate to subscribe to certain online information services that can be browsed for expert knowledge rather than try to incorporate all such expert knowledge directly into the organization's data repository. Ad hoc analysis of information requirements may be done by making a series of observations or by developing use-case scenarios.

Perform a Retrospective Analysis of Decision Making

Performing a retrospective analysis of decision making is another way to approach ad hoc information needs that are difficult to inventory. Whether it is executive management making organizational decisions or providers making clinical decisions, decision makers tend to rely more on instinct and past experience than on factual information. More and more, however, they are realizing that solid data would be of immense help and may even be required for compliance with clinical credentialing. It is difficult for executives or clinicians to identify the types of data they need. Therefore, it can be helpful to have executives and clinicians identify the types of data they would have found helpful in making some recent decisions. This exercise then can populate a set of data that should be captured routinely or provide a means of developing reports from existing data.

Create a Log of Information Requests

All requests for informational reports or access to specific data should be logged and evaluated for new projects.

Compare Functions to Benefits

A good way to conclude the functional needs assessment is to make a list of the benefits cited by the organization in its EHR vision (chapters 4 and 5), identify processes involved in achieving the benefits from the process assessment (chapter 7), and map the processes to the list of functional requirements identified through the preceding processes. Figure 8.7 provides a sample structure for such a comparison.

Conclusion

The EHR is not a single product. Indeed, it may not even be a group of products. Rather, the EHR is the end result of integrating all applications and applying appropriate technology and analytical tools to create information that contributes to improvement of the healthcare delivery system.

Understanding the information infrastructure required to achieve the EHR is critical for everyone involved in the EHR project. The broadest possible scope of what the EHR is should be kept in mind as each component of the infrastructure is addressed.

Figure 8.7. Comparison of EHR functions to benefits

Benefits of EHR	Process	EHR Supporting Functions	Current State	
			Application	Needed
1. Patient safety	*Order entry*	*Clinical and financial decision support*	*Order communication*	*CPOE*
	Formulary	*Managed care contract requirements*	*Automated formulary*	*Match to payer*
	Pharmacy	*Drug alerts*	*Drug–drug*	*Drug–other*
	Medication administration	*Drug identification Person identity verification*	*Point of care support Bar coding*	

Copyright © 2008, Margret\A Consulting, LLC. Reprinted with permission.

The EHR project should begin with an understanding of user needs and functional requirements. User needs are made up of the information content necessary to make executive or clinical decisions. Functional requirements are the means by which data are collected and converted to information to meet user needs.

Most healthcare organizations have undergone considerable automation before undertaking an EHR project. An inventory of what is available and what is needed is critical to building a migration path for the EHR.

References and Resources

American Health Information Community. 2006. (March 19). Harmonized use case for EHR (Laboratory result reporting). http://www.hhs.gov/healthit/usecases/documents/EHRLabUseCase.pdf.

Andrew, W.F., and R.B. Bruegel. 2005 (May). An exclusive look at the EHR system marketplace: 2005 EHR systems review. *ADVANCE for Health Information Executives.* www.health-care-it.advanceweb.com.

Bittner, K. and I. Spence. *Use Case Modeling.* 2002. Indianapolis: Addison Wesley Professional. pp. 2–3.

Certification Commission on Health Information Technology. www.cchit.org.

Dougherty, M. 2005. Practice brief: Understanding the EHR System Functional Model Standard. *Journal of AHIMA.* 76(2):64A–D.

Drury, B.M. 2006. Ambulatory EHR functionality: A comparison of functionality lists. *Journal of Healthcare Information Management* 20(1):61–70.

Health Level Seven. 2004 (Mar.). Press Release: HL7 announces March 18 second ballot opening of electronic health record—System Functional Model Draft Standard for Trial Use. www.hl7.org.

Health Level Seven. 2007. (April 24). Press Release: Emergency medicine to benefit from the HL7's first registered clinical profile derived from the Electronic Health Record System Functional Model standard. http://www.hl7.org/documentcenter/public/pressreleases/HL7_PRESS_20070424.pdf.

Health Level Seven. 2007 (June 18). Press Release: HL7's new legal EHR system functional profile will help reduce administrative burden, reduce costs, and inefficiencies. http://www.hl7.org/documentcenter/public/pressreleases/HL7_PRESS_20070618.pdf.

Institute of Medicine. 2003. *Key Capabilities of an Electronic Health Record System: Letter Report.* Washington, DC: National Academies Press. www.nap.edu/books.

Institute of Medicine. 1997. *The Computer-based Patient Record: An Essential Technology for Health Care,* edited by R.S. Dick, E.B. Steen, and D.E. Detmer. Washington, DC: National Academies Press.

Institute of Medicine. 1991. *The Computer-based Patient Record: An Essential Technology for Health Care,* edited by R.S. Dick and E.B. Steen. Washington, DC: National Academies Press.

Joint Commission. 2008. *Comprehensive Accreditation Manual for Hospitals: The Official Handbook.* Oakbrook Terrace, IL: Joint Commission.

Lumetra. 2005. *DOQ-IT EHR Selection Tools and Resources.* San Francisco: Lumetra.

Thomspon, T.G., and D.J. Brailer. 2004 (July 21). *The Decade of Health Information Technology: Delivering Consumer-centric and Information-rich Health Care—Framework for Strategic Action.* Washington, DC: HHS ONC.

Chapter 9
Data Infrastructure Assessment

Data are the lifeblood of any organization. However, the difference between data in health-care organizations and data in most other industries is that healthcare data are a greater challenge to capture, store, and process because of their textual and contextual nature. Moreover, what is documented in healthcare is often not the raw facts and figures that are typically considered data in the "data processing" sense, but the results of analyzing these data into information (Amatayakul and Cohen 2008). This means that the value of an EHR is highly dependent on the design of its data infrastructure, including its architecture, vocabulary, and quality. Although most commercial EHR products will be based on a proprietary data infrastructure, it is important for those implementing an EHR to have an overall understanding of how the data infrastructure works to ensure the quality of the data and optimize system performance. In addition, many vendors are beginning to adopt standard vocabularies that provide broader adaptability to regional and national reporting structures. This chapter:

- Defines the role of data infrastructure in the creation of a knowledge continuum

- Describes types of data, their formats, and their processing requirements

- Explores vocabulary standards, code sets, and their mapping that support data sharing across the continuum of care

- Distinguishes between types of data architectures, including data sets, databases, data repositories, and data warehouses and how each supports an EHR

- Describes the purpose and construction of a data dictionary

- Describes the purpose and techniques for data modeling

- Emphasizes the importance of data quality and data integrity

Key Terms

Algorithms
Code set
Code
Coding
Controlled vocabulary
Data architecture
Data dictionary
Data infrastructure
Data mapping
Data marts
Data modeling
Data set

Data structure
Database management
    systems
Executive decision
    support
Granular
Health Plan
    Employer Data and
    Information Set
Metadata
Online analytical
    processing

Online transaction
    processing
Optical character
    recognition
Registry
Report writer
Semantics
Smart text
Syntax
Transactions
Value
Variable

Data Infrastructure

The term **data infrastructure** refers to what data are needed to operate an enterprise and how they are structured and processed (architecture), defined (vocabulary), and quality assured.

Data are the raw elements that comprise our communications. Humans have the innate ability to combine data they collect by reading and, through all their senses, produce information to enhance that information with experience and trial-and-error to produce knowledge. This is what affords humans their intelligence and wisdom. This is also referred to as heuristic thought. Computers, on the other hand, are machines that, although they can process data very rapidly and tirelessly, cannot create knowledge without humans programming them with complex structures that attempt to simulate human brain power and heuristic thought. However, when even modest processing structures are in place, computerized sources of data, information, and knowledge can be immensely helpful to humans when having to rapidly collect and process numerous facts and quickly make decisions based on recalling a tremendous volume of information. Computers are now capable of applying sophisticated pattern analysis and other highly sophisticated techniques to, for example, generate a list of favorite medications a given physician tends to order or recognize a person's handwriting and convert it into typed form.

The concept of *knowledge management* is a new discipline that stresses a formalized, integrated approach to managing an enterprise's tangible and intangible information assets. It describes the compilation of an organization's boundless information reserves into one central, mutually accessible database (Haak 1998; Lau 2004).

An industry expert writing in *Oracle Magazine* provides perhaps a more practical definition:

> Knowledge comes from people and their unique experiences. A technology cannot, on its own, provide knowledge. It can merely provide a mechanism that makes it easier for people to capture their insights, experiences, and judgments so that they can record them and others can benefit. Technology that supports the emergence of knowledge lays out information so that people can see unexpected relationships between elements that may seem to have nothing in common and lets them continuously add refinements to the information to increase its value. Thus, although software can play a key role, if you take out the human element, you have lost the spark that ignites the creation of knowledge (Marshak 1998).

Marshak (1998) also describes a knowledge continuum as follows: "data plus content equal information, and information plus experience equal knowledge." Figure 9.1 offers a diagram showing how information technology (IT) can be applied to the knowledge continuum.

Data architecture for an EHR, then, must support the ability of IT to create the knowledge continuum (Harmon 2003). Data architecture for an EHR will be built on an infrastructure that includes various types and formats of data; creation of various structures in which to store and process data; and various measures that ensure data quality and integrity.

Figure 9.1.   Information technology as applied to the knowledge continuum

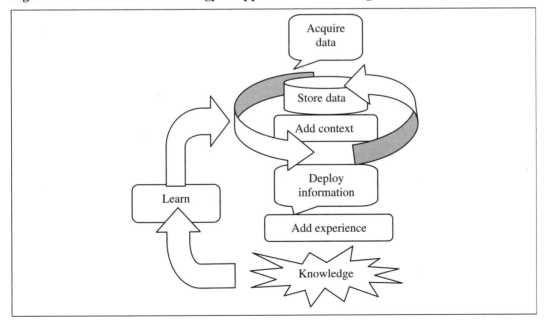

Types of EHR Data

Clinical data come in many different forms. Figure 9.2 illustrates seven different formats of data and gives examples of their various sources.

Essentially, these seven different formats of data are stored in an information system in one of two ways: as an electronic reflection of the original or as a structured data model.

- *Reflections of original data,* often referred to generally as image data, include document images, unstructured text data, video, audio, vectors, and diagnostic images. Image data are stored in an indexed manner and may be recalled from storage using the index. The index is a database that contains the patient's name, medical record number, and, potentially, other identifying information, which may be entered by the person who is operating the document imaging scanner or by bar-coded labels affixed to forms. Generally, the content of the record is performed by applying a barcode to each form type. More **granular** indexing may be accomplished by **optical character recognition** (OCR) applied to components of the forms. Image data cannot be processed by machine beyond the ability to retrieve them by the way they are indexed. The primary value of image data is the ability to rapidly retrieve them from wherever they are stored.

- *Structured, or discrete, data* are stored in databases and can have significant operations performed on them. Structured data are the values associated with variables

Figure 9.2.   EHR data types and their sources

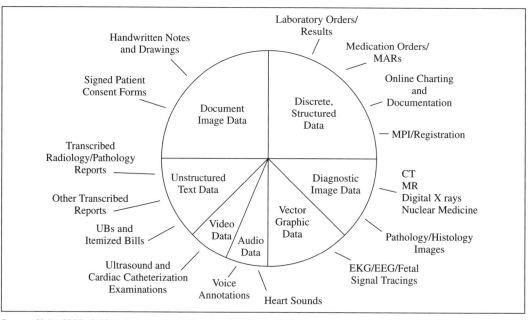

Source: Kohn 2002. © 2001 Deborah Kohn. Reprinted with permission.

that are the important information to be captured about a patient. As in mathematics, a **variable** is a function that may assume any given value or set of values. A **value** is any point in the range of a function. Values for variables in EHRs are generally captured via checklists, pull-down menus, or templates that guide a user in entering the values for each of the required variables. (Refer to figure 1.5 for an example of such data capture techniques.) The ability to enter structured data is one of the key elements that makes an EHR unique from its paper counterpart. For example, temperature is a variable; 99.8° F is one value that may be entered, perhaps at the time of the patient admission. If the patient spikes a fever later in the admission, the value entered at that time may be 101.0°F. Appropriate medication may cause the temperature to lower over time, and these data points may also be captured—in fact, they could be captured through human entry or via a connection to a monitoring device. Because these are entered as structured data, the values of this variable can be graphed automatically by the computer, illustrating the patient's change in temperature. The range of valid values may also be specified and the computer can check that only values within that valid range are entered. In the example of temperature, a valid range can be specified numerically. For values that are narrative, such as drug names, descriptions of pain, and so forth, the values may be limited to a set of predefined terms that are displayed in a checklist or drop-down menu. The basis of all clinical decision support in EHRs is structured data.

Some debate the value of unstructured vs. structured data. However, two important points essentially make the debate moot:

First, both forms of data have an important place in an EHR. For example, it may be equally as important to retrieve a streaming video of a cardiac catheterization as it is to retrieve the discrete values of the last set of vital signs. However, there is somewhat less ability to retrieve individual data elements from document images or from narrative text, although sophisticated indexing and search strategies are making it easier to retrieve data elements from these forms of data types.

Second, the debate usually refers to narrative text keyed in as a stream of human thought as compared to structured data entered into a computer as discrete data elements (such as from pick lists or pull-down menus). Again, there is value to both narrative text and structured data, although the value is different and there are trade-offs in using either format. For example:

- *Narrative text* allows an individual to record context and to convey subtle differences that discrete data entry often does not. The tradeoff is that such data may take longer to enter and be more difficult to process. The time it takes to enter narrative data depends on the volume of data, any available transcription support, and the keyboarding ability of the user. Narrative data are more difficult to combine with other data (for example, on a graph) to form new information.

- *Structured data* can be easily captured and very accurate. Experienced users of an EHR can move rapidly through a series of discrete data collection processes. However, the data collection processes must be well designed and tailored to each user or the process could take longer than keyboarding or dictating. Structured data are generally based on a standard data dictionary, if not a **controlled vocabulary**, that makes use of the data very precise. The ability of the user to select the exact data elements needed for the communication makes the process accurate as well. Structured data also allow data to be processed into graphics for trending and other analyses.

In today's EHR, there are generally combinations of structured and unstructured data; one of the key tasks in implementing an EHR is to determine where and how structured and unstructured data are required.

A significant part of system build during EHR implementation is to construct tables of structured data for use in data capture, and to review how those may be used for various presentation purposes, decision support processing, reporting, and generation of narrative notes. For example, discrete values may be entered for vital signs. Often a range of values is specified as valid values, with anything outside the range generating a flag as part of the system's clinical decision support system. In addition to use in clinical decision support, the clinician may want to see these vital signs trended against the level of medication administered. Pick lists may be used for medications. In this case, everyone who will use the system, including the ordering physician, dispensing pharmacist, and nurse who administers the medication, must agree on the data options that impact the computerized physician order entry (CPOE) system, pharmacy information system, and medication administration record system. Often a clinical vocabulary or nomenclature is referenced to obtain the full complement of a standard set of terms.

Those who are implementing the system must also decide when entering narrative data will be accommodated, for example, at the conclusion of a report of history and physical examination findings to describe a unique situation not accommodated by the data in the selections. In designing CPOE, structured data for medication orders would include not only what data must be accommodated, but also what data are required or optional. For example, a list of drugs may be provided via a pull-down menu. Dose, frequency, and route of administration may be required and accommodated through pick lists. However, special instructions may be optional and could be recorded in narrative format.

In addition to being able to compile a narrative note from discrete data, another form of data combines the concept of structured and unstructured data. For example, a progress note may be created by a series of macros, sometimes called **smart text**. In documenting the progress note, a physician would key in a series of codes representing the desired text. The text may include the place where variable data must be inserted. For example, a procedure performed on the ear would require a place for "right" or "left" to be entered. Each macro must be created by either the system implementer or user. In very sophisticated EHRs, the system may "learn" a user's common phraseology and, after a few times of entering narrative, offer to create a macro for the user. In using such a system, however, it must be recognized that only the fact that a specific set of smart text and the variables within the text are able to be processed. Any element within the narrative that is not a variable is not unique, discrete data. For example, if a pediatrician frequently treated children for otitis media, a macro of "OM" might generate a paragraph, within which there may be variables to identify right or left ear and the appearance of the tympanic membrane. For example, the OM smart text might generate the note that: "The patient has otitis media of the < > ear, with < > tympanic membrane." The system could require each variable to be addresses before the physician could sign off on the note. The system could also limit what may be used as values (such as right or left) or not (that is, the description of the tympanic membrane may be left to the discretion of the physician). The result is that, when searching for the number of cases of otitis media, one could count the number of times such smart text was evoked and, if desired, which ear. One could also generate a list of all tympanic membrane descriptors used, but these would not be standardized such that a valid comparison of appearance with choice of medication could be made.

There are also tools that permit narrative context to be applied to structured data, and to parse unstructured data. Computers can be programmed to wrap narrative text around discrete data elements to form complete sentences. For example, many EHRs contain programs where the history and physical examination for which discrete data were selected can be produced as a narrative report. Entering the patient's age, sex, and response to the level of development and nourishment, the computer can take "3," "F," "younger," and "poor" and create the following sentence: This is a 3-year-old female who appears younger than stated age and poorly nourished. In comparison to the example of the smart text, this narrative reflects fully standardized and discrete data.

Computer programs called natural language processors also can break apart (or parse) narrative text by words or phrases and encode the words and phrases for later processing. This is essentially the reverse of the preceding process. Thus, the sentence would be converted to the respective discrete data elements and stored in a database. Natural language processing (NLP) is still quite immature with respect to being a common function in an EHR system; however, there are a growing number of successful experiments in using NLP for extracting quality data from narrative notes in EHRs. In one study, NLP in an EHR was found to improve the identification of angina pectoris over ICD-9-CM coding (Pakhomov et al 2007). NLP has also been found to enable linking medical text in EHRs to online information resources (Janetzki et al 2004). A survey of five major provider settings (including HealthPartners, Park Nicollet Health Services, Billings Clinic, Kaiser Permanente, and Geisinger Health System) found that using EHRs with a typology for categorizing electronic measures of quality and safety (dubbed *e-indicators*) found much more clinical relevancy to the measures (Fowles et al 2008).

In summary, both structured data and narrative text in an EHR afford much greater access to data than when recorded in a paper record. Discrete data may provide a more automated approach to achieving the knowledge continuum whereas unstructured data rely more on human intervention to achieve knowledge from the data.

Vocabulary Standards

It should be clear from the preceding discussion that it is important to adopt standards to define and structure the language used to supply the values for the data. The primary purposes of using such standards are to reduce inconsistency and ensure understanding.

Unfortunately, in healthcare there are many ways to define, classify, and represent how a language can be structured and used. One way to view the interrelationships among language components is illustrated in figure 9.3.

Figure 9.3.   Interrelationships among healthcare language components

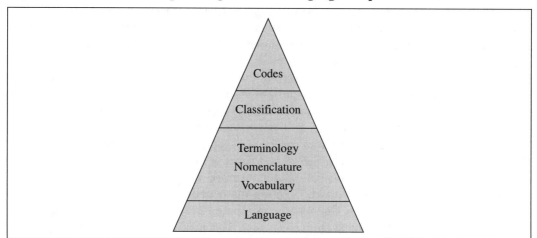

Language

Language generally refers to a system of communication using an arbitrary set of vocal sounds, written symbols, signs, or gestures in conventional ways with conventional meanings. In the schema proposed in figure 9.3, language is the broadest possible set of words available for communication among a group of people.

Often there is reference to "the language of medicine," referring to a subset of words used primarily in medicine. This subset sometimes is referred to as vocabulary and other times as terminology. Dictionaries identify vocabulary and terminology as synonyms. Figure 9.3 suggests that vocabulary is a somewhat broader set of terms than terminology. In addition to the number of terms, a subtle, but important, difference relates to usage of the terms.

Vocabulary, Terminology, and Nomenclature

The term *vocabulary* typically means all the terms that are recognized for communication within the domain. The term *controlled vocabulary* is sometimes applied when referencing vocabulary standards, suggesting that the terms within the vocabulary are carefully selected for their inclusion and terms outside the boundaries of the vocabulary are not acceptable—or in an EHR might not be able to be processed in various applications. Each term has a unique meaning, and there may be explicitly identified synonyms.

In contrast, the term *terminology* often includes a prescribed set of terms authorized for a specific use. For example, the American Medical Association's Common Procedural Terminology (CPT) is a set of terms used for professional billing.

The term *nomenclature* refers to a defined system for naming. The Systematized Nomenclature of Medicine (SNOMED) is the most widely recognized nomenclature in healthcare. It is developed and maintained by the College of American Pathologists. Its current version, SNOMED Clinical Terms (SNOMED CT), is intended to provide a set of concepts and relationships that offers a common reference point for comparison and aggregation of data about the healthcare process. SNOMED CT is often described as a reference terminology (Spackman et al. 1997). SNOMED is discussed in more depth later in this chapter.

For the purposes of this book, vocabulary, nomenclature, and terminology are used as synonyms to mean a body of terms and their definitions.

Classification

A *classification* is a grouping of terms of similar meaning, often for defined purposes. The most widely recognized medical classification is the International Classification of Diseases (ICD); its primary purpose is to categorize diseases for morbidity and mortality reporting. For many years, the United States has used a clinical modification of ICD (ICD-9-CM) for the additional purpose of reimbursement. The World Health Assembly of the World Health Organization (WHO) endorsed ICD-10 in 1990, and WHO Member States began using the classification system in 1994 for both morbidity and mortality reporting. In the U.S., however, it has only been used for reporting mortality since 1999. A clinical modification (ICD-10-CM) for diagnoses and ICD-10-PCS for procedures contains substantial increases in content over ICD-9-CM. Because of the U.S. delay in adopting its version of ICD-10, it is currently unable to compare morbidity data with the rest of the world.

Although the concept of a classification would appear to be straightforward and different from a system of naming, some specialists in medical language use the terms *classification* and *nomenclature* synonymously. This can be confusing, especially with respect to developing a data infrastructure for an EHR. For an information system (IS) whose primary function is charge capture, a classification system is sufficient. For an EHR where clinical decision support rests on very specific data, a classification system is inadequate. However, they can—and should—be coordinated. If a highly granular nomenclature such as SNOMED is used to standardize data capture, it should be able to be mapped into a broader classification system for statistical, reimbursement, and other purposes. In fact, the National Library of Medicine (NLM) maps ICD-9-CM, ICD-10-CM, ICD-10-PCS, and other classification systems to SNOMED (Imel et al. 2004). **Data mapping** is the process of identifying relationships between two distinct data models. As suggested by the example of mapping SNOMED to ICD, mapping may be performed to mediate between a data source and a destination, to consolidate multiple databases, in deidentifying data, and for other purposes.

Codes

In discussing concepts associated with vocabularies and classification systems, the term **code** refers to a representation of words to enable machine processing. Codes may be applied to vocabularies or classification systems. Code systems may have a structure associated with them or be random representations. ICD has a hierarchical structure. **Coding**, in this context, is the term applied when representations are assigned to the words they represent. Coding diagnoses and procedures is the assignment of codes from a code set that follows the rules of the underlying classification or other coding guidelines.

Encoders are computer software programs that assist coders in assigning appropriate codes. EHR systems may include an encoder that helps assign codes. In addition to encoders, many EHRs developed for use by physicians in their offices or clinics incorporate documentation support to help physicians assign the correct evaluation and management (E/M) codes from CPT based on their documentation to support optimal reimbursement. G codes are CPT codes that are used to document quality measures and their assignment also may be supported by EHR logic structures. For example, if a patient who presents with acute myocardial infarction receives aspirin upon arrival in the emergency department, G8006 would be assigned. Codes are used in the Physician Quality Reporting Initiative (PQRI) developed by the Centers for Medicare and Medicaid Services (CMS), for voluntary reporting of 36 evidence-based quality measures (Scichilone and Hull 2006). As another example, G8443-Prescriptions created during encounter were generated using a qualified e-prescribing system is being used for reporting use of e-RX for this incentive (CMS 2008).

Totally automated code assignment also is possible. Natural language processing (NLP) technology can "read" the data contained in the EHR and apply various **algorithms** (rules-based approaches) or statistical approaches to assign codes. If the codes to be applied are highly granular (that is, related very specifically to individual words or short phrases) and include codes for relationships between words (for example, causes), the coding should be successful. Where codes are more reflective of broad classifications (such as ICD or CPT), the quality of the underlying documentation drives the success with which NLP can succeed (Fenton 2002; Schnitzer 2000).

The term **code set** is frequently used to refer to a group of associated codes. The codes may represent individual terms in an inventory or dictionary of terms. (When associated with an entire language or terminology, an inventory or dictionary of terms often is referred to as a *lexicon*.) The codes also may represent classes of terms in a classification, such as ICD. In its Transactions and Code Sets regulation, the Health Insurance Portability and Accountability Act (HIPAA) of 1996 includes medical code sets (such as ICD-9-CM and Healthcare Common Procedure Coding System [HCPCS], including CPT) as well as nonmedical code sets such as revenue codes and claims adjustment reason codes.

Another usage of the terms *code* and *coding* should also be observed: In IT, code refers to the representation of instructions used to direct the processing of a computer. Coding then refers to writing the instructions. This is the software that makes our computers work. Obviously, precision in language matters.

Important Vocabularies in EHR Functionality

Currently, an attempt is underway to create a national standard vocabulary for use in an EHR. The National Committee on Vital and Health Statistics (NCVHS) was tasked under HIPAA to make recommendations for uniform data standards for patient medical record information (PMRI). After several years of analyzing the many candidate terminologies (there is said to be more than 100 different terminologies, of which NCVHS reviewed 46) and hearing public testimony, NCVHS recommended that the federal government recognize a "core set of terminologies" (NCVHS 2003). It further recommended that the Department of Health and Human Services (HHS) provide guidance for industry use of the core set of terminologies, rather than mandate their use by regulation, and that HHS direct government agencies to become early adopters of the terminologies and thus accelerate the process for incorporation of standard terminologies in private-sector information systems. The following terminologies were included in the core set:

- SNOMED CT is a comprehensive clinical reference terminology that allows for consistent capture of detailed clinical information developed and maintained by the College of American Pathologists (CAP). In 2003, CAP signed a contract with the NLM to license English- and Spanish-language editions of SNOMED CT. Starting in January 2004, NLM made SNOMED CT core content and all version updates available free of charge. SNOMED CT and additional supporting tools continue to be available directly from SNOMED International, a division of CAP, in the SNOMED CT structure. (See below for more detailed information about SNOMED CT and NLM.)

- Logical Observation Identifiers Names and Codes (LOINC) laboratory subset is a widely used terminology for representing laboratory data for ordering lab tests and reporting lab test results. It has been further enhanced to include other observational data, such as vital signs. It has now been incorporated as a code set into the proposed ASC X12N standards for electronic claims attachments that supplement the HIPAA claims, eligibility, claim status, remittance advice, and other standards. It is maintained by the Regenstrief Institute and supported in part by grants and contracts from NLM, the Hartford Foundation, and other HHS funding sources.

- RxNorm is a standard notation for clinical drugs developed by NLM, the Veterans Administration (VA), and the Food and Drug Administration (FDA) in consultation with the message standards development organization, Health Level Seven (HL7). It represents drug ingredients, strength, and dose form and includes various relationships to other drugs, such as equivalencies, trade names, and so on. E-prescribing (e-Rx) regulations that grew out of the Medicare Modernization Act require use of the National Council for Prescription Drugs (NCPD) prescription standard (called SCRIPT) if providers use e-prescribing for any prescriptions reimbursed under Medicare Part D. As part of this standard, it is proposed that RxNorm be the standard vocabulary used for the provider to communicate with the retail pharmacy, and it is being pilot tested for that purpose. The RxNorm complements the VA's National Drug File–Reference Terminology (NDF-RT) and commercial drug knowledge bases (such as Multum, Micromedex, First Databank, and Medispan), which are often used in EHR systems as knowledge sources for drug decision support.

- Universal Medical Device Nomenclature System (UMDNS) of the ECRI (formerly the Emergency Care Research Institute) has also been recommended as a core terminology.

In addition to recommending these as core terminologies, NCVHS made several other important recommendations relative to vocabularies, including that:

- Increased funding be provided to accelerate and complete development of federal drug terminologies

- The NLM serve as a central coordinating body to manage the terminology resources and coordinate their ongoing maintenance and distribution

- The core set of terminologies be integrated by creating relationships within the UMLS

- The government recognizes an additional group of terminologies as "important related terminologies" and promotes the creation and maintenance of mappings between these terminologies and the core set. The mapping priorities were cited as: HIPAA medical code sets: CPT, Current Dental Terminology (CDT) from the American Dental Association, HCPCS, ICD-9-CM, and NDC

- Common enabler terminologies including, but not limited to:

  —Diagnostic and Statistical Manual of Mental Disorders (DSM-4) from the American Psychiatric Association

  —Terminologies in private-sector drug information databases (for example, First-DataBank NDDF Plus, MediSpan, Micromedex, Multum Lexicon)

  —International Society for Blood Transfusion (ISBT 128) developed by the International Council for Commonality in Blood Banking Automation (ICCBBA) for describing blood products and tissues

  —Medcin, developed by Medicomp Systems, for structured entry of clinical notes

  —MedDRA for use by international drug regulatory agencies

  —Nursing terminologies not otherwise included in SNOMED CT (See figure 9.4 for nursing terminologies included in SNOMED CT.)

Figure 9.4.   Nursing terminologies included in SNOMED CT

Georgetown Home Health Care Classification (HHCC)
NANDA Nursing Diagnoses: Definitions and Classification, NANDA International (formerly North American Nursing Diagnosis Association)
Nursing Interventions Classification (NIC)
Nursing Outcomes Classification (NOC), The University of Iowa
Perioperative Nursing Data Set (PNDS)
Omaha System

- There needs to be additional work and cooperation to reconcile code sets within the message format standards that NCVHS also recommended as important uniform data standards for PMRI (HL7, DICOM, NCPDP, and IEEE)

- Further research be done to address outstanding content issues relating to dental content, clinical LOINC, and device terminology (for example, Global Medical Device Nomenclature [GMDN] of the FDA)

- There be exploration of incorporation of content from other terminologies, such as the International Classification of Functioning, Disability, and Health (ICF), for coding functional status and terminologies specific to complementary and alternative medicine (such as ABC codes from Alternative Link)

SNOMED CT

As a core terminology for the EHR, SNOMED CT provides a common language that enables a consistent way of capturing, sharing, and aggregating health data across specialties and sites of care. SNOMED CT combines the content and structure of the SNOMED Reference Terminology (SNOMED RT) with the United Kingdom's National Health Service's Clinical Terms Version 3, also known as the Read Codes. This creates an international approach for computerizing terms used by physicians, nurses, and other health professionals for the management of patient records and medical communications. SNOMED CT includes several components, including:

- A concepts table containing 344,000 concepts with unique meanings and formal logic-based definitions organized into hierarchies (See figure 9.5.)

Figure 9.5.   SNOMED CT concepts

Finding	Physical force
Disease	Events
Procedure	Environments/geographical locations
Observable entity	Social context
Body structure	Context-dependent categories
Organism	Staging and scales
Substance	Attribute
Pharmaceutical/biologic product	Qualifier value
Specimen	Duplicate concept
Physical object	

Source: SNOMED International 2004. SNOMED Clinical Terms® Core Content as of January 2004. Available at www.snomed.org. Specific information located under "Concepts" at www.snomed.at/snomedct/documents/Jan04_release_print.pdf. Copyright © 2002–2004 College of American Pathologists. SNOMED and SNOMED CT are registered trademarks of the College of American Pathologists, all rights reserved. Reprinted with permission.

- A descriptions table containing more than 913,000 English- (660,000 Spanish-) language descriptions or synonyms for flexibility in expressing clinical concepts

- A relationships table containing approximately 1.3 million semantic relationships to enable robust reliability and consistency of data retrieval

In addition to its major components, SNOMED CT also cross-maps to ICD and incorporates a number of the nursing terminologies (refer to figure 9.4), concepts for the taxonomic structure of veterinary-focused hierarchies from the American Veterinary Medical Association, extension and clarification of portions of the eye terminology with the assistance of the American Academy of Ophthalmology, terminology to encode four of the updated CAP cancer protocols (breast, colon and rectum, lung, and prostrate) required to meet the accreditation requirements of the American College of Surgeons (ACS) Commission on Cancer, terms within The Bethesda System for coding of Pap smear tests, and the National Quality Forum's Serious Reportable Events (SNOMED International 2004). SNOMED CT has also been mapped to some of the most widely used proprietary vocabularies, including Medcin. This is important because many physician office EHR systems incorporate Medcin as their controlled vocabulary of choice. Many physicians find it a more physician-friendly vocabulary. However, linking it to SNOMED CT as a broader national and international standard vocabulary makes it a viable way to achieve both an easier-to-use language and an adherence to a standard.

Unified Medical Language System (UMLS)

For many years, NLM essentially provided the nation's principal biomedical bibliographic citation database in the form of Index Medicus. Its online counterpart, MEDLINE, is used to search the MEDLARS set of databases of more than 4,500 titles of reference works. (PubMed [pubmed.gov]) is the MEDLINE retrieval service on the Web.) Worldwide users of the MEDLARS indexes are researchers, healthcare practitioners, educators, administrators, and students. To index its journals for the databases, NLM developed the Medical Subject Headings (MeSH) controlled-vocabulary thesaurus. It consists of sets of terms naming descriptors in a hierarchical structure that permits searching at various levels of specificity (NLM 2001–2002).

From its extensive experience in controlled-vocabulary thesaurus development and usage for biomedical literature, NLM designed the UMLS in 1986 to help health professionals and researchers retrieve and integrate electronic biomedical information from a number of sources, not just bibliographic databases. With respect to EHRs, the purpose of the UMLS is to "facilitate the development of computer systems that behave as if they 'understand' the meaning of the language of biomedicine and health" (NLM 2001–2002).

Semantics and Syntax

To help in understanding why NLM with its UMLS should play a coordinating role in terminologies for the EHR, two terms related to the study and use of language should be thoroughly understood: semantics and syntax.

- **Semantics** is the branch of linguistics dealing with the study of meaning, including the ways meaning is structured in language and how changes in meaning and form occur over time. Semantic, then, refers to the meaning of a word or other symbol. For example, the term *attending* may have a general meaning, such as when describing a physician attending to (or taking care of) a patient, in comparison to when the term is used specifically to mean the particular physician designated to be responsible for the care of a specific patient.

- **Syntax** is the study of the patterns of formation of sentences and phrases from words and of the rules for the formation of grammatical sentences in a language. In the example used earlier to describe semantics, it is clear that the pattern (or syntax) in which the terms *attending physician* or *physician attending [to]* are sequenced results in different meanings of *attending* (the first being an adjective that describes a type of physician and the second being a verb that describes what the physician is doing).

For vocabularies to support the language of medicine, both the meaning of terms and how they fit together to form communications must be studied and supported.

Knowledge Sources

To further its goals of serving as the means to retrieve biomedical data from multiple sources, the UMLS develops knowledge sources that can be used by a wide variety of applications programs to help retrieve data caused by differences in terminology and the scattering of relevant information across many databases. There are three UMLS knowledge sources:

- *UMLS Metathesaurus* provides a uniform, integrated distribution format from more than 100 biomedical vocabularies and classifications and links many different names for the same concepts. It supplies information that computer programs can use to interpret user inquiries, interact with users to refine their queries, identify which databases contain information relevant to particular inquires, and convert users' terms into the vocabulary used by relevant information sources. The Metathesaurus is intended for use primarily by system developers but also can be a useful reference tool for database builders, librarians, and other information professionals.

- *SPECIALIST Lexicon* contains syntactic information for many terms, component words, and English words that do not appear in the Metathesaurus.

- *UMLS Semantic Network* contains information about the types or categories to which all Metathesaurus concepts have been assigned and the permissible relationships among these types (for example, virus "causes" disease).

As can be seen from these knowledge sources, the UMLS has a vested interest in controlled vocabularies and ensuring that the many different vocabularies of the different domains of clinical care are not only kept up to date, but also freely available.

Even as NLM through its UMLS project maps vocabularies, mapping at a local level is also an important element of keeping EHRs up to date. Because the EHR in any given healthcare organization frequently uses both proprietary and standard vocabularies and data sets, when any standard vocabulary or data set is updated, the changes must be mapped to the local environment. Organizations should adopt a strategy to ensure that each EHR upgrade also addresses clinical vocabulary mapping (Wilson 2005).

Data Structures

Where data infrastructure refers to what overall data are needed to operate an enterprise and how the data are structured and processed (architecture), defined (vocabulary), and quality assured, **data structure** refers to the more specific way each individual data element is used in the information system. On a practical level for providers seeking to implement an EHR system, a controlled vocabulary would support a data structure that promotes standardization of terms. The vocabulary aids data capture, enhances database management, and helps build a data warehouse for use in executive and clinical decision support. The vocabulary also supports contributions to standard data sets, required either by law or for voluntary participation in research studies, registries, the development of clinical practice guidelines, and many other uses.

Data Sets

Data sets for use in registries have been one of the first ways data have been structured for use in healthcare. A **data set** is a predefined group of data elements to be collected. A **registry** is the actual data collected about individuals in accordance with the defined data set. Tumor registries and immunization registries are examples of healthcare registries. One of the issues with healthcare data sets and registries is that there are so many and none have been mapped to a comprehensive model. As a result, a healthcare organization could be contributing very similar data to multiple registries, which is a burden, but also the data definitions in each core data set may be different (AHIMA Workgroup, 2004).

Each individual standardized data set encourages healthcare providers to collect and report data in a standardized manner. Although they do not necessarily require use of a controlled vocabulary, most data sets make reference to at least some of the standard vocabularies or common code sets in healthcare or may provide a data dictionary that defines data elements for purposes of use within the data set. Some examples of standardized data sets include the following:

- The Uniform Hospital Discharge Data Set (UHDDS) is the core set of data elements that form the basis of the hospital discharge data systems in 34 states. Claim forms are the major vehicle for collecting the UHDDS, and definitions, such as for principal diagnosis and other diagnoses, are consistent with the requirements of HIPAA's Transactions and Code Sets requirements. The National Center for Health Statistics of the Centers for Disease Control and Prevention (CDC) coordinates the state data collection for national survey data (Greenberg 2004).

- The Uniform Ambulatory Care Data Set (UACDS) is similar to the UHDDS and is recommended for use in ambulatory care patient records, with claim forms being the primary vehicle for their data collection.

- The Minimum Data Set (MDS) for Long-Term Care and Resident Assessment Protocols is mandated by the Omnibus Reconciliation Act of 1987 for federally funded long-term care programs. It forms the basis for the resident assessment instrument that requires a comprehensive assessment of each long-term care resident within 14 days of admission.

- The Data Elements for Emergency Department Systems (DEEDS) is a recommended data set published in 1997 by the CDC's National Center for Injury Prevention and Control. This data set was developed in collaboration with the American College of Emergency Physicians, the Emergency Nurses Association, and the American Health Information Management Association (AHIMA). Its specifications have been incorporated into the LOINC database and the HL7 Implementation Guides for Claims Attachments (included in the proposed HIPAA standard transactions) (Pollock 1999).

- The Outcomes and Assessment Information Set (OASIS) was established by HHS for home health data reporting (HHS 2003).

- The **Health Plan Employer Data and Information Set** (HEDIS) was established for managed care accreditation by the National Committee for Quality Assurance (NCQA).

- ORYX was established by The Joint Commission to provide rigorous comparison of the actual results of care across hospitals. Performance measurement using ORYX data helps healthcare organizations support performance improvement and demonstrate accountability to the public and other interested stakeholders through the Joint Commission accreditation process (Joint Commission 2003).

- The Patient Care Data Set (PCDS) is a data dictionary of elements that may be used by nurses to report patient problems and patient care goals. It is not exclusively a nursing vocabulary; some terms relate to other disciplines, such as respiratory therapy and physical therapy (Ozbolt 1999).

- The Core Data Sets for the Physician Practice EHR were developed by AHIMA as model data sets to understand clinical workflows in physician offices in order to enable the best design of an EHR system (AHIMA 2003).

Databases

Data sets are typically collected by providers to be either contributed to an internal form of data structure in their information systems, including a data repository used in an EHR, or submitted to an external entity that stores the data in a data warehouse or database optimized for data analysis (such as for statewide data systems) (Love 2001).

Whether a standard data set has been established by an external entity or a set of data has been captured for internal documentation purposes, the most common data structure for information processing is a file, which contains related records. When considering paper-based systems, a file room houses numerous records. Each record is related to a given patient, and an indexing system helps with record location. Within each record, there is typically some standard content, such as a face sheet or encounter form, problem list, and so on. The forms are used to capture data and also, by their placement in the record or by color coding, to help in finding a certain form or page in the record.

In some cases, the forms guide what is to be captured and may include checklists for structured data recording. Other forms are lined sheets of paper on which certain categories of unstructured data are to be recorded, such as progress notes and orders. Paper file systems are easy and less costly to create than computer systems but are not flexible enough to support relationships needed to describe data in clinical practice. There are limitations to the extent to which their content can be indexed, and, of course, they are accessible to only one person at a time.

Files of records where the content has been scanned into a computer system basically have many of the same limitations as a paper file system of records. However, their indexing capabilities may be more robust so that it is somewhat easier to identify a particular form or page and they make the records accessible to many persons at one time.

To overcome the limitations of files, databases and **database management systems** (DBMSs) were developed. DBMSs are the software and data structures used to support a database. Types of databases include the following (Bontempo and Saracco 1995, 9–18):

- A *hierarchical database* is the oldest form of database structure. Although it is no longer used in the development of new EHR systems, it may be found in existing, legacy systems within healthcare organizations. It is modeled from a treelike structure, with a root, multiple branches, and multiple leaves. Records at a branch level sometimes are referred to as parents, with records at the leaf level referred to as children. Unfortunately, a major constraint of the hierarchical structure is that each child can have only one parent, meaning that multiple copies of the same record may have to be retained to show multiple relationships. Furthermore, programs that retrieve data from hierarchical databases must navigate through the branches from top to bottom to get to the desired record, requiring predefined access paths and slower response time. This structure also is referred to as a "flat file" database.

- A *network database* uses a two-level tree as its basic data structure. This structure supports multiple paths to the same record, thus avoiding the data redundancy found in hierarchical databases. It also supports richer data structures and thus provides more support for logical modeling of complex connections. However, data navigation is still an issue because the selection of the most efficient path can be complex to identify. The network model of database is generally not used in newer applications.

- A *relational database* departs significantly from the first two types and currently is the most common form of database. Relational databases are constructed using tables instead of tree and network structures. The tables do not specify how to retrieve the required data or navigate through predefined paths. Users write queries that reference the data of interest. Software supporting these queries then identifies the tables and specific columns in the tables to retrieve the requested data. Maintenance of the tables is easy. Because rows in a table have no inherent order, they are simply added to as they grow (Mon 2003).

- An *object-oriented database* is the most recent approach to database management, and only a few vendors use a true object-oriented database structure. This type of database is derived from object-oriented programming and has no single inherent structure. The structure for any given class or type of object can be anything a programmer finds useful—a linked list, a set, an array, and so on. Furthermore, an object may contain different degrees of complexity, making use of multiple types and multiple structures. As a result, object-oriented DBMSs emphasize programming language integration rather than programming language independence. Interfacing with the database may mean using object-oriented programming language functions (such as C++) rather than embedding a separate database access language (such as SQL).

Work involving any database used by multiple users must be done within the scope of **transactions**. This means that all processing that logically represents a single unit must be grouped together as a single transaction to ensure all the work is completed and none of it alters the basic database. For example, in retrieving a laboratory result, the request for the result must be accompanied by the result being supplied to a workstation. A request cannot just "hang" in the database without reaching a logical conclusion. The tools used to create and manage the transactions to and from an online database are referred to collectively as **online transaction processing** (OLTP) tools. (Databases may receive and provide data in offline, batch form, but for use in an EHR, transactions must be online, in real time).

Data Repository

Databases typically are created by a particular vendor or data supplier, making them proprietary to the given application. As a result, an organization that has many applications will likely have many databases and there will likely be much duplication of data within those databases. Furthermore, the databases may be unable to communicate with one another (whether they are developed by the same vendor or not). In other words, retrieving data from two different databases may require two different queries. Interfaces may be developed to exchange data between databases, but their programming is time-consuming and the data to be shared must be determined in advance.

A *data repository* is a database designed with an open structure that is not dedicated to the software of any particular vendor or data supplier. It contains data from multiple, disparate application systems so that an integrated, multidisciplinary view of the data can be achieved. A data repository requires the following data integration functions:

- *Data transformation:* This integration function is the process of reconciling and standardizing data content being acquired from numerous data sources. It may be achieved through the application of message standards, SGML/XML languages that define data in documents (chapter 10), off-the-shelf products that make it easier to link and share data between databases, or custom-written interfaces between one vendor's product and another. Clearly, this function would be made easier if there were a standard data model, a data dictionary, controlled vocabularies and coding schemes, and knowledge representation. (See the next section for a discussion of these data management functions.)

- *Data cleansing:* This refers to the detecting and restructuring of bad data to ensure quality and usefulness.

- *Linkage:* This integration function is achieved through an enterprisewide master person index (EMPI).

Data Management

As suggested earlier, data repositories have become extremely sophisticated, to the extent that software has been developed to assist in appropriately structuring and utilizing the data. The basic components of such data management include data modeling, data dictionary maintenance, controlled vocabulary and coding system usage, and knowledge representation.

Data Modeling

Data modeling defines data fields, records of which fields may be a part, and any association or interdependence among records (Freeze 2002). Three primary means of modeling data include the following (Martin and Fuller 1998):

- The entity–relationship model (discussed in detail in chapter 7) illustrates the relationships among a system's different elements (entities).

- The relational model, usually used in relational database design, consists of tables made up of rows describing occurrences of related information and columns providing the attributes that describe a row. Figure 9.6 provides an example of the relational model (Martin and Fuller 1998).

- An object model, used in object-oriented databases, represents static and structural data aspects of a system. Figure 9.7 shows the notations used in object-oriented data modeling, and figure 9.8 provides an example (Coad and Yourdon 1991, 196; Popkin Software 1998). An object is an abstraction of something. For example, "Name" is not a specific patient's name but, rather, a representation or abstraction of a name. Objects may be part of a larger set of attributes and services. This larger set is called a class. For example, the function of "Identification" is a class that includes objects such as "Name," "Birth date," and so forth. Each object has certain attributes. For example, names are alphabetical; dates are numeric and have a certain arrangement. Objects also perform services. Names create new records; a birth date and a current date may calculate an age.

Data Dictionary

A **data dictionary** is used to capture the results of data modeling. In theory, data dictionaries may be compiled as a series of handwritten notes or word-processed documents. However, a database management system is a far better tool to maintain a data dictionary because it can prompt the user to enter all elements of the dictionary, access definitions, and update the dictionary (Duffy 1997).

Figure 9.6.   Relational data model

Health Record Number	Clinical Identifier	Date of Service
100	Primary Care	4/19/2000
101	Telephone	4/20/2000
102	Urgent Care	5/2/2000

Figure 9.7. Object-oriented notation

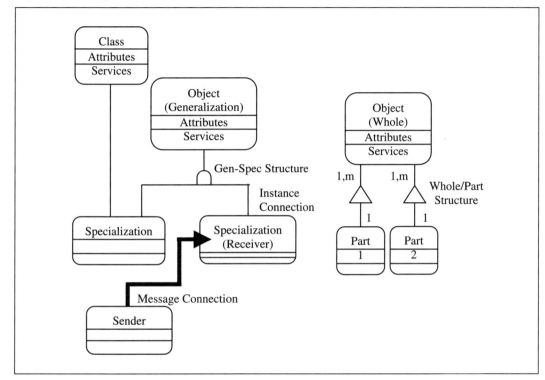

Figure 9.8. Example of object model

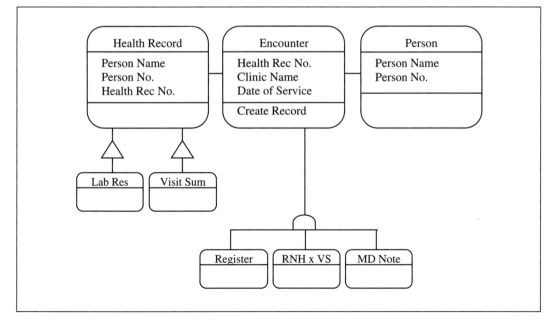

A data dictionary generally is structured around metadata, which are data about data. **Metadata** define all the characteristics about a data element. This information allows different individuals looking at those characteristics to reach the same conclusion about what that data element means and how it is to be used (Nichols and Dolan 1999, 184–187). A data dictionary contains the following:

- Names of entities, tables, and major categories of data elements
- Descriptions of data attributes (Martin and Fuller 1998; Chidley 1998), including:
  —Logical name (the name that would be presented to the user when displayed as a variable for data collection)
  —Physical name/field code name/label (a mnemonic or other code recognized by the computer)
  —Synonyms (aliases, if used)
  —Definition/description (ideally a standard definition from a standard reference— cited below; otherwise the organization or vendor's definition)
  —Reference (source of definition)
  —Source of data (person [and potentially qualifications] or medical device, and through which system application)
  —Format type (alpha, numeric, alphanumeric; calculated or free text; position of characters [for example, mmddyyyy]; and so on)
  —Length (number of characters allowed, if applicable)
  —Allowable range, if any (for example, fixed, variable; number of decimal places)
  —Valid values, if applicable (for which non-valid entry would trigger an alert)
  —Lexicon, if applicable (coding scheme and/or controlled vocabulary)
  —Data restrictions/edits (for example, do not use hyphens)
  —Access restrictions (keyed to organizations security access controls)
  —Authority to change (for example, system administrator)
- Processing rules (usually recorded as a key to the rules retained in a separate database)
- Relationships among entities or classes (from a data model)
- Keys (links to data model)

Figure 9.9 is an example of a part of an entry in a data dictionary.

Most EHR vendors use a proprietary data dictionary in their products and each vendor's data dictionary is specific to its product. However, only some vendors provide access to the data dictionary to the organization acquiring the product. In some cases this is a mat-

Figure 9.9.   Example of a data dictionary entry

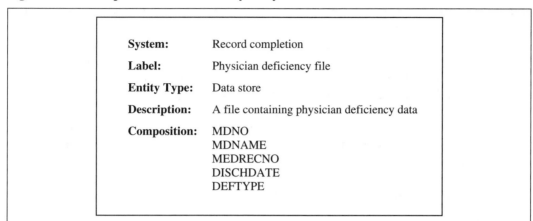

System:	Record completion
Label:	Physician deficiency file
Entity Type:	Data store
Description:	A file containing physician deficiency data
Composition:	MDNO
	MDNAME
	MEDRECNO
	DISCHDATE
	DEFTYPE

ter of competitive advantage, but in many other cases it arises out of concern that the organization may alter the attributes of the data elements in the data dictionary such as to alter the processing capability of the application, with potentially negative affects. For example, if a clinical decision support system relies on five data elements to fire properly, but one data element is often difficult to collect and physicians want to make it an optional rather than a required data element, this change could destroy the ability of the clinical decision support rule to fire correctly. As a result, some vendors offer a wizard that enables limited and controlled changes in the data dictionary.

Because many systems supply data to the EHR and receive data from it, healthcare organizations must be aware that a change to one application may have a ripple effect throughout all other applications. Correcting this may entail countless hours of detailed examination of each application and the interfaces among them. An example was related by Zafar (2008) at Indiana University School of Medicine, in which he described a change to a data element made by a commercial lab. Suddenly without notice, the lab changed a data field originally containing only units, to containing both the units and the unit of measure. The result was thousands of error messages within minutes that literally took 3 months to repair.

However, there may be a need for organizations to compile their own data dictionaries to ensure consistency across disparate systems. The Visible Analyst Workbench is a computer-aided systems engineering (CASE) tool that may be used to manage a comprehensive healthcare organization's data dictionary (Abdelhak, et al. 2001). A comprehensive data dictionary can help address terms that have regularly been found to be inconsistent across systems. Terms such as *patient number, health record number, account number, visit number,* and others may have different definitions. Moreover, definitions of terms such as *attending physician, primary physician, admitting physician,* and so on often have different interpretations within different organizations.

Although a unique set of attributes for each data element would be ideal, it is likely impossible. Generally, it is best not to try to force conformance to a single definition. Thus, the data dictionary must serve as a map to identify such inconsistencies.

Knowledge Representation

Knowledge representation is a growing field of tools for processing data to support clinical decision making (Shams and Farishta 2002).

In summarizing data management within a data repository, it is important to note that although it is possible to provide data integration without a data repository and to provide a view of those data without the multiple functions of a clinical workstation, both the repository and the workstation currently are the primary means of achieving the ability of the EHR to retrieve and process data from multiple sources (Mon and Nunn 1999). However, it also should be pointed out that having a repository does not necessarily mean that an organization has an EHR. It is important to remember that the criteria for what constitutes an EHR include: (1) capturing data from multiple sources (which the data repository facilitates) and (2) using the information to make clinical decisions (3) at the point of care. There is much more to an EHR than a repository alone.

Data Warehouse

In addition to a data repository that is updated in real time, healthcare organizations may want to collect and reorganize data into a format more suitable for ad hoc querying and analytical processing. These secondary, or derived, databases or repositories generally do not participate directly in patient care—they may not even include patient-identifying information. In fact, querying the data repository directly for such secondary uses would have a significant negative impact on system performance. Rather, data are separated into data warehouses. Their use is often referred to as **executive decision support**, although such support may be for health-related management and research as well as administrative data inquiry.

For example, various analytical tools may be used to develop clinical guidelines that ultimately are incorporated into a clinical decision support system. They also may be used by nonclinicians to better manage the organization. Robust queries can be made to evaluate services, make decisions about major capital equipment purchases based on potential for use, and so on. This use of data is often called executive decision support. However the decision support databases are used, when the data are derived from a repository (to which they may have been contributed directly or from multiple databases), they are often referred to as data warehouses. The same types of functions that data undergo for use in a repository are performed by a data warehouse management system (DWMS).

Data warehouses come in several forms, reflecting organizational needs for different kinds of decision-making functions. Some of these forms include (Fox 1997):

- **Data marts** are miniature versions of the primary data warehouse (often referred to as a supermarket). The scope of data managed in each data mart is less than in a typical warehouse, thus suggesting a convenience store, or mart, that holds focused data within a limited subject area or business function.

- The operational data store (ODS) is the most real-time-sensitive, operationally oriented form of data warehousing. It retains small amounts of key indicators from operational systems. Based on what is essential in running day-to-day processes, key indicators are captured and quickly made available to operating managers.

- The data warehouse report center is used in compiling data for repetitive reporting, report production, and distribution.

Data warehousing can be a cost-effective way to achieve a consolidated view of the healthcare enterprise and the trends affecting it. Data warehouse applications have been primarily used as follows:

- In *revenue management,* no single transaction system can address all the different contractual and regulatory reimbursement formulas that the typical integrated delivery system is subject to. With revenue based on a mix of fee-for-service, capitation, and risk pooling, a data warehouse is often necessary to obtain a picture of the organization's revenue stream and the factors controlling it.

- *Clinical management* provides one of the greatest returns on investment for warehouses, where day-to-day patient data can be fed into highly sophisticated analytical applications to contribute to best practices and to identify areas of excessive variation from best practices.

- *Outcomes management* goes a step beyond clinical management in which factors such as treatment regimens and response to treatment are studied in order to develop best practices and contribute to improved clinical outcomes.

- *Operations management* refers to the management of administrative functions. For example, cost accounting, case-based budgeting, and variance analysis help improve the healthcare organization's operational efficiency.

- *Population management* contributes to proactively managing the health of a group of individuals, such as the members of a health plan, by predicting healthcare utilization and identifying at-risk members requiring case management.

Inference Engine (Analytical Tools)

To accomplish the preceding functions with data warehouses, a number of analytical tools may be used. A simple query tool and **report writer** are common ways to access data in any database structure. Spreadsheets may be created from the data to use in manipulating them, and various statistical analyses may be performed via the spreadsheet or other software. Two other tools, data mining and **online analytical processing** (OLAP) are key to sophisticated utilization of data warehouses for decision support (Fickenscher 2005).

Figure 9.10 provides a pictorial view of the concepts of local databases, clinical data repositories (CDRs), and data warehouses.

Data Quality Management

Because data drive all the functions of data repositories and data warehouses, they must be as accessible, accurate, consistent, current, comprehensive, defined, granular, relevant, pre-

Figure 9.10. **Data architecture**

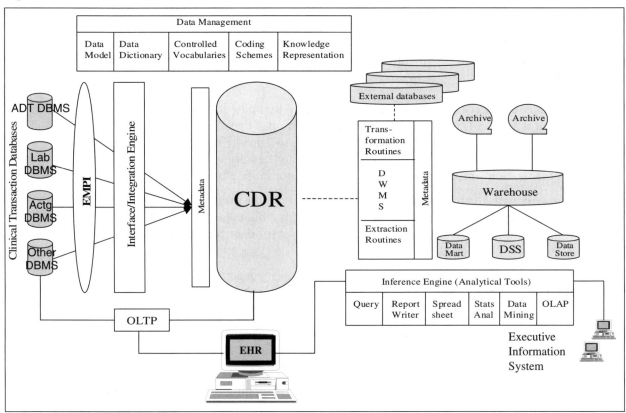

cise, and timely as possible. AHIMA's 1998 Data Quality Management Model (figure 9.11) establishes principles for managing the quality of health data in their collection, analysis, application, and warehousing. (See appendix C.1 on the enclosed CD.)

Interestingly, although the quality of the data used to support quality of care delivery and to measure quality of care delivered is critically important, little has been written about health data quality management as a process outside of the health information management (HIM) profession, whereas an increasing body of knowledge is growing concerning data quality management in other fields. For example, Geiger (2004) writes "Data Quality Management: The Most Critical Initiative You Can Implement" and observes that corporations have increasingly come to realize that [customer and business] data is an important corporate asset. At a conference of the Financial Executives International, it was observed by chief financial officers that data quality/information integrity is the top technology issue for the second year running (Herin 2008). *DM Review Magazine* (Loshin 2004) estimated that the cost of poor data quality to U.S. businesses exceeds $600 billion each year.

Although data quality management has come to be recognized as critical to U.S. businesses, data quality has only just begun to be raised as in issue broadly in healthcare. The

Figure 9.11.   AHIMA's Data Quality Management Model

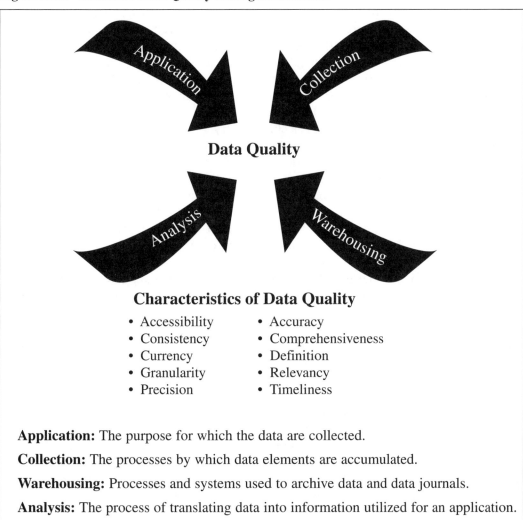

Data Quality

Characteristics of Data Quality

- Accessibility
- Consistency
- Currency
- Granularity
- Precision

- Accuracy
- Comprehensiveness
- Definition
- Relevancy
- Timeliness

Application: The purpose for which the data are collected.

Collection: The processes by which data elements are accumulated.

Warehousing: Processes and systems used to archive data and data journals.

Analysis: The process of translating data into information utilized for an application.

National Committee on Vital and Health Statistics included data quality in its stewardship framework (2008). Although the challenges in healthcare data quality are somewhat different than in general industry, data quality for healthcare data must look to clinical data standards (Fenton et al 2007), data content defintions (Kallem et al 2007), and processes to verify that the data *values* as they are entered into an EHR meet the principles outlined in AHIMA's Data Quality Management Model.

Today, companies are developing software to better manage data quality in customer databases. They are able to profile, monitor, and actively manage the quality of enterprise data. They can integrate and standardize data across multiple systems and business units. Data correction rules can be defined that are organizational specific and used to cleanse and standardize data. In healthcare, evaluation of data validity, reliability, completeness, and timeliness may be accomplished through a combination of human and machine processes, although the subjective nature of some data make even this difficult.

For example, data editing rules can be established that validate data entries into the EHR. For example, if the value for a data element is to be between .1 and .10, a value of 11 entered by the user would be flagged for action. However, if a value of 4 is entered, there is no way to know with certainty that it is a correct entry. In fact, if the variable for which this data was being entered was a pain scale, 4 could have been considered a severe pain (on a categorical pain scale of 1, none, to 4, severe) that would likely have triggered administration of pain medication such as morphine, or only a moderate pain (on a numerical scale of 1 to 10) that might have triggered only an extra-strength aspirin. Without correlating other information that may or may not have been documented in the record and appreciating the professional judgment of the clinicians involved, it would be impossible for anyone to judge the accuracy of this information after the fact, despite the importance of monitoring and attending to patients' pain (Haig 2007).

Data integrity is another tool that can be used to evaluate data quality. Data integrity refers to alteration of the representation of the data in electronic systems. Data integrity is obviously a critical component of the technical design of an EHR. For example, if a data edit rule was for the data to be between .01 and .10, and the user entered .1, but the representation of the entry was altered somehow by the equipment to be 1, this error is just as critical as if the user had entered the invalid value. It might even be more critical because the data-editing rules will not catch a machine error. As a result, data integrity controls must be in place to ensure that data are not altered after they are entered. Data integrity problems can arise from poor data integration, where data from multiple systems are not properly synchronized. Programming errors can contribute to data integrity issues where processes can produce erroneous data. Human error in keystroking can produce unintended commands that alter data. Exposure of equipment and media to excessive heat, strong magnetic fields, or other mechanical problems may corrupt data. Finally, viruses and other malicious codes may threaten data integrity (Amatayakul, et al 2004).

Conclusion

The data infrastructure for an EHR system presents special challenges. IT in healthcare is perhaps more challenging than it is in any other industry because of the unique focus in healthcare on narrative information. In most other industries, IT processes discrete data elements, such as wind speed, weight, interest rate, time, and so on; and these data then are processed into information that contributes to knowledge. In healthcare, however, the context of the original data is as important as the context that surrounds the resultant information to produce knowledge. This distinction makes it essential to model and define data precisely. The healthcare industry has developed a number of vocabularies in its attempt to standardize the meaning of words and phrases. Unfortunately, competing and proprietary interests have resulted in more than one standard, although the industry has begun to address coordination of vocabularies.

Overall, data architecture for an EHR system consists of individual databases contributing to a central data repository from which data may be either drawn directly to supply the EHR workstation or sent to a warehouse that performs sophisticated analysis on data to supply decision support. How well the quality of these data structures is managed will determine the quality of the knowledge that can be supported with an EHR. AHIMA's Data Quality Management Model is an outstanding tool to ensure data accuracy, accessibility, consistency, comprehensiveness, currency, definition, granularity, precision, relevancy, and timeliness.

References and Resources

Abdelhak, M., et al. 2007. *Health Information: Management of a Strategic Resource,* 3rd ed. St. Louis. Saunders Elsevier.

AHIMA Data Quality Management Task Force. 1998 (June 15). Practice brief: Data Quality Management Model. *Journal of AHIMA* 69(6). Available online from ahima.org.

AHIMA e-HIM Workgroup on EHR Data Content. 2006 (Feb.). Guidelines for developing a data dictionary. *Journal of AHIMA* 77(2):64A–D.

AHIMA Workgroup on Core Data Sets as Standards for the EHR. 2004 (Sept.). Practice brief: E-HIM strategic initiative: Core data sets. *Journal of AHIMA.* 75(8):68A–D.

Amatayakul, M. 2003. *HIPAA Made Simple,* 2nd ed. Marblehead, MA: Opus Communications.

Amatayakul, M and M. Cohen. 2008 (May). Rewiring the Brain. *ADAVANCE for Health Information Executives.*

Amatayakul, M., S.S. Lazarus, T. Walsh, and C.P. Harley. 2004. *Handbook for HIPAA Security Implementation.* Chicago. American Medical Association: AMA Press.

American Health Information Management Association. 2003 (Oct.). Practice Brief: Core data sets for the physician practice electronic health record. *Journal of AHIMA.* 74(10).

Bontempo, C.J., and C.M. Saracco. 1995. *Database Management Principles and Products.* Upper Saddle River, NJ: Prentice-Hall.

Chidley, E. 1998. Data dictionaries: What are they and why. *For the Record* (June): 14–18.

Coad, P., and E. Yourdon. 1991. *Object-Oriented Analysis,* 2nd ed. Englewood Cliffs, NJ: Yourdon Press.

Copenhaver, M.S. 1998. Where's the data? *ADVANCE for Health Information Executives* 2(8):27–32.

Duffy, P.G. 1997. Data dictionaries: An overview. *Journal of AHIMA.* 68(2):30–34.

Fenton, S.H. 2005 (May). An Introduction to the Unified Medical Language System. *Journal of AHIMA* 76(5):60–62.

Fenton, S.H. 2002. Clinical classifications and terminologies. In *Health Information Management: Concepts, Principles, and Practice,* edited by K.M. LaTour and S. Eichenwald. Chicago: American Health Information Management Association.

Fenton, S.H., et al. 2007. Data Standards, Data Quality, and Interoperability. *Journal of AHIMA.* 78(2).

Fickenscher, K.M. 2005 (Oct.). The new frontier of data mining. *Health Management Technology*, 26–30. www.healthmgttech.com.

Fowles, J.B., et al. 2008 (May). Performance Measures Using Electronic Health Records: Five Case Studies. *The Commonwealth Fund: Health Policy, Health Reform, and Performance Improvement*, 92.

Fox, C. 1997. Data warehouse and CDR essentials. *ADVANCE for Health Information Executives* 1(7):16–22.

Freeze, Wayne S. 2002 (May). Digital Database Design. Microsoft Office Solutions. http://www3.ca.com/Files/IndustryTrends/microsoft_office_solutions.PDF.

Fyffe, K. H. 2007 (June). Recommended Requirements for Enhancing Data Quality in Electronic Health Records, Final Report Executive Summary, RTI International.

Geiger, J.G., Intelligent Solutions, Inc., 2004 (May). Data Quality Management: The Most Critical Initiative You Can Implement. www2.sas.com/proceedings/sugi29/098-29.pdf.

Greenberg, Marjorie. 2004 (Jan. 7). Unpublished interview with author.

Haak, B. 1998. Taking control of knowledge. *ADVANCE for Health Information Executives* 2(11):97–98.

Haig, S. 2007 (Feb. 20). How Real Is Your Pain? *Time*.

Hardin, J. Michael. 2002. Expert systems and decision support. In *Health Information Management: Concepts, Principles, and Practice,* edited by K.M. LaTour and S. Eichenwald. Chicago: American Health Information Management Association.

Harmon, Paul. 2003 (Jan.). Developing an enterprise architecture. *Business Process Trends*. Available online from edtn.bitpipe.com.

Health and Human Services. 2003 (Feb. 10). Press Release: HHS to provide home health quality information to improve quality of care provided by home health agencies. www.cms.hhs.gov.

Herin, J., Computer Sciences Corporation. 2008 (May 6). Chief Financial Officers Cite Data Quality/Information Integrity as Top Technology Issue for Second Year. *PR Newswire*.

Imel, M., K. Giannangelo, and B. Levy. 2004 (Oct.). Essentials for mapping clinical terminology. *2004 IFHRO Congress and AHIMA Convention Proceedings*. Chicago: American Health Information Management Association.

Janetzki, V., et al. 2004. Using Natural Language Processing to Link from Medical text to Online Information Resources, MEDINFO 2004, *IOS Press*, Amsterdam.

Joint Commission. 2003. *Shared Visions—New Pathways*. Oakbrook Terrace, IL: Joint Comission.

Kallem, C., et al. 2007 (July). Data Content for EHR Documentation. *Journal of AHIMA* 78(7): 73–76.

Kohn, Deborah. 2002. Informatics in healthcare. In *Health Information Management: Concepts, Principles, and Practice,* edited by K.M. LaTour and S. Eichenwald. Chicago: American Health Information Management Association.

Lau, F. 2004 (Sept. 20). Toward a conceptual knowledge management framework in health. *Perspectives in Health Information Management* 1:8.

Lee, F.W. 2002. Data and information management. In *Health Information Management: Concepts, Principles, and Practice,* edited by K.M. LaTour and S. Eichenwald. Chicago: American Health Information Management Association.

Loshin, D. 2004 (April). Issues and Opportunities in Data Quality Management Coordination. *DM Review Magazine*.

Love, D. 2001. Statewide data systems: Entering a new era. *Journal of AHIMA* 72(10):40–46.

Marshak, R. 1998 (May/June). Knowledge: The human touch. *Oracle Magazine*, pp. 11–12.

Martin, T., and S. Fuller. 1998. Components of the EHR: An overview. *Journal of AHIMA* 69(9):58–64.

McBride, S., et al. 2006 (Feb.). Data mapping. *Journal of AHIMA* 77(2):44–48.

Mon, D.T. 2003. Relational database management: What you need to know. *Journal of AHIMA* 74(10):40–50.

Mon, D.T., and S. Nunn. 1999. Understanding the EHR architecture: An HIM professional's guide. *Journal of AHIMA* 70(2):30–37.

National Committee on Vital and Health Statistics. 2003 (Nov. 5). Letter to the Honorable Tommy G. Thompson. www.ncvhs.dhhs.gov.

National Committee on Vital and Health Statistics. 2008 Report: Enhancing Protections for Uses of Health Data: A Stewardship Framework. www.ncvhs.dhhs.gov.

National e-prescribing Conference Centers for Medicare and Medicaid Services. October 6 & 7, 2008. Healthcare IT leaders kick off government's e-prescribing drive.

National Library of Medicine. 2001–2002. Fact Sheets: Unified Medical Language System, UMLS Metathesaurus, Medical Subject Headings (MeSH). www.nlm.nih.gov/pubs/factsheets.

Nichols, J.C., and P. Dolan. 1999. Data dictionaries: Enterprise tools for EHRs. In *Electronic Health Records: Changing the Vision,* edited by G.F. Murphy, M.A. Hanken, and K.A. Waters. Philadelphia: W.B. Saunders.

Ozbolt, J. 1999. Patient Care Data Set. www.ncvhs.dhhs.gov/990518t3.pdf.

Pakhomov, S., et al. 2007. Epidemiology of Angina Pectoris: Role of Natural Language Process of the Medical Record. *American Heart Journal* 153(4): 666–673.

Pollock, Daniel A. 1999 (May 17). Data Elements for Emergency Department Systems (DEEDS). Testimony to National Committee on Vital and Health Statistics.

Popkin Software. 1998. Modeling Systems with UML. www.popkin.com.

Rynberg, S. 2004 (Oct.). Data dictionary standardization in a single or multi-hospital system. *2004 IFHRO Congress and AHIMA Convention Proceedings.* Chicago: American Health Information Management Association.

SAS Data Quality Solution, Ensuring Information Excellence Through Data Quality Lifecycle Management, Fact Sheet.

Schnitzer, G.L. 2000. Natural language processing: A coding professional's perspective. *Journal of AHIMA* 71(9):95–98.

Scichilone, R.A., and S.M. Hull. 2006. G codes for quality measure reporting. *Journal of AHIMA* 77(2):82–84.

Shakir, Abdul-Malik. 1999. Tools for defining data. *Journal of AHIMA* 70(8):48–53.

Shams, Kam, and Mehnaz Farishta. 2002. Knowledge management. In *Health Information Management: Concepts, Principles, and Practice,* edited by K.M. LaTour and S. Eichenwald. Chicago: American Health Information Management Association.

SNOMED International. 2004. SNOMED Clinical Terms Core Content as of January 2004. www.snomed.org.

Spackman, K.A., et al. 1997 (Oct.). SNOMED RT: A reference terminology for healthcare. *Proceedings of the American Medical Informatics Association Annual Symposium.* Nashville, TN: AMIA.

Vogenberg F.R., and S. Hull. 2006. Coding for medication therapy management services. *Journal of AHIMA* 77(2):74–76.

Warren, J.J., and S. Bakken. 2002. Update on standardized nursing data sets and terminologies. *Journal of AHIMA* 73(7):78–83.

Wilson, P.S. 2005 (Oct.). Maintenance and update issues for clinical vocabulary mapping. Clinical Vocabulary Mapping Methods Institute, 77th AHIMA Convention and Exhibit.

Zafar, A. MD. 2008 (March 27). Associate Professor of Medicine, Indiana University School of Medicine, Affiliated Scientist, Regenstrief Institute, Inc., and Academic Staff, AHRQ, National Resource Center for Health IT. Presentation on HIE Architectures, Health IT Certification.

Chapter 10
Information Technology and Systems Infrastructure Assessment

Albert Einstein is quoted as having said, "Everything should be made as simple as possible, but no simpler." Current EHR technology is by no means simple in its technical infrastructure but should appear simple to the user. Information technology (IT) and systems infrastructure refer to how hardware and software work together to deliver EHR functionality to users. Technology is constantly changing, and so the primary goal of this chapter is to serve as a technical primer that points the reader in the right direction to continuously monitor emerging technology trends. This chapter:

- Discusses the scope of EHR system architecture

- Identifies the primary processing, storage, input/output (I/O), network, and other hardware associated with EHR systems

- Identifies the types of software that support EHR systems

- Describes standards for integration/interface among applications

- Identifies system reliability, and privacy and security considerations

- Suggests strategies for addressing emerging technologies

Scope of EHR System Architecture

When applied to the overall EHR system infrastructure, architecture refers to the technical building blocks that support the functions of the EHR. The inputs, processes, and outputs of information systems must be carefully constructed. Just as a house or other building has a structural design, so too must an information system have a structural design, or architecture.

Key Terms

Central processing unit

Client/server
  architecture

Clinical document
  architecture

Ethernet

Extranets

Firewall

Flash drives

Interface

Interface engines

Intranet

Language

Medical identity theft

Messaging standards

Platform

Scripting language

Source code

T-lines

Thin clients

Topology

Virtual private network

Web services
  architecture

Hardware Architecture

Every computer system operates with hardware, or equipment, that serves to capture data (input), save and manipulate the data (process), and present it to the user (output). Although the fundamental architecture of a computer should be well known to any reader of this book, special considerations of the input/output, storage, and processing capacity for EHRs will be addressed in turn.

Input/Output Devices

Input/output (I/O) devices include keyboards (for entering text), display screens (for viewing), navigational devices (for selecting objects such as mouse, touch pad, light pen, and so on), speech recognition, optical character recognition (for handwriting recognition), optical scanners (for document imaging), bar code scanners, radio frequency identification devices (RFID), picture archiving (for images), voice input (for navigational commands), voice output, speakers, printers, and more. Because many of these devices serve both input and output functions, they are typically described together, although obviously some only serve input (for example, keyboard) or output (for example, printer).

In general, I/O devices are considered peripheral devices because they are separate from the central processing unit of the computer, even if they are housed in a single casing (for example, a notebook computer or personal digital assistant [PDA] will have a keyboard, display screen, and navigational device physically in the same casing as the central processing unit).

When computer users whose primary function is not IT are expected to use an EHR, the term workstation or human–computer interface may be used to convey that the I/O device should support humans' work and be as seamless to use as pen and paper.

The term *workstation* was originally used to describe a stand-alone computer system for performing moderate amounts of computations, but relatively high-quality graphing, such as for engineering applications, desktop publishing, and software development. Now, the distinction is blurring between what once was a specific type of computer and what is now a generic term used to refer to any single-user computer, including personal computers (PCs) of many different types and that often are linked together to form a local area network (LAN). Multimedia workstations containing cameras and video players to incorporate sound, still images, and animated video sequences along with the data used in traditional information processing were often characteristic of high-end stand-alone computers. Today, such features can be found on cellular phones, high-quality cameras, and other such devices, and they play an important role in telehealth applications.

Another term whose definition was blurred in the past but is becoming clearer is *desktop*. Originally, desktop computers were considered less powerful workstations, but now the term is generally used to distinguish between a computer that remains on a desk and is generally not portable and notebooks, laptops, tablets, and PDAs that are truly portable, often called mobile devices. Sometimes the term *intelligent workstation* is used to distinguish a desktop computer from the furniture (also sometimes called a workstation) on which a computer may be placed.

Determining what type of I/O device or devices should be acquired for use in an EHR system is a critical component of the overall EHR system architecture. Although one size does not fit all, too many different types of devices can be a nightmare for the IT department to maintain. There are definitely economies of scale that must be considered. Still, because of the variety of work performed, especially in different parts of a care delivery organization, some variety of devices may be needed.

Some of the considerations for selecting I/O devices include their source of power, network connectivity, portability, screen size and resolution, and navigational devices.

Source of Power

Power supply is critical issue. Although most desktop computers are connected directly to a power supply, portable devices require a battery for their power, which is perhaps one of their main drawbacks for use in a 24/7 environment, or even in an 8-hour day. Most portable computers still do not have sufficient battery power to last even a full 8 hours. Some organizations address this issue by supplying each location where the portable device may be used with a power cable. Hospitals may use carts on which a portable device is mounted. The cart can carry a more powerful battery pack as well as other peripheral computer equipment, such as bar code readers for medication administration, and medical devices. Moreover, there is an added measure of security for the computer devices when secured to such carts. Carts with computers have been dubbed "computers on wheels," or COWs. However, even these are not without their problems, as the battery packs must be recharged. As the devices are fairly large and hospitals generally have not been built with "parking lots" or charging stations for such devices, putting them in hallways was found to be a fire department violation in at least one hospital. In another, the carts became unwieldy to maneuver in very small rooms, and had to be temporarily parked in hallways, disrupting traffic flow.

Network Connectivity

Network connectivity is another issue. Again, a desktop computer generally has a hardwire connection to the organization's network, even if it is mounted to a wall or ceiling. However, portable devices also need a connection to the network to access data. Although it is possible to dock a portable device to a network station to download all the information needed for the day, or shift, and then dock again to upload new information, this is not satisfactory as more robust clinical decision support processing is demanded, which requires significantly more data than what would be downloaded for a day's work. As a result, many healthcare organizations are adopting wireless network technology. There are also challenges here as well. Special considerations must be made to the building architecture to identify potential dead zones. In addition, wireless technology tends to be a bit slower than wired technology, although this is being addressed by wireless standards organizations.

Portability
Portability is especially important when a clinician needs his or her hands free to care for a patient. Considerations include the weight of the I/O device, hot spots on tablet computers, ability to balance the device while attempting to use a keyboard, and where to put the device when examining the patient. All these considerations help to explain why many hospitals have migrated to COWs. In clinics, providers like the ability to move around and stay logged on with their devices. In this case, they might need to consider shelving or special pull-out drawers in examination rooms.

Screen Size and Resolution
Monitors come in a variety of sizes, forms, and resolutions. The size of the screen is often referred to as the screen's "real estate." One reason for the popularity of tablets is that the screen real estate is large enough to view an amount of data essentially equivalent to what is viewable on a sheet of paper. The screen real estate on PDAs is often considered too small to be useful except for occasional reference purposes.

The amount of resolution in a monitor determines the ability to clearly view the content. Resolution is measured by pixels. Generally, there are three categories of monitor resolution. A good way to understand their difference is in reference to the ability to see detail on an x-ray. High resolution ($2,000 \times 2,500$ pixels) is used to replace the conventional view box for diagnostic interpretation of x-rays. Most radiologists report that this is not only sufficient resolution for diagnostic purposes, but the ability to rotate, zoom, and create a three-dimensional image enhances diagnostics even more. Medium resolution ($1,200 \times 1,600$ pixels) generally is used for viewing x-rays for reference purposes, such as in an intensive care unit, operating room, or conference room. Low resolution (512×512 pixels) is reserved for casual reference in the office or for some teleradiology applications where cost is too great to transmit higher-resolution data. Such resolution is adequate for viewing text.

Navigational Devices
Workstations also have a variety of navigational devices, including keyboards, handwriting recognition pads and pens, voice recognition microphones, and so on, associated with them for data entry and retrieval as well as various token slots, biometrics, and other devices for security. Anything that can be separated from the device is subject to loss. Many organizations find they need to either tether pens and microphones to the devices or keep an extra supply on hand.

Many physicians consider speech recognition the panacea to avoid keyboarding, yet find it awkward to speak into these devices in front of patients and often distracting when they must do their own correction. Both speech and handwriting recognition devices tend to be slower than normal dictation devices or even keyboarding by a moderately skilled individual. These technologies appear to be useful primarily in circumscribed areas, such as radiology, where the clinician is not using the speech device at the point of care and uses a relatively circumscribed amount of vocabulary, or in an emergency department where short notes might only supplement templates with pick lists and checkboxes.

Storage Devices

Storage devices are peripheral devices in the same manner as I/O devices. Although there is some storage in the same "box" as the **central processing unit** (CPU), virtually all EHR applications, with their large quantities of data, require "mass storage" devices, which are frequently separate units and may even be separate networks. In addition to the main storage, back-up storage and remote disaster recovery capability must also be considered. Magnetic media such as magnetic tapes and disks have been the most popular forms of storage. Optical disks have also become popular, although are not totally replacing cheaper yet often faster magnetic disks.

Devices for storing data sometimes are referred to as secondary storage because they hold the data and software to be used in an application, as compared to memory in the CPU, which is considered primary storage and holds the permanent machine instructions and just the data and instructions currently being operated on. Secondary storage may be available continuously (online) to the CPU for real-time access to data or physically separated (offline) and require online loading to be connected to the CPU. The term *drive* is often used to describe the device that runs the secondary storage medium.

Secondary storage media include the following:

- *Magnetic tape* is an older storage medium now used for offline storage for back-up and archival purposes, although not as frequently as in the past even for these purposes. It can store a fairly large amount of data, but access to data is sequential so that the time to access a particular data element on magnetic tape is relatively slow. Magnetic tape is removable from the tape drive.

- *Magnetic disks* come in a variety of forms. With the exception of the hard disk within a workstation, magnetic disks are frequently used where speed of access is essential but the ability to write over data is not. A workstation's hard disk is a magnetic disk encased in a protective material and placed within the system unit, forming the hard drive. It is used in stand-alone PCs as the primary source of continuous online data and programs. External hard drives are used primarily for system backup.

- *Optical disks* are a newer alternative to magnetic disks. They may be write once, read many (WORM) or erasable and are particularly well suited for storing multimedia information, including images, sound, and motion (video). Optical disks started out being used in healthcare to store images of documents and clinical data such as x-rays; now they are replacing most magnetic media. Optical disks may be stacked in sets (called a jukebox) for continuous, online access or come in a compact disc (CD) form and be used for offline storage. Older CDs are read-only memory (CD-ROM) and so are used to store computer programs. Newer CDs can be written to and used to store data. Digital versatile disks (DVDs) are still newer optical disk technology, and holographic DVDs add a three-dimensional effect. Optical disks can be miniaturized and stored in a device with a USB port adapter. These devices, and even those containing computer circuitry for storing data, go by different names, such as **flash drives** or USB drives. About the size of a car key, they are highly portable and often come with a ring to attach to a key chain. Because of security concerns, many organizations are disabling the USB port of desktops and portable computers. Although most EHR applications are written to avoid direct download capability to such a local drive, there are concerns that screen prints or cut-and-paste functionality can be used to copy data. Although this has been true for other forms of local storage media, the size of USB drives makes them particularly vulnerable.

Although not a form of media per se, configuration of media is an important part of storage. One configuration that is commonly used is called redundant arrays of inexpensive (or independent) disks (RAID). RAID comes in different levels; although the names of the levels are not standardized, there are typically from two to five levels described. Usually the first level uses multiple drives to increase throughput or the ability of data to be read more rapidly. The second level is called disk mirroring, which means that each set is composed of two disks that are exact duplicates of each other. Thus, if one disk breaks down, the other can take its place. This level of RAID should be considered the minimum requirement for an EHR system. The highest level of RAID uses sets of three disks to address some of the shortcomings in lower-level RAID devices and is preferred in EHR systems that are truly paperless.

Storage and backup for mission-critical functions, such as the EHR will become when it replaces all or most of the paper chart, should be planned carefully. Although the cost of storage media is getting inexpensive, the cost of managing storage is becoming much more expensive. Entire networks are being created to manage the storage of data, and multiple types of storage are being used depending on the nature of what is stored, how frequently it is accessed, and whether its purpose is to support current use or archive data. For example, images of x-rays can be stored on media that are read-only because the image would never be altered in the course of its being viewed. (It may be enlarged, rotated, or zoomed, but these are functions of the presentation layer and monitor, not the media used to the store the image.) Read-only media are less expensive than media that would be written to, such as where the radiology report would be stored and signed. Storage area networks and storage management, then, are becoming critical aspects of EHR architecture and maintenance.

Processors

The CPU, sometimes called the processor, is the area of the computer where data in machine-readable form are processed, according to specific instructions (software) that also are in machine-readable form. Processors are made of semiconductor material etched on a small electronic device called a (silicon) chip or an integrated circuit. Chips may contain from 100 to more than 1 million components. Data and instructions for their processing are converted into binary form, representing the two states of electrical pulses on/ off, the combination of which is what machines can read. The two states are commonly represented as 0 and 1, and are called bits. Sequences of bits, called bytes, are used to represent each character in any language. When describing the size of any component of a computer, reference is made to the number of bytes that can be stored or processed in the component. Sizes may be expressed in kilobytes ([KB] roughly one thousand bytes), megabytes ([MB] roughly one million bytes), gigabytes ([GB] roughly one billion bytes), or even terabytes ([TB] roughly one trillion bytes).

When a computer is first turned on, internal functions are activated ("booted") and diagnostics are performed to check for potential electronic problems. The special instructions that perform these functions are kept in a section of the CPU called read-only memory (ROM). When the computer is turned off, the contents of ROM are retained. ROM does not have to be large, the size depending on the size of random access memory (RAM), number of processors, and processing speed.

RAM is sometimes just called memory or central memory. The memory section of the CPU houses the data and instructions being processed at any point in time. It is volatile, meaning that when the computer is turned off, anything in RAM is lost. The size of RAM relates to the amount of data that can be processed at one time and contributes to the speed with which processing of data can take place. The speed of the CPU is getting faster and faster. A megahertz (MHz) is one million cycles per second. Some CPUs can process cycles of instructions at gigahertz (GHz) speeds. One GHz is equal to 1,000 MHz.

The arithmetic-logic unit (ALU) is the location in the CPU that performs the actual processing of the data held in memory. The ALU also may be referred to as registers. As the name implies, the ALU is where addition, subtraction, multiplication, comparisons, and so on are performed.

The CPU also may contain cache (pronounced *cash*) memory, which is used to accelerate transfer of data and instructions between the registers and central memory. A memory cache is made of high-speed static RAM instead of the slower dynamic RAM used for main memory. Memory caching speeds up the process of accessing data and instructions that are used repeatedly. Disk caching is a similar concept, but it uses conventional main memory. The most recently accessed data from an application is retained in the disk cache. When a program needs to access data, it first checks the disk cache to see if the data are there. (If the needed data are not in the disk cache, the program needs to go to the computer's hard disk or on a special computer called a storage server.) Disk caching makes data retrieval faster when the most recent data are needed repeatedly. Because of disk caching, however, portable devices that connect to a network for only short periods of time and then are used elsewhere should have the data stored in cache erased as a security measure in the event the device is lost or stolen. Wireless devices provide this erasing capability when the device is moved a certain distance away from a wireless access point. (It should be noted that there is a database product called Caché (pronounced *cash-á*) that has nothing to do with memory or disk cache.)

The CPU components are connected by tiny wires through which the data and instructions are passed. The collection of wires is often called a bus.

Finally, because the CPU is being called on to perform so many tasks, seemingly simultaneously, many organizations are buying computers with dual processors, or even dual-core or multicore processors. Dual processor refers to two separate physical computer processors, running in parallel. Dual-core or multicore processors combine two or more processors onto a single integrated circuit. Such technology boosts the computer's multi-tasking capability.

Computer Categories

Although every computer operates in much the same way as described earlier, there are some significant differences. Some of these are suggested here:

- A *supercomputer* is a fast computer, usually dedicated to the performance of specialized applications that require an enormous amount of computation.

- *Mainframe computers* utilize a single large computer with many terminals directly connected to it and sharing the resources of the single computer. When first introduced, mainframe terminals had no processing capability of their own. Most mainframe computers have disappeared. However, a surprising number of hospitals still have an AS/400 computer system, which is an IBM mainframe introduced in 1988, now upgraded (as the iSeries) to support client/server and Web-based applications. The extent to which any AS/400 has migrated to these newer architectures depends on the extent to which upgrades have been performed on the hardware.

- *PC* is a term coined by IBM and adopted by vendors who made similar machines. Computer purists would quickly point out that such computers also may be patterned after the Apple Macintosh. In general, however, a PC is a stand-alone computer system. PCs have been beefed up to serve as powerful computers supporting other computers as servers in a client/server network architecture and skinnied down to serve almost as if they were terminals in a mainframe environment (in which case they may be called dumb terminals).

- *Portable computers,* often in the form of notebook computers, laptops, or tablets, are smaller in size but may be as powerful as a PC. Tablet computers are characterized by a writing slate. Tablets that do not come with a keyboard are referred to as slates, and those that do come with a keyboard are referred to as convertibles.

- *Handheld computers* or PDAs are small enough to be carried in a pocket, purse, or briefcase. Many are approaching PC capability.

- *Network computers* (NCs), also called **thin clients** (discussed under client/server network in the next section), are low-cost PCs with minimal processing capability of their own.

Communications and Network Architecture

Whenever two or more computers need to communicate with each other, a network is needed. Whether this is connectivity to the biggest network of all, the Internet, or simply to one other computer in a LAN, many of the same principles of network architecture apply. Networks have different configurations, or architectures, and an entire set of hardware devices, cabling, and protocols associated with them.

Two primary types of architectures currently are used to communicate among computers in a healthcare organization: client/server and Web-services architectures.

Client/Server Architecture

Client/server architecture is the predominant form of computer architecture used in healthcare organizations today. In client/server architecture, certain computers (servers) have been configured to perform most of the processing and resource-intensive tasks, while other computers (clients), which are generally less-powerful computers, capture, view, and perform limited processes on data.

A server can range in cost from as low as $500 to more than $100,000. It is generally dedicated to providing a specific service to client computers on a network. For example, servers provide database services, application services, file-sharing services, print-sharing services, fax services, e-mail services, and many other specialized services such as authentication. They may be centralized in one location or distributed throughout a network. When grouped together, the collection of servers is sometimes called a server farm. Blade servers are the newest configuration, where a number of server computers, or blades, occupy the space typically occupied by a single computer.

Servers have their own operating systems, which may be Windows-based, a variety of UNIX and Linux versions, a Mac version, or one of the more technical operating systems provided by other vendors.

Client computers are PCs, which may be desktops or portable devices. They generally need, and have considerably less, power (at less cost) because they derive their functionality from the server. When client computers are stripped of most of their processing and storage capabilities, they are called thin clients or network computers. Although thin clients may be attractive because of their cost and security, many EHR applications will not run on them because of their intense processing and response time requirements.

Web Services Architecture

Web-based, or **Web services architecture** (WSA), uses the technology concepts of the Internet and World Wide Web for local area (intranet) or wide area (extranet) network design. Although this is the latest form of computer architecture, it is still not widely used for EHR systems. Its use, however, is increasing and is often combined with the client/server architecture. WSA is more widely used in other parts of the world where there were no legacy systems to be replaced. (A legacy system is any system based on less than the most currently available architecture. Once an organization uses one architecture extensively, it is a costly proposition to convert all of its applications to a new architecture.) WSA uses programs that act as Web browsers. These programs transfer multimedia-based information among computers; support interactive services, allowing users to request information and receive immediate feedback free from the traditional time and space constraints of other media; and use a **standard markup language** to preorganize and structure the form of narrative text (W3C 2004).

Network Configuration

Networks may be configured in a variety of ways, depending on what systems need to be included. Figure 10.1 displays a diagram of some of the concepts described in this section. For healthcare organizations, the most typical private network configurations are:

- *Local-area network (LAN)*: A group of computers typically connected within a relatively small geographic area, such as an office, building, or campus. Connectivity is generally achieved through dedicated cable.

- *Wide-area network (WAN)*: A group of computers that connect across great geographical distances, often using telephone or cable services for connectivity.

- *Wireless local-area network* (WLAN): A group of wireless devices that connect to a LAN via radio waves.

Figure 10.1.   Diagram of network concepts

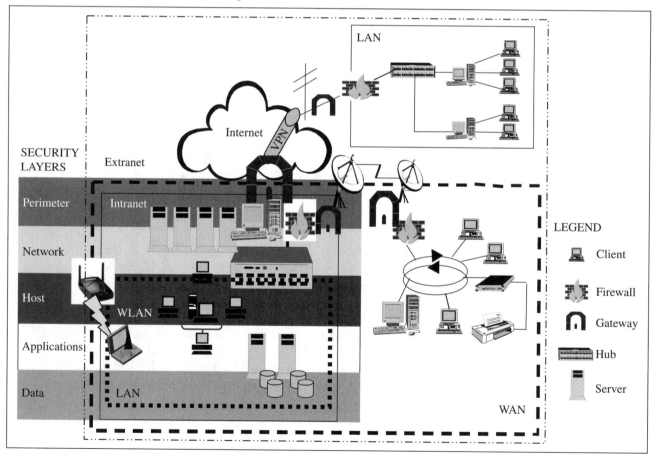

- *Virtual private network (VPN)*: A special kind of WAN that uses a private tunnel through the Internet as the transport medium between locations rather than privately owned cable or leased lines. A VPN reduces networking costs significantly because much of the maintenance is performed by an Internet service provider (ISP).

In addition to these private network types, network configurations using Internet technology (while restricting access to authorized persons) are also used in healthcare organizations.

An **intranet** is a network located within an organization (separated from the Internet by a **firewall**) that uses Internet technologies to enable users to find, use, and share documents and Web pages. Intranets use traditional Internet protocols to transfer data but reside behind a **firewall** (special hardware or software that provides a security barrier between networks and the Internet [MAI]) for security so that they are accessible only to authorized users. **Extranets** are networks that connect a given organization to its customers and business partners or suppliers (business associates in healthcare). Although extranets send information over public networks, requiring a greater level of security, access to them is still restricted to the services and persons authorized.

Topology

Topology refers to the arrangement of the network. There are two types of topology: physical and logical.

Physical Topology

A physical topology is the way in which network devices are connected. Networks are generally arranged in one of three physical topologies:

- *Bus topology* is the simplest network topology, connecting one device to another along a "backbone." In a bus network, all computers on the network receive the same message at the same time. However, only one computer at a time can transfer information; thus, if one segment of the network goes down, the entire network is affected.

- *Star topology* connects individual computers through a central hub that serves as a traffic cop for the data. (This is illustrated in figure 10.1 within the LAN.)

- *Ring topology* connects computers via a cable arranged in a ring. Information is sent through the ring to get from one computer to another, and special kinds of signals are required to direct the data. (This is illustrated in figure 10.1 within the WAN.)

Logical Topology

A logical topology describes how data are transmitted through the physical devices. An **ethernet** is a family of frame-based computer networking technologies that currently is the most widely used topology for LANs. It defines the wiring and signaling standards for the physical transmission of data. Ethernet is standardized as IEEE 802.3 (pronounced *eye-triple-E)*. IEEE is the Institute of Electrical and Electronics Engineers, the leading developer of international standards that underpin many current telecommunications, IT, and power generation products and services. An ethernet utilizes a combination of twisted pair cables for connecting end systems to the network and fiber optic cable for site backbones.

Network Components

Every network must have at least three components to operate: a network operating system (NOS), a network interface card (NIC) or other form of adapter, and cabling or some other form of transmission medium (Derfler and Freed 2000).

Network Operating System

A NOS is a family of programs that run the networked computers. The most common NOS currently in use in healthcare are Windows- or UNIX-based, although a few EHR vendors have created their own operating system. (See the discussion of operating system software later in this chapter.)

Network Interface Card

The NIC, LAN adapters, or wireless access card creates the connection between a computer and the transmission medium. NICs create packages of data that enhance the strength of low-powered digital signals inside a computer to enable the packages to travel through a transmission medium.

Transmission Media

Transmission media carry data through a network and vary by cost, type of service, amount of potential interference and signal degradation, and bandwidth (the maximum speed at which a given device can transmit data). Transmission media for a LAN include:

- Hardwire cables, with speed depending on the size and type of cable, which may be coaxial (with speeds up to 10 MB per second), unshielded twisted pair (up to 100 MB per second), shielded twisted pair (up to 150 MB per second), or fiberoptic (which uses light signals to transfer information through a core of glass or plastic and is capable of moving more than 2 GB per second). Fiberoptic cable is expensive and often reserved for the main cable, or backbone, of a network.

- Infrared light (for example, Bluetooth) also may be used to carry information between devices in a network. It is popularly used between PDAs and cell phones to "beam" data from one device to another, and in healthcare between medical devices and information systems.

- Radio waves and microwaves handle transmissions in a wireless network.

For a WAN, transmission media are often included under the domain of telecommunications. Telecommunications refers to communication over long distances and includes telephone, radio, telegraphy, television, voice-over Internet protocol (VoIP), cellular service, data communications, and computer networking. For constructing a WAN in the healthcare environment, the most common media remain different forms of telephone service:

- Plain old telephone services (POTS) requires a modem to convert analog to digital signals. Although certainly no long popular, many remote areas of the country still rely on POTS.

- Frame relay is another connection service that is easy to use, but less efficient because it does not use a clear channel to pass along data. Data must be formatted into data packets called frames.

- Integrated services digital network (ISDN) is another connection alternative that can transmit data at speeds of 128 KB per second at considerably lower cost.

- Trunk lines (**T-lines**) are the backbone of long-distance, packet-switched network transmission that transmits data in digital form. They come in a variety of speeds and may also carry voice. Many WANs use T1 lines with speeds of 1.544 MB per second (usually costing several thousand dollars per month for usage) or even T3 lines, which are many times faster and more expensive.

- A digital subscriber line (DSL) is at least as fast as a T1 line and runs over standard telephone wire.

- Satellite systems relay signals from satellites at varying bandwidths depending on the system and are costly.

Other Network Devices

In addition to the three main components of a network, a variety of other devices may be used to serve various other purposes in the network. The device used depends on the network topology, the transmission medium, and the standards to which the device manufacturer adheres (Whitehead 1997, 58–76). These devices include:

- *Hub*: The central location where cables on a network come together.

- *Bridge:* Enables computers on individual networks or separate parts of a network to exchange information.

- *Routers*: Connectors used to link different networks together. These devices can automatically determine the best route for information given the amount of traffic on a network.

- *Switch*: Similar to a hub, but newer. It is applied to networks that have many users. The switch is beginning to take the place of bridges and routers.

- *Gateway*: Links two different network types together.

- *Multiplexor*: Traditionally used to divide a long-distance, high-speed telecommunications line so that it can be shared by many users. High-end routers that can interface directly with wide-area communication services are reducing the need for multiplexors.

- *Modems*: Enable computers on a network to exchange information across telephone lines by translating the information from digital form to analog form.

Network Protocols

Network protocols are the rules for sending and receiving data across a network. If the physical topology of a network is the base of the network and the logical topology is how data are transmitted through the base, network protocols establish rules of communication.

The rules are based on a standard called the open-systems interconnection (OSI) model, developed by the International Standardization Organization (ISO). The OSI model consists of seven layers, each of which is responsible for a particular aspect of communication. For example, one layer may be used to specify how information is addressed and another to check errors during transfer.

When data are being transferred over a network, they must pass through each layer of the OSI model. As this happens, information is added to the data to help ensure consistency of communication. When the data reach their destination, they again must pass through the layers of the OSI model so that the information previously applied can be removed at each level (Whitehead 1997, 146–158). Figure 10.2 shows the layers of the OSI model and their purposes.

Protocols are the actual hardware or software components that carry out the OSI model guidelines for transferring information on a network. Most of the protocols are generic across the industries using them and specific only to the different operating systems and network architectures employed.

TCP/IP is a collection of protocols used to allow the communication as described in the OSI model to occur among networks with different types of computer systems. It also is what is used on the Internet. The collection of protocols in TCP/IP include, among others:

- *Transmission control protocol (TCP)*: Used to transfer information between two devices on a network.

- *Internet protocol (IP)*: Responsible for addressing information.

Figure 10.2.   OSI model

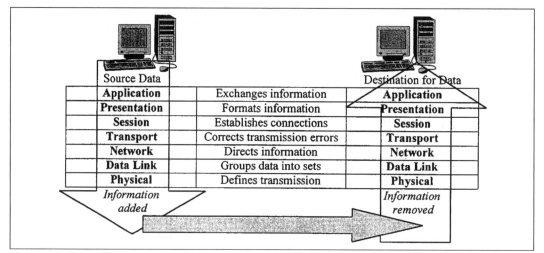

- *File transfer protocol (FTP)*: Used to transfer documents between different types of computers.

- *HyperText transfer protocol (HTTP)*: Used to transfer information from Web servers to Web browsers.

At the application level of the OSI model, industries often create their own standard protocols for communicating (sending messages/exchanging data) between applications. (See the applications integration/interface section in this chapter.)

Physical Plant

The physical plant of the healthcare organization should be included in any technical infrastructure assessment. This ensures the building construction is capable of supporting the electrical power, cabling, and other hardware needs. This is not a trivial consideration, especially as new technology is applied to older buildings.

Software That Supports EHRs

Software refers to the instructions, or programs, that direct the processing of data in computers. Individuals evaluating EHR systems should be concerned about two primary types of software: operating system software and application software. The nature of the operating system and application software language will help determine much of the ability to program and thus support various EHR functions. For example, if an EHR vendor does not use a **scripting language** designed for writing programs to be executed on the Internet, it will be difficult to incorporate intranet technology with the EHR system.

Operating System Software

Operating system software is considered the **platform** on which application programs work. Operating systems perform basic tasks such as recognizing input from the keyboard, sending output to the display screen, keeping track of files and directories on a disk, and controlling peripheral devices such as disk drives and printers. The system acts as a traffic cop, ensuring that different programs running at the same time do not interfere with each other. In addition, the operating system is responsible for many security functions. Operating systems may be proprietary, developed by one vendor for its equipment and applications, or nonproprietary, intended to be used by many vendors.

An example of a nonproprietary (open) operating system is UNIX. UNIX is the trademark name for operating system software originally designed for mainframe computer systems. Because it was written in the nonproprietary programming language called C, it operates well on many different types of computers, although it lacks a graphical user interface (GUI). Linux is a free, newer version of UNIX available on the Web (linux.org) or through some low-cost distributors. UNIX was fairly popular in healthcare computing platforms; Linux is becoming more popular as it becomes more stable and better supported.

Individual PCs have operating systems that permit just the one computer to use various application programs. When computers are networked, the operating system must support multiple users, tasks, and processes. NOSs support such activities. Various Microsoft Windows operating systems for networks are very popular operating systems for client/server environments. Macintosh computers have their own operating system, although the latest Macs are using Intel processors that now support both the Mac operating system as well as Windows.

MUMPS (Massachusetts General Hospital Utility Multi-Programming System) was an operating system created in 1965, specifically for medical information systems. Revisions are still currently being used in some applications under the name of M Technology.

Application Software

Application (or high-level) software makes applications perform their functions. The language in which this software is written provides the algorithms, which are rules or instructions that define a path that guides a process to a logical end point. A variety of application programming languages are currently used in EHRs. Java, Visual Basic (VB), C, and C++ are the most common. Databases also require programming, and database management systems use languages such as SQL, Oracle, and others. As programming for the Internet became prevalent, various programming tools emerged for writing browser-based applications. Although each language has different purposes, Java, JavaScript, ActiveX, Dreamweaver, and ASP.NET are commonly used in EHR systems (Andrew and Bruegel 2003).

As mentioned earlier, creating documents on the Web is becoming an extremely important part of developing an EHR. Standard Generalized Markup Language (SGML) is an international standard for organizing and tagging elements of a document. It does not specify any particular formatting requirements for documents but, rather, specifies the rules for tagging elements contained in them. These tags then can be interpreted to format elements in different ways.

HTML is an authoring language used to create documents on the Web. Similar to SGML, it defines the structure and layout of a Web document by using a variety of tags and attributes. Hundreds of tags are used to format and lay out the information in a Web page. Additionally, tags are used to specify hypertext links that allow Web page developers to direct users to other Web pages by clicking a link.

eXtensible Markup Language (XML) is actually a metalanguage for describing markup languages. It provides the means to define tags and structural relationships between them. Because anyone can define tags, it is helpful for an industry to adopt standards. Health Level Seven (HL7) v3 (discussed in the next section) uses XML to create XML documents incorporating HL7 message content, to generate messages from document content, and to exchange and process messages and documents among disparate systems. XML may use document type definitions (DTDs) to help create XML tags for healthcare information. HL7's clinical document architecture replaces the need for such tags.

In addition to the programming languages, the service-oriented architecture (SOA) is a software architecture where functionality is grouped around business processes and packaged as interoperable services. WSA (previously described under hardware architecture) can be used to implement SOA. A variety of languages support SOA (He 2003).

Source Code

Application software that has been created using one of the application software languages is called **source code** because it is the source of instructions for the application. Generally, the developer of the software owns the source code. This allows the developer to sell the program to multiple consumers. However, healthcare organizations sometimes want to have a copy of the source code. For example, if the developer goes out of business, it may be difficult to maintain the application without this source code. Some healthcare organizations, particularly academic and other large institutions, want to customize an EHR system extensively and often have the staff and expertise to make modifications in the source code.

Organizations wanting the source code may find it difficult to acquire. Some are able to buy rights to a copy of the source code so they can maintain and enhance it themselves or codevelop it with a vendor and maintain interest in it. When the consumer obtains a copy of the source code, vendors often will no longer support it when it does not function properly or when upgrades or patches do not work on it.

Application Integration/Interface

Different applications whose software has enabled them to be designed together and work together with no required intervention are said to be integrated. This means they should exchange data among the various applications seamlessly. Perhaps the best example of this is Microsoft Office. Word, Excel, Access, PowerPoint, Outlook, and other components of the suite all look the same and exchange data easily (although any power user knows that even in this case the programs do not work exactly the same).

When application programs are written independently of one another, they do not have the same look and feel. They may even operate exclusively on different platforms. When data are to be exchanged among these disparate applications, an interface must be built. An **interface** is the hardware, software, data definitions, and standard messaging protocols required for data to be exchanged among separate computing systems (Siwicki 1998).

Creating an interface can be expensive and time-consuming, and the interface may never work as well as a fully integrated system. In purchasing systems that require interfacing, the organization must consider the tradeoff between a less-than-completely-smooth connection and the advantages of the newly introduced system. Vendors are becoming much more experienced in writing interfaces, and new technology, called **interface engines**, is helping as well. Still, interfacing can be an arduous process.

In healthcare, some of the traditional hospital information system (HIS) vendors have created highly proprietary applications that work extremely well together (such as those for master person index [MPI], registration–admission/discharge/transfer [R-ADT], HIM department functions, and order communication). Because these have not been built on an open architecture (using common standards), they are difficult to interface. Of course, this

may have originally been done on purpose as a marketing ploy to get the healthcare organization to buy all the components from one vendor.

Because healthcare computing has expanded to virtually every information area, many
of the vendors have been unable to keep up the development pace and address all the information system needs. In many cases, vendors have bought companies and tried to integrate
their respective products to round out their product lines. Some of these efforts have been
more successful than others.

One important consideration in buying an EHR product is how well it will work with
the rest of the organization's applications. One way to ensure more integrated data is to use
a data repository to which data can be sent and integrated for retrieval at an EHR workstation. (Data repositories are discussed in chapter 9.) New Web-based products using XML
can achieve data access that simulates integration, although many of the analytical processes for clinical decision support are unavailable without a repository.

Standard Messaging Protocols

Within healthcare, standard protocols that support communication between nonintegrated
applications are often referred to as **messaging standards**, also called interoperability
standards or data exchange standards. Messaging standards provide the tools to map proprietary formats to one another and more easily accomplish the exchange of data. However,
because the standard protocols developed to date have often had a lot of optionality, full
interoperability is still not completely assured.

Some of the standards development organizations (SDOs) are starting to reduce the
optionality in their standards and are also incorporating semantic interoperability, which
means they are making accommodations for embedding standard vocabularies as well as
standard syntax (format) in their messages.

Figure 10.3 provides examples of the different types of messaging standards used in
healthcare, and which are discussed next.

Figure 10.3.   Messaging standards

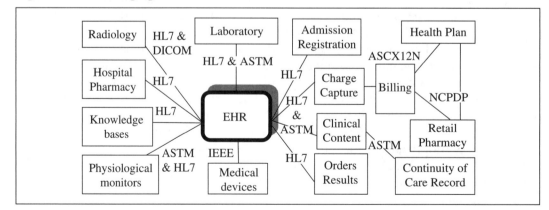

Copyright © 2008, Margret\A Consulting, LLC. Reprinted with permission.

Health Level Seven

HL7 is the most common healthcare application level standard that helps ensure communication across information systems. HL7 is the name of both the SDO and the standard it produces. The standard consists of rules for transmitting demographic data, orders, and patient observations, such as laboratory results and historical and physical examination findings. It also has message rules for appointment scheduling, referrals, problem list maintenance, and care plans. HL7 currently supports v2.3, v2.4, and v2.5 for order entry, scheduling, medical record/image management, patient administration, observation reporting, financial management, and patient care. HL7 v3 was developed in 1999 and adopted an XML schema for use in a WSA. Unfortunately, it is not backward compatible with the HL7 2.x versions, and so few vendors for the U.S. market have incorporated it in their product development. It has been recommended that the federal government stimulate acceleration of development and implementation of HL7 v3 through various incentives and early adoption by government entities.

In addition, HL7 has been at the forefront of incorporating semantic and lexical understandings of the message content relative to message syntax specification. It uses an object-oriented methodology, including the Reference Information Model (RIM), to identify all data content relevant to HL7 messages. It is an essential part of the development of HL7 v.3. HL7 also has recognized the need to adopt the "language of the Web" in its standards. That is, it has taken the lead in creating a document markup standard for the structure and semantics of exchanged "clinical documents." This standard is the **clinical document architecture** (CDA) and the first nationally certified XML-based standard for healthcare (NeoTool n.d.; Shakir 1997).

Digital Imaging and Communications in Medicine

The Digital Imaging and Communications in Medicine (DICOM) standard supports retrieval of information from imaging devices and equipment to diagnostic and review workstations and to short-term and long-term storage systems. Originally developed by the American College of Radiology/National Electrical Manufacturers Association, DICOM is now an independent, and international, SDO.

Integrating the Healthcare Enterprise

Although not an official SDO, Integrating the Healthcare Enterprise (IHE) is an initiative by healthcare professionals and industry to improve the way computer systems in healthcare share information. IHE promotes the coordinated use of established standards such as DICOM and HL7 to address specific clinical needs in support of optimal patient care. IHE develops integration profiles to provide a reliable way of specifying a level of compliance to existing standards sufficient to achieve truly efficient interoperability. Systems developed in accordance with IHE integration profiles communicate with one another better, are easier to implement, and enable care providers to use information more effectively. Physicians, medical specialists, nurses, administrators and other care providers envision a day when vital information can be passed seamlessly from system to system within and across departments and made readily available at the point of care. IHE is designed to make their vision a reality by improving the state of systems integration and removing barriers to optimal patient care.

National Council for Prescription Drug Programs

National Council for Prescription Drug Programs (NCPDP) standards are widely adopted by pharmacies and payers for exchange of retail pharmacy payment information. The NCPDP Telecommunication Standard Implementation Guide, Version 5, Release 1, and equivalent NCPDP Batch Standard Batch Implementation Guide, Version 1, Release 0, were specified in the HIPAA Transactions and Code Sets regulation (August 2000) for use for retail pharmacy claims, eligibility verification, and payment and remittance advice. Their NCPDP SCRIPT standard communicates prescription information (including new prescriptions, refill requests, fill status notifications, and cancellation notifications) between prescribers and pharmacies and has been regulated for use under the Medicare Modernization Act (MMA) of 2003, Medicare Part D e-prescribing. It should be noted that MMA does not require e-prescribing, but requires use of the NCPDP standard if e-prescribing is used. Pending legislation may change this and require e-prescribing, at least for all Medicare Part D prescriptions, in which case, both e-prescribing in general and the NCPDP SCRIPT standard in particular will become much more widely adopted.

Institute of Electrical and Electronics Engineers

IEEE standard IEEE 1073 is a set of medical device communications standards, also promulgated by the ISO and known as ISO 11073. These standards communicate patient data from medical devices such as patient monitors, ventilators, infusion pumps, and so on. IEEE was also previously mentioned in describing networking standards, although these are not unique to healthcare.

American National Standards Institute–Accredited Standards Committee X12-Insurance Subcommittee

The American National Standards Institute–Accredited Standards Committee X12-Insurance Subcommittee (ANSI–ASC X12N) provides messaging standards for electronic data interchange (EDI) of financial and administrative transactions. Their transactions for institutional (837I), professional (837P), and dental (837D) claims, coordination of benefits (837), eligibility inquiry and response (270/271), claims status inquiry and response (276/277), payment and remittance advice (835), and referral certification and authorization (278) in v4010A1 were required for adoption by those using electronic transactions under HIPAA. An upgrade to v5010 was proposed in 2008.

Another set of X12N standards (277/275) is under development for health plans to request, and providers to send, claims attachments electronically. The X12N 275 will embed an HL7 message containing electronic content, either as discrete data using LOINC codes (discussed in chapter 9) to encode the message or the in clinical document architecture (CDA) format. Currently available are messages for ambulance services, rehabilitation services, medications, laboratory results, clinical reports, and emergency department services.

ASTM International

One other messaging SDO of note for healthcare is ASTM International. Formerly the American Society for Testing and Materials, this organization has developed standards for healthcare data security, standard record content, and protocols for exchange of laboratory data. Recently,

ASTM worked with the American Academy of Family Physicians (AAFP), the Massachusetts Medical Society (MMS), and the Health Information Management and Systems Society (HIMSS) to create the Continuity of Care Record (CCR) standard. The CCR standard was developed in response to the need to organize and make transportable a set of basic patient information consisting of the most relevant and timely facts about a patient's condition.

The CCR standard is not intended to be a standard for all of the EHR but, rather, to provide a minimum data set for making patient referrals, transferring the care of patients to other providers, ensuring that discharge information (such as from an emergency department or urgent care center) goes to a primary care physician, and serving as a personal health record (PHR) (ASTM 2003).

Since development of the CCR, HL7 has collaborated with ASTM International to incorporate the CCR into the HL7 CDA format to create the Continuity of Care Document (CCD) standard, which incorporates both the content standards of the CCR and the message formatting of the CDA (HL7 2007). The CCD is being used as the basis for a number of PHR structures.

Standards Development Organizations

No discussion of healthcare standards would be complete without a brief note about the organizations that create standards and their processes. The American National Standards Institute (ANSI) is the body that accredits SDOs for all types of standards in the United States. Its accreditation process ensures that standards are developed in an open, voluntary, consensus-building manner to which, ideally, all parties to whom the standard is important have contributed. What this means is that anyone is free to join an SDO (usually a nominal membership fee is charged for administrative purposes) and contribute to the standards development process by offering ideas, writing (pieces of) the specifications, and voting on standards ballots. Standards frequently go though several ballots before they are approved. The ideal outcome is something that everyone can live with; at a minimum, it is something that is usually respected by most of the key parties.

Standards may be created in other ways. The government may create standards and regulate their use. For example, the NIST, an agency of the Department of Commerce, creates many of the federal government's security standards, which are mandated for use in government agencies and often by their contractors. When the government mandates standards for use in the private sector, it attempts to adopt standards that have been developed in the private sector under the auspices of ANSI accreditation. For example, the HIPAA Transactions and Code Sets regulation adopted the ASC X12N and NCPDP standards. Where standards do not exist, however, the government may create its own (such as in the HIPAA Privacy Rule and Security Rule).

In addition, there are industry de facto standards. These are protocols or specifications that become standards because of their widespread adoption. Microsoft products are a de facto standard in many respects.

Healthcare Information Technology Standards Panel (HITSP)

One other important organization that must be recognized in discussing health information standards is the Healthcare Information Technology Standards Panel (HITSP). In the fall of 2005, the U.S. Department of Health and Human Services' (HHS) Office of the

National Coordinator (ONC) for Health Information Technology awarded multiple contracts to advance President Bush's vision for widespread adoption of interoperable EHRs within 10 years. The contracts targeted the creation of processes to harmonize standards, certify EHR applications, develop nationwide health information network prototypes, and recommend necessary changes to standardized diverse security and privacy policies. The ANSI, in cooperation with strategic partners HIMSS, Booz Allen Hamilton, and Advanced Technology Institute, were selected to administer the standards harmonization initiative. The resulting collaborative, known as the HITSP, brings together experts from across the healthcare community—from consumers to doctors, nurses, and hospitals; from those who develop healthcare IT products to those who use them; and from the government agencies who monitor the U.S. healthcare system to those organizations who actually write the standards.

The Panel's objectives are to serve and establish a cooperative partnership between the public and private sectors to achieve a widely accepted and useful set of standards that will enable and support widespread interoperability among healthcare software applications in a nationwide health information network (NHIN) for the United States; and to harmonize relevant standards in the healthcare industry to enable and advance interoperability of healthcare applications, and the interchange of healthcare data, to ensure accurate use, access, privacy, and security, both for supporting the delivery of care and public health. The result of HITSP's work to date has been the federal government's recognition of 30 standards within interoperability specifications for three of the American Health Information Community (AHIC) use cases (EHR/Lab, Consumer Empowerment, and Biosurveillance). It is currently working on interoperability specifications for additional AHIC-specified use cases.

System Reliability, Privacy, and Security

System reliability and security often come last in discussions of information system functionality. However, this should not cause their importance to be misconstrued but, rather, should reflect their underlying and cross-functional nature. Reliability and security relate to all aspects of EHR system functionality, from the policies and procedures that address confidentiality and data integrity to the nuts and bolts of hardware and software that both safeguard data from compromise and ensure system performance.

Reliability

In a computer system, reliability refers to the ability of a system to perform its functions without errors, crashes, or performance problems.

Errors

Errors occur because of a system performance issue or lack of security. A system performance issue may result from overloading the system with data and actions beyond its capabilities, poor maintenance, physical breakage (such as someone dropping a PC or accidentally cutting a cable), or other technical difficulties. In the description of network architecture, it was noted that techniques are used to prevent the collision of data. Such an occurrence would be a technical difficulty. Errors also occur, however, because someone or something has caused them to occur. Security features are intended to safeguard against such potential harm, although obviously there is not 100 percent protection.

Errors are extremely critical in healthcare because they can result not only in added cost (in terms of correction or liability), but also in the death of a patient. Moreover, they are not always immediately identifiable. Constantly monitoring systems and the routines that check for errors and reviewing output are important activities in identifying and tracking the causes of errors.

Crashes

Crashes are caused by many of the same system performance issues or breach of security issues that errors are, but rather than produce an error, they cause the system to stop functioning altogether. In a mission-critical IS such as the EHR, full-redundancy backup must be in place to ensure that the system operates 24 hours a day, 7 a week. However, full-redundancy backup does not negate the need for disaster recovery planning and emergency mode operations procedures (that is, contingency planning) because a backup system is intended only to serve in the event of emergency.

Performance Problems

Performance problems are produced by many of the same events that cause errors and crashes but are more likely to be annoyances, such as slow response times in data entry or retrieval. Performance problems also can be associated with insufficient processing power and size of hardware. System monitoring should identify when the volume of data and number of transactions are beginning to be too much for the capacity of the system.

Moreover, performance can be a human issue, related to the number of workstations, printers, and other devices needed to operate the EHR. Without an adequate number of workstations (including desktop, portable, and handhelds), the EHR will not be used to its full extent.

Privacy and Security

Although healthcare has always been concerned with patient privacy and the confidentiality of health information, prior to HIPAA there were no national standards to ensure equal privacy protections among all providers or a baseline of security to provide confidentiality, data integrity, and availability. HIPAA includes several important provisions for covered entities (health plans, healthcare clearinghouses, and providers who conduct administrative and financial transactions in electronic form) and other entities with which they do business. HIPAA addresses qualifications for health insurance and brought about the fraud and abuse regulations that have led to the creation of corporate compliance initiatives.

The HIPAA's Administrative Simplification provisions require use of standard transactions and code sets for the electronic exchange of financial and administrative transactions (see section on ASC X12N in this chapter), and complementary privacy and security provisions.

The Privacy Rule

HIPAA's Privacy Rule addresses uses and disclosures of protected health information (PHI) and individuals' rights in their PHI, including the right to a notice of privacy practices, access to their health information, and the right to request amendment, restrictions and confidential communications, and accounting for disclosures. The Privacy Rule also has administrative standards that require the designation of an information privacy official (IPO), the provision of training, the handling of complaints, and the application of appropriate sanctions against members of the workforce who fail to comply with privacy requirements. These requirements also require the entities covered under HIPAA to mitigate the harmful effects of a use or disclosure violation, refrain from retaliation, and have in place policies, procedures, and documentation in support of compliance.

The administrative standards of the Privacy Rule also include a requirement for administrative, technical, and physical safeguards to protect the privacy of PHI. Sometimes this standard is referred to as the minisecurity rule. It is important because HIPAA's Security Rule addresses PHI only in electronic (ePHI) form.

It is also important to recognize that state law preempts HIPAA where state law is more stringent than the HIPAA Privacy Rule. This is particularly applicable in the area of consents and authorizations for uses and disclosures. The final form of the Privacy Rule permits—but does not require—consent for use or disclosure of PHI to carry out treatment, payment, or healthcare operations (§164.506(b)). Many states, especially when setting up requirements for health information exchange (HIE), are incorporating a consent requirement for participation.

Health Information Security and Privacy Collaboration

Recognizing the "crazy quilt" of state laws and the impact lack of harmonization may have on a nationwide health information network, the federal government supported the Health Information Security and Privacy Collaboration (HISPC) to assess and develop plans to address variations in organization-level business policies and state laws that affect privacy and security practices that may pose challenges to interoperable HIE. HISPC is a partnership consisting of a multidisciplinary team of experts and the National Governors' Association (NGA). A set of reports developed under the Privacy and Security Solutions for Interoperable Health Information Exchange project has been released. The reports summarize the work and plans generated by 34 states and territories engaged in the project, sponsored by the Agency for Healthcare Research and Quality (AHRQ) and conducted under contract by RTI International. They also provide guidance for ensuring the safety and security of electronic HIE (HISPC 2007).

The Security Rule

The HIPAA Security Rule includes standards for administrative, physical, and technical safeguards, as well as requirements for policies, procedures, and documentation. The specific security standards are discussed in the next section.

HIPAA's Administrative Simplification provisions also include two other important requirements. The first requirement relates to organizational issues, including how covered entities relate to one another as (1) affiliated covered entities, where there is common ownership or control; (2) organized healthcare arrangements, where there is data sharing for quality or utilization purposes; and (3) hybrid entities, where a company has healthcare components (such as a retail pharmacy in a grocery store or a faculty practice plan in a university). Covered entities also exchange data with a significant number of business associates (BAs), and business associates frequently use agents to perform work for them. Because HIPAA could not regulate nonhealthcare entities directly, it requires covered entities to have contracts with its BAs to ensure that they and their agents follow the same set of standards with respect to PHI.

As more and more uses are made of PHI, deidentified health information, and personal health information (that is, information compiled outside of the HIPAA construct of covered entities and business associates), especially in light of new HIE organizations and the concept of the NHIN privacy and security controls become increasingly important. The National Committee on Vital and Health Statistics (NCVHS), which is a statutory advisory body to HHS tasked within HIPAA to provide oversight, was asked by the ONC to recommend practical solutions for protecting current health information usage. Among its recommendations on data stewardship are tighter contract provisions between covered entities and BAs, as well as extension of HIPAA principles to PHR vendors. While not carrying the force of law or regulation, this guidance is being widely adopted by HIE organizations (NCVHS 2007).

Threats to Security

The HIPAA Security Rule is risk-based. This means the standards provide general requirements for security safeguards, but the organization must decide, through a risk analysis, what specific controls will afford those safeguards.

A *risk analysis* is a process in which the organization analyzes its vulnerabilities or weaknesses in security controls, and threats that might exploit them. Controls to thwart threats to vulnerabilities should consider the size, complexity, and capabilities of the organization; the organization's technical infrastructure; the costs of security measures; and the probability and criticality of potential risks to ePHI. Figure 10.4 illustrates the risk analysis process.

Figure 10.4.   Risk analysis process

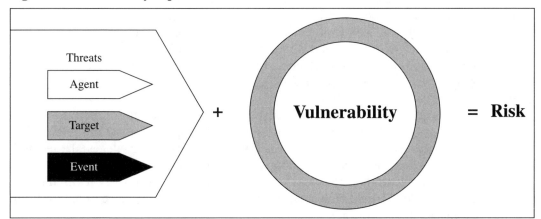

Threats are typically considered to be composed of agents, targets, and events. An agent is usually an individual with the motivation and resources to carry out a threat (for example, a computer-savvy disgruntled employee or a thrill-seeking hacker with a password cracker). Targets are the objects of a threat. HIPAA identifies data confidentiality, integrity, and availability as the objects to be concerned about. Many add accountability to this group. Events are the results of the threat. In general, four types of events can occur (and each is related to one of the types of targets):

- *Unauthorized access and disclosure* is a threat to confidentiality in which data are accessed inappropriately or revealed to an unauthorized person.

- *Modification, alteration, or destruction of data* causes a data integrity problem and often a data availability problem as well.

- *Denial-of-service attacks* prevent the system from performing its functions and may render data unavailable.

- *Repudiation* is a situation in which a user or system denies having performed some action, such as modification of information. There is no accountability for the action.

Vulnerabilities are weaknesses, or gaps, that occur in administrative processes, the physical facility, and the technical infrastructure. Lack of policy or policy enforcement is a common vulnerability. In healthcare, a wide-open campus with unguarded doors is a vulnerability. Viruses and other malicious software can attack any computer system, but as computers become more networked and especially use the Internet for communications, they are much more vulnerable to all forms of attack.

Security Controls

There are many tools on the market that can be purchased to thwart attacks, and as rapidly as new forms of attack are being designed, new tools are being created. To fully understand an organization's security needs and invest wisely in security, it is important to consider HIPAA's requirements not only to identify threats and vulnerabilities, but also to understand how likely they are to occur and what impact they will have. If a network has minimal attempts at attack, an intrusion detection system will not be needed. Alternatively, if a hospital's employees are uncomfortable seeking care at the hospital, weak access controls could be a reason worth investigating.

Moreover, technical tools are not the only, or necessarily the most effective, control. The strongest possible authentication measures and audit logs may exist in the organization, but if management does not support sanctions for misuse of privileges, the technology cannot be effective. In December 2006, CMS, which has jurisdiction for enforcing the Security Rule, released its first Security Guidance document, primarily focused on the physical security of devices and media, clearly recognizing the importance of policy, training, and risk management strategies.

Even more recently, CMS initiated proactive, HIPAA security on-site investigations and compliance reviews. The first such review was conducted in March 2007, at Atlanta's Piedmont Hospital (Vijayan 2007).

Most security experts believe that a layered approach to security is critical, which means two things:

First, there is an entire system of security in which:

- A solid base of management support understands and can articulate its risk posture that establishes the level of controls desired.

- A thorough applications and data criticality analysis, as well as a vulnerability assessment, has been performed that supports understanding of a potential threat's impact.

- Executive management has approved policies that reflect the organization's risk posture and are available to all members of the workforce and procedures that provide detailed instruction for carrying out controls (some of which may be sensitive information that should be safeguarded to the same or even greater extent than PHI).

- Responsibility for security is part of everyone's job, but the organization also needs to designate an ISO to provide oversight.

- Administrative, operational, and physical controls support technical controls, and these all have been appropriately implemented and tested, and changes managed effectively.

- Users have been thoroughly trained on security, with follow-up provided via ongoing awareness building and reminders.

- An ongoing auditing and monitoring process serves continuously as a feedback loop to enhance controls, where necessary.

Second, a layered approach to security also refers to the logical and physical structure of controls that are implemented. These were illustrated in Figure 10.1 in relationship to the overall network architecture. There should be controls from the outermost layer of the network (perimeter layer controls), throughout the network (network layer controls), at each device (host layer controls), in the applications (application layer controls), and to the data (data layer controls). For example, HIPAA includes implementation specifications relative to encryption for data at rest (that would be applied at the data layer) and for transmission security (that would be applied at the perimeter layer and possibly the network layer). Access controls and authentication mechanisms may be specific to data, to the application, or to the network. Figure 10.5 illustrates a layered approach to security.

Figure 10.5.   Layered approach to security

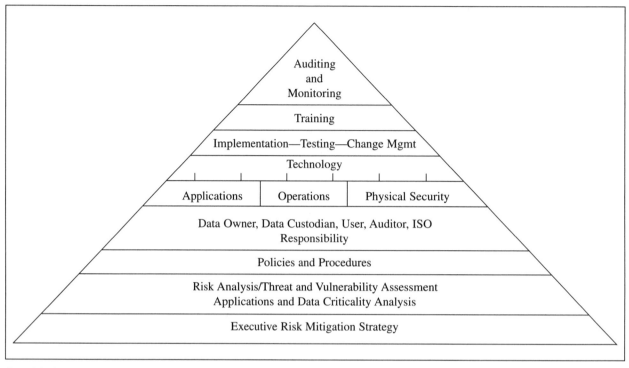

HIPAA Security Rule Standards

Table 10.1 provides a summary of the HIPAA Security Rule standards. All federal regulations are filed in the Code of Federal Regulations (CFR) by section number. In addition to the standards, the Security Rule includes implementation specifications that are either required (R) or addressable (A). Required implementation specifications must be implemented. Addressable implementation specifications must be implemented or an alternative measure should be implemented, if reasonable and appropriate. Any deviation from implementing the specification must have an explanation documented.

Authentication Requirements

It should be observed that the HIPAA Security Rule, while requiring user identification and making encryption and decryption addressable for access control and requiring person or entity authentication, does not specify the exact nature of signature requirements a healthcare organization should use. Three general types of authentication currently may be used in information systems to replicate the "wet signature" in a paper environment (Health IT Certification 2008):

- *Digitized signatures* are representations of a wet signature made by a person signing onto a signature pad, the scanned image of which is stored in the information system in association with the information that is signed. Although this is generally

Table 10.1.   Summary of the HIPAA Security Rule standards

Security Standards	CFR Sections	Security Implementation Specifications (R) = Required, (A) = Addressable
Administrative Safeguards		
Security Management Process	§164.308(a)(1)	Risk Analysis (R) Risk Management (R) Sanction Policy (R) Information System Activity Review (R)
Assigned Security Responsibility	§164.308(a)(2)	(R)
Workforce Security	§164.308(a)(3)	Authorization and/or Supervision (A) Workforce Clearance Procedure (A) Termination Procedures (A)
Information Access Management	§164.308(a)(4)	Isolating Health Care Clearinghouse Function (R) Access Authorization (A) Access Establishment and Modification (A)
Security Awareness and Training	§164.308(a)(5)	Security Reminders (A) Protection from Malicious Software (A) Log-in Monitoring (A) Password Management (A)
Security Incident Procedures	§164.308(a)(6)	Response and Reporting (R)
Contingency Plan	§164.308(a)(7)	Data Backup Plan (R) Disaster Recovery Plan (R) Emergency Mode Operation Plan (R) Testing and Revision Procedure (A) Applications and Data Criticality Analysis (A)
Evaluation	§164.308(a)(8)	(R)
Business Associate Contracts and Other Arrangements	§164.308(b)(1)	(R)

(continued)

Table 10.1.   (Continued)

Security Standards	CFR Sections	Security Implementation Specifications (R) = Required, (A) = Addressable
Physical Safeguards		
Facility Access Controls	§164.310(a)(1)	Contingency Operations (A) Facility Security Plan (A) Access Control and Validation Procedures (A) Maintenance Records (A)
Workstation Use	§164.310(b)	(R)
Workstation Security	§164.310(c)	(R)
Device and Media Controls	§164.310(d)(1)	Disposal (R) Media Re-use (R) Accountability (A) Data Backup and Storage (A)
Technical Safeguards		
Access Control	§164.312(a)	Unique User Identification (R) Emergency Access Procedure (R) Automatic Logoff (A) Encryption and Decryption (A)
Audit Controls	§164.312(b)	(R)
Integrity	§164.312(c)(1)	Mechanism to Authenticate ePHI (A)
Person or Entity Authentication	§164.312(d)	(R)
Transmission Security	§164.312(e)(1)	Integrity Controls (A) Encryption (A)

Source: 45 CFR 164 Appendix A, Security Standards: Matrix.

considered a weak form of signature in information systems, it is acceptable under the Electronic Signatures in Global and National Commerce Act (ESIGN), which was signed into law in June 2000. ESIGN defines an electronic signature as: "an electronic sound, symbol, or process, attached to or logically associated with a contract or other record and executed or adopted by the person with the intent to sign the record." Such a signature is widely used in retail stores. In healthcare, digitized signatures are being used to capture patient signatures on authorization forms, consents, and other documents when presented electronically.

- *Electronic signature* is the use of a password, token, biometrics or some combination of such to create a logical manifestation of a signature. (The stronger the component and the more components used, the stronger the authentication becomes. In other words, a password is not as strong as biometrics, and a password and token together is even stronger. When two components are used together, this is referred to as two-factor authentication.) It should be noted that a UserID is technically not part of the authentication, but is used to identify the user for purposes of triggering the access controls. Organizations may impose specific policies around how one may obtain a UserID, including requiring presence in person and specific credentialing. For instance, in order for a user to write a prescription for controlled substances, the user must have on file a Drug Enforcement Administration (DEA) number. The electronic signature may be invoked when the user logs on to the system with UserID and whatever components of electronic signature are required; many healthcare organizations require an additional "click," or acknowledgment of action for certain functions. For example, in signing a transcribed document, the system may require that the user log on, but the document will not be considered signed until the end of the document is reached and the user clicks an icon signifying acceptance of the document. The electronic signature is the most commonly used means to authenticate information electronically today in health record applications.

- *Digital signature* is the term reserved to describe a process of encryption and non-repudiation. Encryption provides the means to protect the content of a message from being revealed (whether the message is a signature only or content and signature). Encryption is a form of cryptography where an algorithm is used to scramble the content so that only an equivalent algorithm can be used to decrypt the message. Nonrepudiation is substantial evidence of the identity of the signer of a message and of message integrity, sufficient to prevent a party from successfully denying the origin, submission, or delivery of the message and the integrity of its contents.

    There are many mathematical algorithms that have been used to create various forms of digital signature. The NIST has a Digital Signature Standard (DSS) that has become a Federal Information Processing Standard (FIPS 186-1). This standard enables the use of the RSA (Rivest-Shamir-Adleman) digital signature algorithm or the DSA (Digital Signature Algorithm) to digitally sign messages. RSA is the most popular digital signature, used in many Web browsers and with the Secure Sockets Layer (SSL) protocol. When integrity of the data within the message is required, the Secure Hash Algorithm (SHA-1) can be added. Hash, also called a *message digest*, is a number generated from a string of text. It is substantially smaller than the text itself, and is generated by a formula in such a way that it is extremely unlikely that some other text will produce the same hash value.

Table 10.2.   How PKI Works

To do this . . .	Use
Send an encrypted message	Receiver's public key
Send an encrypted signature	Sender's private key
Decrypt an encrypted message	Receiver's private key
Decrypt an encrypted signature (and authenticate the sender)	Sender's public key

Source: SearchSecurity.com October 2006.

Public Key Infrastructure

Public key infrastructure (PKI) is the set of policies, procedures, standards, and practices that enable use of a digital signature. PKI consists of a certificate authority (CA) that issues and verifies a digital certificate (using the X.509 digital certificate standard) that identifies the individual, a registration authority (RA) that acts as the verifier for the CA before a digital certificate is issued to an individual, one or more directories where the certificate and their public keys are held, and a certificate management system. The process of digital signature works with a combination of public key and private key cryptography, as illustrated in table 10.2.

Currently there is no requirement within HIPAA or any other federal law for use of a digital signature.

Identity Theft

According to the Federal Bureau of Investigation (FBI) and Consumer Sentinel, the federal government's Web site focusing on the fight against fraud, identity theft has been identified as one of the fastest-growing crimes in the U.S., affecting as many as 10 million people each year.

Misuse of credit cards accounts for half of all forms of identity theft. There are certainly many things individuals and organizations can do to reduce the risk of such theft. Healthcare organizations that accept credit cards for payment should already be aware of the Payment Card Industry (PCI) Data Security Standard (DSS) that was developed by five major credit card associations to protect customer information through the global adoption of consistent data security measures. It is currently mandated that all online and brick-and-mortar merchants and service providers meet certain security standards when storing, processing, and transmitting cardholder information. The regulations are complex and require significant reporting to guarantee the privacy and integrity of customer data. Even the American Medical Association (AMA) has warned physicians of identity theft issues in general and medical identity theft in particular—especially as such theft is often an "inside job." Cited in a recent AMA newsletter (Wilson 2008) was a report from the World Privacy Forum, a nonprofit research and consumer education organization, about an employee of a provider organization who pled guilty to selling information involving more than 1,000 patients and which resulted in $7 million in Medicare fraud—despite the organization having browser controls to limit the number of records employees could view.

In June 2008, the ONC for Health Information Technology has awarded a contract for the assessment and evaluation of the scope of medical identity theft in the U.S. (HDM 2008) **Medical identity theft** is the inappropriate or unauthorized misrepresentation of individually identifiable health information for the purpose of obtaining access to property or services, which may result in long-lasting harm to an individual interacting with the healthcare continuum. Medical identity theft accounts for 3 percent of identity theft crimes according to the Federal Trade Commission (FTC). Examples of medical identity theft include situations wherein an individual accesses medical services in another individual's name to obtain benefits for which the individual is not eligible, obtain services for which the individual will not pay, or perpetuate other fraud or illegal activity, such as erroneous billings or drug-seeking behavior for personal use or illegal distribution. AHIMA has published a practice brief on how to prevent, investigate, and mitigate the damages caused by medical identity theft (AHIMA 2008).

Emerging Technologies

Obviously technologies and their uses are rapidly evolving. It is said that technology changes every 18 months. Although healthcare may not always appear to be at the forefront of adopting new technology, understanding trends in emerging technologies is critical to making the right choices about what new technologies to adopt and when.

New technologies for healthcare are not unique to information systems. In fact, healthcare often adopts new technologies more rapidly in the clinical arena than in the IS arena. Everything from smart bandages that can differentiate among bacteria, new contamination-detection technology that can alert someone that his or her hands are not clean enough, RFID tags that can be implanted under the skin, digital pens, to radio-surgical technology to enhance radiography and radiation therapy have been identified.

Monitoring publications and Web sites is critical in the development and use of EHR systems. Even if you already have an EHR system, understanding what new technology is being created can help you anticipate upgrades, push for adoption of new technologies from your vendor, and respond to challenges from those who want to adopt new technology you do not have yet.

Another important aspect of monitoring emerging technology is the ability to plan for new technology. Many healthcare providers have bought system components from a single vendor because the components were well integrated. This strategy of buying from one vendor is called buying "best of fit." But as IS capabilities have expanded, some of these vendors did not support some of the newer functionality or, in some cases, purchased functionality from other companies that was not as interoperable. This has left many providers considering their options: Do they wait for their vendor to support new technology for their older systems? Do they buy an interface engine or the best interface programmers possible to adopt a best-of-breed strategy? Do they replace their aging systems? Obviously, there is no one right answer. However, to the extent that new systems are being acquired, it behooves the organization to buy as openly architected systems as possible so they can plug and play with many new technology components and to plan for obsolescence.

Conclusion

When a healthcare organization sets out to "buy" an EHR, it is essentially buying hardware and software to integrate data from multiple sources and to enable the functionality of information flow and knowledge support to be brought directly to the user.

From the perspective of users, the design of workstations for data capture and retrieval is critical. These human–computer interfaces should be as comfortable and intuitive to use as possible, help computer use integrate seamlessly into the workflow of the healthcare setting, and support the manner in which clinicians retrieve data.

Considerable functionality is unique to the EHR that organizations must decide on when developing their functional specifications. This chapter has attempted to categorize the functionality, to both ensure completeness and reflect the migration path of sophistication. The major categories chosen for this purpose include data access, data capture and retrieval and results management, communication/connectivity and patient support, administrative processes and workflow with order entry/management, decision support, and reporting and population health. Additionally, special attention must be given to system reliability and security because the EHR is a mission-critical system in which confidentiality, data integrity, and availability must be ensured.

References and Resources

AHIMA Practice Brief: e-HIM Workgroup on Medical Identity Theft: Mitigating Medical Identity Theft. 2008. *Journal of AHIMA* 79(7): 63–69.

American Health Information Community (AHIC). http://www.hhs.gov/healthit/community/background.

American Society for Testing and Materials. 2003. The Concept Paper of the Continuity of Care Record (CCR), Version 2.1b. www.astm.org.

Andrew, W.F., and R. Bruegel. 2003. 2003 CPR systems market summary. *ADVANCE for Health Information Executives* 7(4):59–64.

CMS. HIPAA Security Guidance. 2006 (Dec 28). www.cms.hhs.gov/SecurityStandard/Downloads/SecurityGuidanceforRemoteUseFinal122806.pdf.

CMS, Sample Interview and Document Request for HIPAA Security Onsite Investigations and Compliance Reviews, http://www.cms.hhs.gov/Enforcement/Downloads/InformationRequestforComplianceReviews.pdf.

CXO Media. 2000–2006. Executive Guide on Intranet/Extranet. www.guide.darwinmag.com.

Derfler, F.J., and Freed, L. 2000. *How Networks Work*. Indianapolis: Que Corporation.

Dubin, J. 2006 (March 20). PKI, *Information Security*. www.searchsecurity.com.

Featherly, K. 2005 (Jan.). Emerging technologies. *Healthcare Informatics*, 25–34.

Featherly, K. 2004 (Jan.). Emerging technologies. *Healthcare Informatics,* 29–38.

Federal Register. 2005 (Nov. 7). E-prescribing and the prescription drug program, final rule. 42 CFR Part 423, 67568–67595.

Federal Register, 2008 (June 27). Electronic Prescriptions for Controlled Substances; Proposed Rule. 21 CFR Parts 1300, 1304.

Federal Trade Commission, What Is Identity Theft? www.ftc.gov.

45 CFR 164. Appendix A. Security standards matrix.

HDM Breaking News 2008 (June 12). Medical Identity Theft Study Launched. www.healthdatamanagement. com/news.

Health Level 7 2007 (Feb. 12). Press Release: Continuity of Care Document, a Healthcare IT Interoperability Standards, Is Approved by Balloting Process and Endorsed by Healthcare IT Standards Panel. www.hl7.org.

He, H. 2003 (Sept 30). What is Service-Oriented Architecture. O'Reilly XML.com.

Healthcare Information Technology Standards Panel (HITSP). www.hitsp.org.

Health Information Security and Privacy Collaboration (HISPC). https://privacysecurity.rti.org.

Health IT Certification, LLC. 2008. Legal and Regulatory Aspects of HIT, EHR, and HIE, V6.0.

IEEE 802.3 2002 standard. www.standards.ieee.org/getieee802/download/802.3-2002.pdf.

iHealthBeat. 2007 (Dec. 14). DEA Takes Steps to Allow E-Rx of Controlled Substances.

iSeries home page. www.ibm.com/eserver/iseries.

National Committee on Vital and Health Statistics. 2007. Report on Enhancing Protections for Uses of Health Data: A Stewardship Framework.

NeoTool Development. n.d. Company Brochure: HL7 Desktop Reference Guide. Plano, TX: NeoTool.

PCI Security Standards Council. www.pcisecuritystandards.org.

Shakir, A.M. 1997 (July). HL7 reference information model: More robust and stable standards. *Healthcare Informatics.* www.healthcare-informatics.com.

Siwicki, B. 1998 (Feb.). Systems integration. *Health Data Management,* 75–86.

Telecommunications Industry Association. www.tiaonline.org.

Vijayan, J. 2007 (June 19). HIPAA Audit: The 42 Questions HHS Might Ask, *Computerworld.* http://www. computerworld.com/action/article.do?command=printArticleBasic&articleId=9025253.

W3C Working Group Note 11, Web Services Architecture, February 2004.

Welch, J.J. 1999. Virtual private networks. *Journal of AHIMA* 70(1):18–19.

Whitehead, P. 1997. *Teach Yourself Networking Visually.* Foster City, CA: IDG Books Worldwide.

Wilson, B. 2008 (March 3). Medical Identity Theft Is Often an "Inside Job." www.amednews.com.

Chapter 11
Return on Investment

An article discussing EHR and the return on investment (RIO) asked, "Is healthcare IT ROI an oxymoron?" (HIMSS 2003). A growing number of healthcare executives understand that there are significant projected benefits for EHR (C!TL 2003) and that acquiring such is becoming a cost of doing business in healthcare (Goldstein and Groen 2006). However, the price tag of an EHR project remains high and executives need to know the expenditure will, in fact, make a positive contribution to the organization's bottom line. Some organizations may require a strict financial impact analysis. Others may want to see a strong business case that incorporates various forms of value, including both financial results and quality benefits as described in chapter 5. This chapter:

- Distinguishes among various forms of financial impact analyses

- Identifies risks in conducting financial impact analyses

- Describes data collection processes for conducting financial impact analyses

- Explains how to compile a pro forma cost–benefit analysis to determine the feasibility of, and budget for, the EHR project

- Provides financial models for evaluating return on investment of EHR projects

- Identifies the advantages and pitfalls of performing a benefits realization study to evaluate the impact of the EHR

- Identifies potential sources of funding for an EHR project

Forms of Financial Impact Analysis

Three basic types of financial impact analysis may be performed for an EHR project. The terms associated with these analyses may vary somewhat. For instance, the term *return on investment* (ROI) may be used generically to describe financial impact analysis in general, or may refer to a specific type of financial impacts. The following terms and their definitions are used in this book to help distinguish between financial analyses with respect to timing and purpose:

- **Pro forma cost–benefit analysis**: An estimate of costs and benefits conducted before vendor selection to determine the feasibility of, and budget for, the EHR project. It is based on rough estimates and often is performed to prioritize capital investments or to establish a strategic plan to acquire financial resources. It may be accompanied by pro forma financial statements to predict the impact of the EHR expenditure on the organization's assets, liabilities, and fund balance. A pro forma cost-benefit analysis typically answers a CEO's question of "Will an EHR contribute to increased revenues as much as a new wing, parking lot, or medical device?" It has been observed that in the past 10 years, the nationwide average age of physical plants has increased 20 percent. Add to that capacity issues at many hospitals, and as one observer noted, "you've got the perfect storm of capital expenditures coming" (Solovy 2005). It is in this environment that an EHR project must compete.

- **ROI analysis**: An economic analysis that uses fairly firm cost and benefits estimates from finalist vendor candidates. The result of comparing costs and financial benefits given the specific product's functionality is evaluated against the organization's required **payback period** or **internal rate of return** (IRR) threshold criteria. It is one of the final steps in vendor selection, and its purpose is to justify the expenditure. A time-phased budget also may be prepared to estimate the project's impact on cash flow and to help identify financing requirements.

- **Benefits realization study**: An evaluation of the benefits that have accrued from the EHR investment. It may be performed at specific milestones in the life of the project and used to help in future systems planning, designing, and implementing. If either cost–benefit analysis or ROI, or both, is performed, benefits realization also can identify where deviations from projected benefits are so that corrective measures can be taken. Returning to questions a CEO might be considering include the fact that to date, the healthcare profit center has been the hospital and capital projects have been seen as a way to shore up that profit center. However, the EHR often results in fewer inpatient days and less hospital utilization, resulting in lowered profit. Furthermore, many industry watchers observe that healthcare is moving to ambulatory and home care, which to date have not been profit centers for hospitals. How, then, would an EHR make economic sense for a hospital? The key is to have a vision that creates a migration path for *both* profitable care delivery via new modalities *and* knowledge management that will likely support an EHR that extends across the continuum of care. This will carry the organization through today's transition to new forms and locations of care and into the recognition that "clicks, not bricks" make the difference. A CEO should be able to look at the balance sheet after an EHR has been implemented and understand that it was impacted by the EHR, even though there is no line item that says "EHR." Instead, every department or business unit will have been improved through use of the EHR.

Risks in Conducting Financial Impact Analysis

The following is a sample of recent articles describing EHR benefits that highlight some of the risks in attempting to conduct a financial impact analysis:

- *A Pilot Study to Document the Return on Investment for Implementing an Ambulatory Electronic Health Record at an Academic Medical Center* (Grieger, et al 2006) found a 16-month RIO and total annual savings in the first year of $14,055 per provider at the University of Rochester's five ambulatory offices with 28 providers.

- *Study: The Value of Electronic Health Records In Community Health Centers: Policy Implications* (Miller 2007) where quality improvement gains were found at six community health centers, while five of the six incurred ongoing, substantial net financial loses as a result of implementing EHRs.

- *Return on Investment Does Not Drive EHR Adoption in Hospitals* (Wise 2007) describes how there is a real business case to be made for EHRs, but the word has not gotten out. Cited in the report was a $2.5 million increase in revenue at Evanston Northwestern Healthcare in Chicago because of improved charge capture, and $775,000 savings in transcription costs at North Fulton Family Medicine in Georgia because of adopting EHRs.

- *Electronic Health Record Use and the Quality of Ambulatory Care in the United States* (Linder et al 2007) describes a study conducted on data from the 2003 and 2004 National Ambulatory Medical Care Survey and found no significant difference in performance [on quality indicators] between visits with vs. without EHR use.

How can studies be so far apart in their findings? In responding to the essence of this question, Jeffrey Linder and Blackford Middleton, who lead the Center for Information Technology Leadership (C!TL), both of whom are affiliated with Brigham and Women's Hospital and Harvard Medical School, made some important observations:

- During the period of their study (Linder et al 2007), many of the EHRs in use "were basically replacements for the paper chart." As a result, they did not reengineer processes or incorporate important features for quality and safety in their applications.

- "Even in the best EHRs, doctors hardly turn on the decision support function in the full complement of ways it can be turned on."

At least for this study where it is recognized that a fully comprehensive EHR was not being utilized, there was really no difference between a practice with or without an EHR, hence, how could one expect to find a difference in outcomes.

In addition to type of EHR and utilization considerations, it should be observed that most ROI studies have been conducted in ambulatory practices. It is difficult to experience true cost savings when only fractions of staff members' time can be saved by an EHR. Furthermore, without studying the continuum of care, it is difficult even to determine impact on quality.

However, while improved quality, medication safety, enhanced compliance efforts, utilization of evidence-based best practices, and patient satisfaction are all qualitative benefits, the long-term impact of these benefits can be financial, especially if a critical mass of full engagement of comprehensive systems occurs (Sarasohn-Kahn 2007). Richard Clarke, President and CEO of the Healthcare Financial Management Association (HFMA), has observed that "universal implementation of EHRs will produce a profound societal return, both in improving the quality of healthcare in our country and in reducing healthcare costs."

As a financial impact analysis is performed, it is important to understand the nature of the EHR being planned, the nature of financial gains that are truly feasible, the full impact of quality on cost, and the extent to which the organization believes it will gain full adoption of the EHR. In fact, many organizations are developing ROI analysis for different scenarios along their migration path.

Data Collection for Impact Analysis

Whatever form of impact analysis is performed, certain basic data must be collected. Essentially, these are cost data and benefits data.

Cost Data

Data to determine the cost of an EHR project must be obtained for hardware, software, implementation, maintenance, and support. The set of all costs associated with EHR is referred to as the **total cost of ownership**. Some vendors will only quote prices for software or software and their installation support. This skews the cost low because the organization will still have to acquire hardware (potentially including modifications to furnishings and other equipment), frequently require interfaces and other utilities not provided by the EHR vendor, may often need additional staff support for implementation, and must budget for ongoing maintenance and support as the EHR requires continual updating, tailoring, and upgrading.

Some of the costs will be one-time, and others will be ongoing. Some of the costs will be fixed, and others will be variable. The time period over which a cost–benefit analysis is performed, and thus the ongoing costs are projected, may be preestablished by management or an estimate of the investment's payback period.

Costing an EHR project is part psychology and part financial analysis. Some organizations try to attribute only costs directly associated with the EHR to the project in order to keep them initially within some preconceived notion of a budget. However, they then often find lack of support for acquiring the less-direct, but still necessary, components. In the end, not anticipating such costs puts the project over budget, or results in less success because the additional expenditures could not be made. For example, some organizations do not enhance their network sufficiently or provide ubiquitous human–computer interfaces and then wonder why users are unhappy with response time or refuse to use the system because they have to wait for a workstation. Many organizations do not initially invest in sufficient disaster recovery or other security services, only to find problems with downtime later.

Alternatively, organizations that attribute all costs to the EHR project to ensure its success must deal with the sticker shock up front. This may delay the project or elongate the migration path. This actually may be an appropriate solution, however, especially in comparison to a failed project due to cost overruns or inadequate expenditures.

Even when a total cost of ownership is attempted to be compiled, many organizations find they underestimate the cost of the EHR project. This is partly because they underestimate the level of effort needed to configure the system to their needs, maintain it, and properly train and support users. However, this also happens because of the pervasive nature of a comprehensive EHR project. Frequently, the impact of the EHR on other systems and associated operations is not fully anticipated. That is why development of a migration plan that clearly lays out the various associated strategies is so critical to the success of an EHR project. For example, although a computerized provider order entry (CPOE) system may be able to be implemented within the existing ancillary system environment, an organization may find that lack of bidirectional interfaces from the laboratory and pharmacy systems results in less than fully comprehensive clinical decision support that provides the value to the clinician in using it. A migration path also contributes to the psychology of costing the project, as executive management and the board of directors understand how the pieces tie together and the ongoing commitment necessary to keep the project up to date. For example, any time there is an upgrade to one system, the interface (for both systems) must be checked and potentially reworked.

The following descriptions help identify all the costs associated with the EHR. How costs are categorized is not as important as ensuring that all costs are considered. However, care should also be taken not to include the same costs twice.

Hardware Costs

Hardware costs include the cost of computers, network devices, workstations (of all forms), printers, scanners, and any other equipment associated with the project. Sometimes hardware costs also include special furniture or remodeling. Hardware is usually a one-time, fixed cost unless the equipment is leased, in which case the cost of the lease is spread over time.

The cost of the hardware also may be spread over time if not all required hardware is purchased at once. For instance, a large organization may phase in its EHR system over a period of a few years and not buy all workstations initially (although this may result in foregoing some quantity discounts). Hardware that is purchased also is generally depreciated. This has an impact on the organization's financial statements. Finally, hardware upgrades and additions should be planned. Even though hardware is generally considered a one-time cost, planning for obsolescence and additions should be identified across the entire budget period.

Software Costs

Software may or may not be a one-time cost and is often variable. Some vendors price the EHR software as a one-time cost that is essentially a license through perpetuity; others sell it as a license that must be renewed periodically, at which time the cost will likely increase.

Some vendors license EHR software for a given number of users or according to some other pricing structure. For physician offices, many vendors price the license per provider and include a ratio of support staff to the provider (for example, four or five support staff to every physician). Thus, software pricing varies considerably.

As the healthcare organization grows, the organization may have to acquire additional licenses. Software includes not only the software licensed by the EHR vendor, but any other software that may be needed to make it work, such as the operating system, database management system, interfaces from other systems, an interface engine, a data repository, rules engines, and so forth. Another common addition is a license fee for access to special utilities, such as report-writing software, the CPT codes, drug knowledge databases, pharmaceutical formulary information, and benchmarking data. Additional fees may be associated with using network transmission media. Some EHR vendors include many of these additional licenses in their overall license; others price them separately, or do not include them at all and leave the organization to negotiate for such licenses.

Any organization doing cost–benefit analysis for an EHR project must decide what hardware and software costs will be attributed to the EHR project and what costs will be attributed to basic infrastructure. For example, some organizations include only the EHR software itself, attributing operating system software, networking fees, and other such costs to basic IT infrastructure. This also may be the case for certain hardware costs, such as upgrading a network. Although additional bandwidth may be required for the EHR, it may be considered an infrastructure cost that supports the organization as a whole, including its e-mail and other uses. Organizations may or may not attribute the cost of knowledge bases to the EHR, depending on whether it can be attributed to a specific department or set of users. For instance, benchmarking software enabled by the EHR may be attributed to the EHR itself or to a quality improvement department or marketing department. A medication administration record function may be attributed to nursing or the EHR. Although these are important considerations in association with the EHR project, they are all costs and, ultimately, need to be evaluated in light of the organization's capital budget.

Implementation Costs

Implementation costs are primarily one-time costs. They generally include installation, training, and testing.

Installation Costs

Implementation of an EHR includes many different tasks. At a minimum, a vendor installs the software that is licensed and provides some basic training on the system. Internal staff then may have to manage the rest of the implementation aspects, including installing the hardware in preparation for the software installation, performing the system build to configure the product for its own use, writing or hiring other programmers to write interfaces, conducting testing, and training all end users. In other cases, components of implementation beyond the basic installation of software may be purchased from the vendor as additional services. Still other vendors actually do not sell a system without providing all such services and routinely include these costs in the basic price. Understanding what is being bought is important in understanding the price of a product. An initially low price may add up to be a high cost if all such services are priced separately.

For an EHR, system build is often the most time-consuming part of implementation, and the part that requires the most user input. **System build** is the configuration of the system to meet the organization's specific needs. It includes creation of master tables with the organization's information, such as its physician list, employee list, names of departments, formulary, protocols for workflows and processes, and much other organization-specific information. It also includes the design and documentation of screens and their drop-down menus, pick lists, and customization of other data capture tools. Additionally, it includes construction of rules logic, clinical protocols, incorporation of knowledge bases, and other decision support factors. Although most EHR products come with a default set of such system characteristics, the more customization desired, the higher the implementation costs.

Other implementation costs will vary with how much internal staff have the time and expertise to perform various tasks. For example, there may be costs associated with setting up workstations, plugging in printers, running cable for the network or setting up wireless access points, designing storage systems, installing redundant back-up systems, and enhancing security measures. If the EHR includes a Web portal, home pages need to be designed and implemented, and content needs to be acquired and loaded. Moreover, implementation must include thorough process redesign and testing. A significant body of literature has started to be developed on EHR components that have not worked well or have contributed to medical errors because processes associated with the systems were not evaluated and tested thoroughly. Training and user support during go-live, when the system is first rolled out for use, also are areas where many organizations do not budget fully. Many believe the systems to be sufficiently intuitive or that super users will be available to help others, but such availability of support is often not practical in a busy healthcare environment. Implementation also requires a comprehensive set of documentation to support the system.

Implementation costs also may include monies paid for interfaces, data conversion, project management, and other special aspects required to implement the EHR system. As previously noted, consultants who are experts in project management are frequently hired to guide and oversee installation. This relieves existing staff to conduct the actual implementation. External support also can be especially useful when multiple vendors require coordination, such as when special interfaces have to be written. The third party can serve as a neutral party to gain cooperation. Many times, organizations find it less expensive to hire expert consultants for implementation when the IS department lacks the staff or expertise but is able to maintain it thereafter. This is often referred to as outsourcing the implementation.

Additional operational costs also are common and these generally extend beyond the implementation phase. Organizations may hire additional specialists in information management, including a **medical director of information systems** (MDIS) or chief medical informatics officer (CMIO), a nurse informaticist, health informaticists, and other clinical, or business, and technical analysts.

Training Costs

The importance of training cannot be emphasized enough. Training costs are both one-time and ongoing costs, as well as direct and indirect costs. Training may be conducted in a variety of ways, but typically, a set of super users are trained, often by the vendor and at a direct cost.

These individuals then train trainers who train end users. The cost of train-the-trainer includes not only vendor fees, but also potential travel to a vendor training site. In addition, the costs of staff training must consider staff time. In many cases, staff must be replaced during their training experience. Overtime or replacement staff costs may be incurred whether training is conducted away from the work environment or on site. If training can be performed directly on the job, the costs may be minimized, but not altogether dropped.

Some costs may be associated with outfitting a training room, buying training materials, or establishing a training or demo system. An alternative is to hire temporary staff to train and support users during their initial work with the system. If temporary staff are used, however, a sufficient number of staff must be available to train newcomers in the future. In some instances, training manuals must be prepared. Most EHR products come with online "help," but some organizations prepare a basic set of EHR training materials for all new users, customized to the organization's requirements. The initial training effort will be large, but ongoing training of new members of the workforce as well as reinforcement of training should not be forgotten in ongoing costs.

Another consideration is reimbursement of physicians for their training time. In physician offices, there also may be reimbursement for, or at least accounting for, loss of revenue if the physicians' schedules have to be altered to accommodate the learning curve.

Testing Costs

Testing and its costs also are often not adequately budgeted. It is essential to create an entire test environment so not only the initial component development can be performed and tested, but so fixes, patches, upgrades, and their associated interfaces can be tested without impacting the production systems. Many organizations already have test environments, but some do not and others may be insufficient to accommodate EHR testing. Some organizations consider using third parties to validate testing to ensure that systems are truly ready for production.

Finally, the cost of planning for the EHR project may be factored into the implementation cost. Although staff time for planning generally is not attributed to a project, special costs associated with hiring a consultant to help with the cost–benefit/ROI analysis and vendor selection may be included in overall project costs. Other costs associated with project planning also may be included. Some are trivial, but others can be significant, such as site visits to conduct due diligence on vendor products.

Maintenance Costs

Ongoing maintenance costs generally include the maintenance of hardware and software. Software maintenance agreements include regular upgrades, certain enhancements, and the ability to obtain help from the vendor when problems occur. Most vendors have a flat fee, which can be anywhere from 15 percent to 20 percent of the software licensure, but others have a fee schedule based on usage, which may be described as a **service-level agreement** (SLA). Such SLAs may be based on the nature of the service to be provided, the time during which service may be available (for example, 24x7 or only certain hours of operation), or volume of service calls.

Support Costs

Support costs are generally ongoing costs associated with keeping the system running well and up to date. The upgrades provided by the vendor under the maintenance agreement may have to be loaded and tested by IT support personnel. There will be ongoing support of trainers, testers, and clinicians to continuously review clinical decision support systems and keep tables current with the latest medical knowledge, vocabularies, drugs, and so on.

Often healthcare organizations use one or more physicians to champion the EHR project and reimburse them for their time, which can be anywhere from 1 day a week to full time (although most physicians prefer to retain some practice time). In hospitals and large clinics, physician champions can spend as much as half their time assisting in all phases of planning, selection, implementation, and ongoing maintenance of templates, practice guidelines, and so on.

Sources of Cost Data

Where to obtain the various estimates for cost data depends, in part, on the timing of the impact analysis. The organization will not have firm cost data for a pro forma cost–benefit analysis, but only fairly broad estimates. A few vendors may be invited to review the organization and provide a rough estimate. Because the vendor will not have done a comprehensive evaluation of the organization's present systems, and because the organization may not yet have a comprehensive set of functional requirements, both parties are somewhat "blind." Moreover, at this time, the vendor will not be providing any discount or incentive pricing. However, these rough estimates will give a good idea of the type of hardware required for the type of system being considered and a range of prices for the software. The fact that the estimates are not discounted probably is in the organization's favor because discounted costs might contribute to an underestimation of the true cost.

On the other hand, if the organization is conducting an ROI analysis, it will want to obtain a firm quote from the vendor or vendors of choice for the specific configuration desired. At this time, the organization may have already begun to negotiate some form of discount, incentive, or financing and can factor these costs in as well.

In both scenarios, it is important to ensure that as many of the costs as can be identified have been covered adequately. The organization should be realistic but not underestimate the potential for unplanned costs. Because the EHR project is truly a strategic investment, on par with bricks and mortar projects with which it regularly competes, contingency costs are common and should be anticipated by those with final authority to approve it. It is not unusual to include the costs of dealing with labor issues, unexpected shortage of materials, and so on in a building or renovation project, and so contingency costs also should be included in the EHR project. Some organizations budget as much as 30 percent for contingencies, especially when they are new to implementing clinical systems and are planning implementation of a large array of components.

Benefits Data

Quantifiable benefits are achieved basically through one of five ways: cost savings, productivity improvements, revenue increases, contribution to profit, and cost avoidance. All these depend on the organization's process redesign efforts and the likelihood of compliance with changes. These are not trivial factors. Organizations that implement EHR systems must anticipate and manage for a significant level of change. Conducting a financial impact analysis clearly identifies the benefits that must be achieved to pay for the system. Some organizations will not expect a full ROI for this infrastructure project but, instead, will consider its strategic contribution to the overall goals of the organization. Still, a benefits analysis or benefits realization study can motivate the necessary changes and maximize their opportunity for achievement.

Cost Savings

Cost savings are direct reduction in expenditures. Some of these can be significant, whereas others are trivial. For example, if the EHR will eliminate a large proportion of dictation through the use of templates, transcription expenses would be eliminated. This would include both transcriptionists who are on staff—if their positions are eliminated, and outsourced transcription services. For an ambulatory environment, this can be a significant benefit. However, most hospitals will find such savings a long time in coming. Most will want their physicians to continue dictating discharge summaries, operative reports, and consultations. Although it is feasible to reduce the cost of transcription of history and physical examinations, x-ray reports, and potentially emergency department reports, even these can be a hard sell. Another cost savings is paper chart supplies. Again, this is common in the ambulatory environment and much less common in hospitals. Hospitals often find their paper processing costs go up—as they either will not eliminate filing paper (and often find the volume of paper generated by an EHR to be more than in a paper-based environment) or will find themselves printing to paper only to scan back into an electronic document management systems (EDMS); and then find the need to print from such systems when end users do not like viewing the images online. Another potential cost savings area is chart archiving, and here both hospitals and clinics find they can reduce costs if they scan all paper.

Productivity Improvements

Productivity improvements through EHR are real, but may or may not result in actual financial savings. Most productivity improvement benefits have to be projected through process redesign efforts. Each area affected by the EHR should identify specific goals and the functionality that will assist in achieving those goals, and then commit to seeing the goals realized.

Several different sources of data may be used to anticipate productivity improvements. The process assessment performed by the organization should be the primary resource. The experience of vendors with implementations at similar institutions can also be helpful in directing the organization to look for additional benefits. Moreover, the body of literature is solid and fairly extensive on EHR benefits and can be invaluable in benchmarking how realistic impacts may be.

When a process redesign effort has been conducted, it is important to quantify the results for use in the impact analyses. Figure 11.1 displays a tool that combines a simple systems flowchart with metrics to measure the steps in the flow of the process. The example used in the tool is that of the flow of a request to a clinic by a patient for a prescription refill and through to the pharmacy prior to EHR implementation. A similar flowchart would be created to illustrate the anticipated changes with an e-prescribing function in the EHR, and then the metrics would be compared.

Figure 11.1.   Process redesign quantification

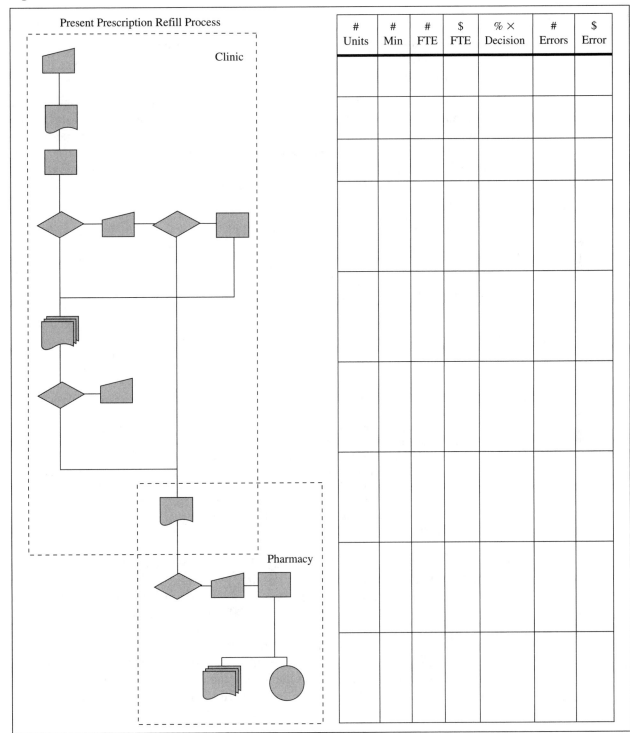

# Units	# Min	# FTE	$ FTE	% × Decision	# Errors	$ Error

The example illustrated in figure 11.1 uses the following metrics to quantify the steps in the process:

- *Number of units performed:* Generally, this is captured per day, although if the number of units performed per day is small, it may be appropriate to use weekly or monthly figures. The goal is to summarize the data on an annual basis.

- *Number of minutes it takes to perform the step:* Generally, this is an average number of minutes. If the step takes a highly variable amount of time, the minimum, maximum, and most common time can be recorded. Also, if certain tasks are performed only on certain days of the week or month, care should be taken in performing subsequent calculations. In addition to actual minutes to perform the step, some process redesign analysts may include the number of minutes of elapsed time between steps. This helps illustrate the delay factor.

- *Number of full-time equivalents (FTEs) to perform the step:* Generally, this is not how many FTEs but, rather, the percent of each FTE's time. For example, if 10 refill calls from patients are received per day, and each takes 5 minutes on the phone (the first task), that might represent 10 percent of a person's time. This is calculated in the following manner:

  > Assuming that 480 minutes are in a workday (60 minutes/hour times an 8-hour workday), if ten units take 5 minutes each, 50 minutes is spent on this process per day. The total number of FTEs this represents is 50 minutes divided by 480 minutes, or 0.10, or 10 percent. Be aware, however, that many process redesign analysts use a percent of the workday rather than the full workday as the basis for the calculation, assuming that everyone needs to take breaks. This is called a person's productivity rate. This productivity rate could be calculated for each worker or class of worker through an observational study, or an industry average could be used. Typically, a productivity rate of 86 percent is used in healthcare (Dunham-Taylor and Pinczuk 2005). If that were the case, recalculating the number of FTEs would be 50 divided by 413 minutes per day, or 12 percent.
  >
  > It should be noted that in the illustration, multiple tasks are shown on the same "line," as if these were performed simultaneously. If tasks are truly performed simultaneously by the same person, this is acceptable. However, because the goal of process redesign is to reduce the total number of tasks or to shift tasks to lower-paid workers, it may be best to separate the tasks.

- *Cost of FTE per year:* This is the salary plus benefits earned by the person performing the task multiplied by the percent of time performed on the task. If a nurse earning $45,000 (salary and benefits) takes the call, the cost of the FTE performing that task per year is 10 (or 12) percent of $45,000, which is $4,500 (or $5,400).

Caution must be exercised when identifying productivity improvements as financial benefits of the EHR project. Although this example clearly illustrates how to calculate potential financial benefits in staff time, remember that unless the staff time can actually be reduced or staff members eliminated, this is still a "soft" benefit, not a financial benefit. Most organizations attempt to redeploy staff where they can, and where there are fractional gains, establish expectations for how the time should be spent. For example, the 10 percent or 12 percent of nurse time could be redeployed to perform patient call-back. This may result in increased patient satisfaction, which is good, but not a financial benefit. However, such an activity could result in one additional patient visit per day. If that is anticipated, the result is a *revenue increase*.

Revenue Increases

Financial benefits through revenue increases are often feasible. An increase in revenue is the ability to add income through use of EHR. An example of a direct source of benefits for both hospitals and clinics is from improved coding. In clinics, physicians have been conservative in their evaluation and management (E/M) coding in the ambulatory setting and often can generate an increase in revenue through more accurate coding. Other sources of revenue may derive from improvement with compliance for medical necessity certification, increased referrals, and other forms of increased volume such as described earlier. For example, hospitals that have a high occupancy may find the communications capabilities of the EHR can reduce length of stay, improving bed turnover, and resulting in not having to divert patients to other facilities. This may also be experienced similarly in the emergency department. Although more focused on the academic setting, the ability to participate in clinical trials can also generate revenue.

Cost Avoidance

Cost avoidance is the ability to not have to make a planned expenditure, such as renting a warehouse to house paper charts. Many productivity improvements lead to cost avoidance. For example, it is possible to reduce overtime if the same amount of work can be performed in less time. (This can also lead to increased revenue because an increased volume of work, such as laboratory tests, can be performed in the same amount of time.)

Many quality benefits also contribute to cost avoidance. For example, many estimate that the cost of a medication error to a hospital includes additional days' stay. Although some of these costs have been passed off to insurance companies, heightened scrutiny at contract time could result in less than ideal discounting if there is a history of extended stays or revisits due to errors. For physicians, an actual cost savings may accrue from their malpractice carrier, or there may be avoidance of an increase due to improvements in quality and patient safety. Most healthcare organizations will work with risk management to decide an average cost per type of error. This average usually is based on the frequency with which each of the types of consequences occurs. The following may be helpful ways to find such consequences:

- *Percent of times a particular decision must be made* (represented in the systems flowchart in figure 11.1 by a diamond shape): The percent of time a particular decision must be made can represent a potential for error. Although not always having a monetary amount associated with it, it is a metric to investigate further to describe the potential financial impact. In the example, one of the decisions to be made with respect to prescription refills may be to recall from memory the patient and patient's prescription in the event the chart cannot be found immediately. The risk, of course, is that memory is not perfect and the chart may reveal a reason for the patient to be seen prior to refill or that the refill dosage or amount needs to be changed. The metric will likely be reported as "number of times refill decisions are made because the chart cannot be found."

- *Number of errors:* The number of errors is the actual number of errors. It is unlikely that every task will have a figure in this column. But it should be possible to attribute any errors to a specific task that was performed incorrectly or could not be performed. For example, if a clinic knows three medication errors occurred last year because charts were not reviewed, this number of errors should be posted on the same line as the decision task described earlier. After all metrics are quantified, it may be appropriate to review the task list to determine if all known errors have been accounted for. If they have not, the task associated with the error should be incorporated into the chart and the metrics.

- *Cost of errors:* Many factors contribute to the cost of an error of any kind. If the organization has kept risk management data, the total cost of all actual errors (of each type) can be recorded here. However, this should be carefully studied, as previous experience is not always an indicator of future events. In the case of medication errors, the following consequences could occur:

  —Revisit(s) to clinic

  —Additional or repeat diagnostic test(s)

  —Loss of revenue if patient chooses to get healthcare elsewhere

  —Cost of consultation/specialist visit(s)

  —Cost of hospitalization(s)

  —Impact on malpractice insurance

  —Cost of lawsuit

  —Settlement amount of lawsuit

Contribution to Profit

A final category of financial benefit is contribution to profit—where there is the ability to turn added income into profit. Using less expensive medications, avoiding repeat diagnostic tests, and also reducing length of stay contributes to profit. The American Hospital Association estimates that a reduction in 0.5 days on average length of stay can generate $150,000 per month; it suggests that the range of benefit is from 0.5 to 1.5 days on average (AHA Solutions). Retrospective clinical denials and other revenue cycle management benefits may also be classified here.

Source of Benefits Data

As with many costs, there are many ways to achieve financial benefit through the EHR. How these benefits are categorized is less important than accurately identifying all that are reasonable. However, it must be stressed that benefit is achieved only through a change in behavior; it cannot be achieved through technology alone.

In addition, it cannot be emphasized enough that benefits are both tangible and intangible, and both are equally important. Arlotto (2003) has suggested that it is rare to "find anything so 'soft' that it refuses to be quantified." But quantification does not necessarily mean in monetary terms. A reduction in medication errors by 10 percent is quantifiable and important, but if monetary gains do not result, the benefit cannot be placed on a ROI calculation. To ensure that false expectations are not established, it is prudent to use only directly quantifiable monetary benefits in a financial ROI analysis, while ensuring that what Chaiken (2003) calls "clinical ROI" accompanies the financial analysis. For example, the following benefits may have been identified in a vendor's cost–benefit analysis (which many vendors will gladly perform):

> Most of hospital A's source systems were automated. Nursing documentation had been implemented in the critical care units. The final step was to implement the EHR, extending nursing documentation to all units, adopting bar code medication administration, and introducing structured data entry and decision support for computerized provider order entry and progress notes. The vendor estimated a time savings of 1.5 hours per nurse per shift, at considerable financial savings. However, the hospital recognized that it could not add these hours together to eliminate nurses or send nurses home after 6.5 hours of work. Unless the time savings is in overtime that can be eliminated as a result of the EHR, it cannot be used in calculating costs savings for a financial ROI.

This is not to say that the qualitative benefit in this illustration should be ignored. In fact, it should be highlighted as a tangible benefit (Chaiken's "clinical ROI"). It then becomes incumbent on the nursing department to demonstrate value through quality improvement measures for the additional time now available. For example, more time spent in patient instruction may result in increased patient satisfaction or even better outcomes. Although these may not be able to be translated into financial benefits, they are important and should be documented as part of a value proposition, or business case.

Impact Analysis Results

Conducting a financial impact analysis on the EHR system involves collecting cost data, capturing process redesign results, and summarizing the findings. Figure 11.2 is another example of a process redesign and associated metrics. It also shows a prescription refill process but uses the flow process chart tool. It illustrates only the steps in the clinic, shows both before and after EHR implementation, and provides quantitative benefits for before, after, and the difference.

As suggested in figure 11.3, for every group within the organization that reviews the impact analysis, different levels of detail will also be desired.

The detail with which the process redesign teams document their observations, redesigned processes, benefits calculations, and assumptions is certainly not the detail sent forward to any of the groups to which the teams report. But the detailed documentation should be retained in the event it is needed to substantiate or recalculate summary reports and for when a benefits realization study is performed.

The steering committee relies on the process redesign teams to ensure that all functionality required to achieve the process redesign and quantitative benefits is identified in a

Figure 11.2.   Example of process redesign and benefits metrics

Process: Prescription Refill   **Department: Nursing**   **Date:**

T = Time in number of days   U = Number of units   ? = Potential for error, see explanation below

Current Process	Description	T	U	?	Proposed Process	Description	T	U	?
●⇨□D▽	Pt calls for refill		10		●⇨■D▽	Pt calls for refill		10	
●⇨□D▽	Clerk takes message		10	a	●⇨□D▽	Clerk enters message		10	a
O➡□D▽	Clerk puts in MD slot	½	10		O➡□D▽	Routed to RN or MD		10	
O⇨■D▽	RN reviews message		10		O⇨■D▽	RN/MD rev & rec	½	10	
●⇨□D▽	Calls pt if incomplete	1	2		O➡□D▽	To pharmacy		10	
●⇨□D▽	Requests record	1	5	b	O⇨□D▽				
O⇨■D▽	RN follow protocol?		10	c	O⇨□D▽				
O➡□D▽	Puts in MD slot	½	8		O⇨□D▽				
O⇨□D▼	RN/MD record		10	d	O⇨□D▽				
O➡□D▽	To pharmacy		10		O⇨□D▽				
		3					½		

Summary: O 4, ⇨ 3, □ 2, D 5, ▽ 1

Summary: O 2, ⇨ 2, □ 2, D 1, ▽ 1

Quantitative Benefits:

	# Units /Day	# Min. /Unit	Tot # FTEs	Tot $ FTE/Yr	Material $/Unit	Tot $ Mat/Yr	# Errors /Yr	Ave $ /Error	Tot $ Error/Yr
Present					$0.02	$50	75	$60	$4,500
Clerk	10	5	0.125	$2,600					
RN	10	15	0.313	$11,719					
Total		20		$14,319					
Proposed					$0	$0	0	0	0
Clerk	10	10	0.25	$5,200					
RN	10	5	0.10	$4,773					
Total		15		$9,973					
Savings					$0.02	$50	75	$60	$4,500
Clerk		(5)		($2,600)					
RN		10		$6,946					
Total		5		$4,346					

(Continued)

Figure 11.2.   (Continued)

Assumptions:

There are 250 days that the clinic is open in which calls for prescription refills are received from patients. All employees work 8 hours per day and are paid for 2,080 hours per year. The clerk makes $10 per hour, and the RN makes $18 per hour.

Summary of Quantitative Benefits

Although there are fewer steps to the process and less of the RN time reviewing message and medical records, this did not equate to one actual staff person. The $4,346 savings therefore cannot be realized in impact analysis.

Cost savings in materials come about through not recording on a form sent to the medical record. Although this is a real cost savings, most organizations do not track cost savings this small.

There is potential for reduced errors. The organization previously did a quality assurance study that demonstrated that there were 75 errors out of 2,500 refills (3%) due to information not being available or other operational considerations. It was estimated that each error resulted, on average, in 1 additional visit to the clinic, priced at $60 per visit, for a total of $4,500 in loss to profit in a capitated environment. This $4,500 is the quantitative benefit in contribution to profit.

Description of Potential for Error and EHR Improvement

a. Clerk may get the patient's name wrong, in which case there is a delay in waiting for the patient to call back and potential for the patient to be dissatisfied. Using an EHR, the clerk calls the patient and while on the phone verifies accuracy of patient name and phone number. The frequency with which this happens is minimal.

   Clerk may get patient name correct, but wrong telephone number, requiring check that delays processing with MPI if the patient must be contacted. The frequency with which this happens is moderate.

   Clerk may not get complete information necessitating RN review of message and call to the patient, constituting a delay and potential for patient to be dissatisfied. The frequency with which this happens is moderate to often. With an EHR that calls up the current medications and prompts the clerk to check off requested refill, opportunity for error is greatly reduced (although still possible for clerk to check off wrong medication).

b. In half of the instances, the medical record is required for checking other medications the patient is currently taking, resulting in a significant delay. It is possible, however, that the medical record does not have the desired information or is not requested due to oversight.

c. The RN may not follow protocol for whatever reason. The frequency with which this happens is minimal. The EHR will automatically check that there is an RN protocol and route the request to the RN if so, or the MD if not. There is still some delay in that the RN or the MD probably does not clear the in-basket constantly.

d. The RN or the MD may err in writing the refill, although there is the potential for error in the EHR. The frequency with which an error in writing happens is minimal; the potential for error through the EHR is considered even less.

   The record of the refill may also not make it to the applicable medical record. The frequency with which this happens is minimal to moderate. This would be totally avoided in the case of the EHR.

Figure 11.3.   Level of impact analysis detail

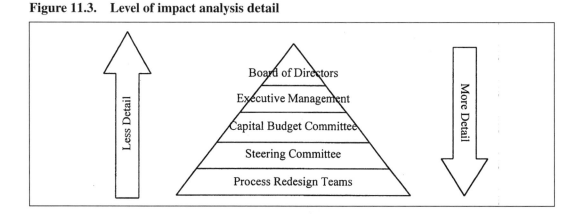

request for proposal from vendors. For example, the functional requirements that would be derived from the illustration in figures 11.1 and 11.2 would include the following:

- Clerical staff members who answer the phone would be able to access patient demographics and insurance information to ensure that the clinic continues to have the most current information.

- The system would be able to provide a template to initiate all prescription refill calls that would serve as a workflow tool until the prescription refill request has been completed.

- When the nurse reviews the request initiated by the clerk, the system would be able to display the most current prescriptions and also provide a medication history based on the clinic's experience with the patient. In addition, any alerts that had previously been entered with respect to the refill (for example, to diminish a leading dose or to monitor dosage in relationship to laboratory values) could be displayed. Information about pertinent clinical information in accordance with the medication protocol also could be provided. A link to the patient's insurance eligibility could be provided so that the medication could be screened by an up-to-date formulary that is consistent with the patient's pharmacy benefits. Finally, suggestions for any new and comparable drugs that may be more efficacious or lower in cost could be offered. Based on the nurse's authority, the nurse may be able to authorize the refill or send it to the physician for approval.

- An in-basket feature would be present in the system to notify the physician of a prescription refill waiting to be approved.

- Upon review of the information presented, the system would be able to generate a legible and accurate prescription refill by authorized personnel to be sent electronically to the designated pharmacy.

- When the pharmacy receives the prescription refill request from the clinic, it should be able to merge the request with its medication history file to determine whether any prescriptions from other sources would contraindicate the request. If the physician needed to be contacted regarding potential contraindications, the pharmacy could use an autodial function. Eligibility for insurance benefits would be verified when the refill request had been finalized. The prescription refill request would enter a workflow queue to be filled, and autodial would be used to inform the patient that the refill was ready. Tailored instructions could be generated for the patient. The clinic could be notified when, or if, the patient has picked up the refill.

Cost–Benefit Analysis

The steering committee is the group most likely to be the recipient of a cost–benefit analysis. The cost–benefit analysis example in table 11.1 is a summary of all costs and the value of all benefits as defined by the process redesign teams. *Net impact* is costs less benefits. In this example, the first year's net impact is the total cost of the EHR and its implementation,

Table 11.1.   Cost–benefit analysis

$M	Year 1	Year 2	Year 3	Year 4	Year 5	Total
Costs						
Hardware	1.30	0.50	0.25	0.00	0.00	2.05
Software	1.20	0.00	0.10	0.00	0.00	1.30
Installation and Training	0.50	0.10	0.00	0.00	0.00	0.60
Maintenance	0.00	0.75	0.75	0.75	0.75	3.00
Support	2.60	2.15	1.80	1.80	1.80	10.15
Total	5.60	3.50	2.90	2.55	2.55	17.10
Benefits						
Charge Capture	0.00	0.22	0.58	1.20	1.45	3.45
Clinical Trials	0.00	0.00	0.10	0.50	0.75	1.35
Decision Support	0.00	0.10	0.50	0.75	1.00	2.35
Diagnostic Studies	0.00	0.20	0.75	1.10	1.50	3.55
Financial Management	0.00	0.10	0.20	0.20	0.20	0.70
Med Record Operations	0.00	1.50	4.00	4.50	4.50	14.50
Nursing Department	0.00	0.00	0.30	0.50	0.60	1.40
Referral Management	0.00	0.20	0.50	0.70	0.80	2.20
Total	0.00	2.32	6.93	9.45	10.80	29.50
Net Impact	−5.60	−1.18	4.03	6.90	8.25	12.40

or $5.6 million. Over the 5-year period for which the cost–benefit analysis is constructed, some benefits are realized in the year following EHR implementation, but most are not realized until the next year. After 1 year, most benefits become fairly stable.

Some practical considerations in presenting a cost–benefit analysis such as this include simple issues such as naming the years. Some organizations prefer to consider the year of implementation to be year 0, with the first year of benefits being year 1. Obviously, an EHR implementation may not take 1 year. It may take less time in a small or medium-sized physician office but will generally take more time in small hospitals and certainly more time in medium to large-sized hospitals.

Another consideration is that the benefits are described by type. This is often not how a provider's financial statements look. Income statements and balance sheets are based on revenues, and expenses and assets and liabilities, respectively. Some providers would like to see pro forma income statements and balance sheets to determine the impact the EHR has on them. Pro forma means "provided in advance." Generally, the accounting staff or finance officer incorporates the cost–benefit analysis data into a pro forma income statement and balance sheet.

For example, with regard to the income statement, a cost–benefit analysis projection of $220,000 of benefits in charge capture in year 2 means that there is $220,000 increased revenue in year 2. Referral management was to yield $200,000 worth of benefits. The accountant would need to evaluate this benefit and decide whether it represents an increase in revenue to the organization or a decrease in cost, which would reduce expenses. (This depends on whether the provider is reimbursed for its services through discounted fees for service or capitated reimbursement.) The medical record operations category (of $1,500,000) is clearly a cost savings that would reduce expenses.

ROI Financial Models

The capital budget committee is likely to want both pro forma financial statements, especially the balance sheet, and ROI measures. The **balance sheet** describes an organization's overall financial position with respect to its total assets and total liabilities. From a pro forma balance sheet, the capital budget committee can study the impact of a large expenditure. Various forms of financing can be considered with respect to their impact on the balance sheet.

In addition to the pro forma financial statements, specific financial measures can be calculated. The most common are the payback period, the internal rate of return, and **net present value**. It should always be remembered, however, that the numeric variables used to compute any of these ROI measures are imprecise. Bauer (2003) observes that one of the most serious problems in performing these calculations is absence of consistency.

Payback Period

The payback period is the number of years it takes to recoup expenditure. It is typically calculated by dividing the total cost of the project by the annual incremental cash inflows. However, if the annual cash inflows are variable, as in the example in table 11.1, the payback period is more readily calculated by dividing the total net impact by the total cost. For the example, this would be $12.40 million divided by $5.60 million, or 2.2 years.

Although the data in table 11.1, when presented as a table, are intuitive to some, it is often helpful to plot some of this information on graphs for visual effect. Such graphics are useful for presentations to executive management and especially boards of directors (Kian et al. 1995). The graphs depicted in figures 11.4 and 11.5 clearly show the point in time at which benefits begin to outweigh costs. This payback period also may be considered the break-even point.

Some of the major pitfalls of the payback period financial analysis are that it ignores both costs and benefits that occur after the break-even point and the time value of money. By ignoring future costs, it may reflect an accelerated payback period. Figure 11.6 illustrates this concept; it considers the cumulative impact of the EHR, where the cumulative effect

Figure 11.4.   Projected EHR costs and benefits graph

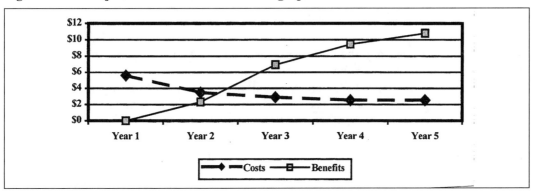

Figure 11.5.   Net impact of the EHR

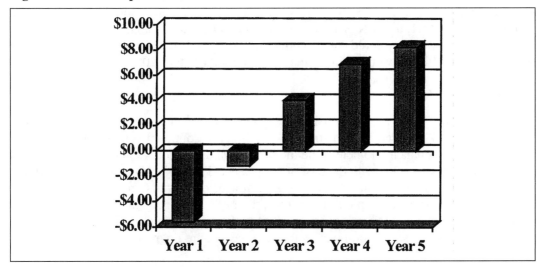

Figure 11.6.   Cumulative impact of the EHR

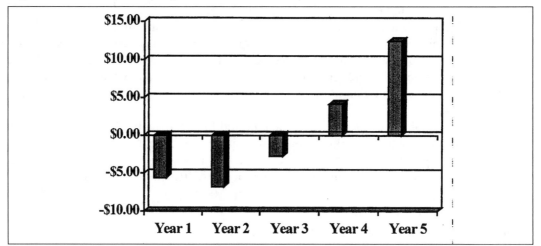

of both the project costs and the ongoing costs are not offset until year 4. Some financial analysts will use this as the payback period, instead.

By ignoring future benefits, the analysis ignores potential profitability. By ignoring the time value of money, it ignores the issue of how funds to make the expenditure are paid for or what the difference would be if the funds were invested in another way.

Internal Rate of Return

Internal rate of return (IRR) is a financial measure that considers the time value of money. Its strict definition is the interest rate that makes the net present value calculation equal zero. What this means is that it is the interest rate at which the present value of the projected cash inflows equals the initial investment. To calculate the IRR, a financial calculator, table of present values for an annuity, or a spreadsheet with IRR function should be used. For the example in table 11.1, the IRR is 42 percent. In general, financial analysts would compare this rate with the rate they could earn on other investments. If it is higher, investment in the project is good. If it is lower, the investment is not good (Anthes 2003).

Net Present Value

Net present value (NPV) is often considered the most precise method of cash flow analysis, although typically reserved for investments of long term, continual value. It uses the organization's cost of financing to determine the present value of incremental cash inflows and compares the present value with the cost of the project. The project is considered favorable if the NPV is positive. Again, a financial calculator or other tools are needed to perform the calculation. For the example in table 11.1, the NPV at 12 percent cost of financing is $13.92 million, which is favorable (Dunn 1999). NPV is not often used for EHR projects because the EHR is a set of components that change and are upgraded over time.

Benefits Realization Studies

As described in chapter 5, a benefits realization study is conducted after the EHR has been implemented to determine that the benefits described in the cost–benefit analysis or ROI analyses have been met. The same tools and the same metrics used to conduct healthcare process assessment should be used to conduct the benefits realization study. This is both the benefits realization study's strength and weakness.

An impact analysis performed after EHR implementation without a baseline set of values relies on guesswork and is often influenced by satisfaction or dissatisfaction with the EHR. However, if a baseline set of values exists, comparison should be relatively straight-forward. Unfortunately, the timeline for EHR selection and implementation is frequently anywhere from 2 to 5 or sometimes 10 years, depending on the migration path. Proponents of benefits realization studies suggest conducting the studies at designated milestones if the migration path is expected to be lengthy. In this case, interim ROI analyses also should be calculated as baselines. Even so, the biggest drawback to the accuracy of the benefits realization is the presence of confounding variables. Anything from a new physician leader to a new disease and everything in between, including changes in reimbursement structures, different accreditation processes, new legislation, and so on, can intervene and interfere with the accuracy of the calculations.

If it is found that an organization is not interested in a benefits realization study, it may be appropriate to consider conducting EHR benefits surveys that assess user satisfaction, overall financial performance, productivity improvements, quality improvements, and patient satisfaction. Such surveys do not depend on time-consuming quantification processes but can reveal successes and problems to be addressed.

Many healthcare organizations do not conduct benefits realization studies, often citing lack of time or skills to do so and the many intervening variables that may play a role in results. For example, when implementing a CPOE system, the implementation strategy may be to gradually introduce alerts, so as to avoid alert fatigue. It may also be recognized that some members of the medical staff have EHRs of their own and probably are more inclined to use the hospital's CPOE system when first implemented than those members who do not have an EHR; however, over the course of a few years, the number with EHRs may grow. The result then is that the CPOE itself and its potential users are continually changing, making it difficult to assess the results. Still, Classen and others stress the importance of continual evaluation of such systems. CPOE systems, in particular, have invited considerable scrutiny after some notable failures and unintended consequences. Benefits realization studies, if nothing else, will ensure that appropriate utilization of these systems is monitored (Classen et al 2007).

Healthcare is not alone in its challenge to perform benefits realization. Several studies of IS managers conducting benefits realization studies in all industries have found that, although quantifiably measuring and reporting the benefits of IS projects is considered important, evaluating project benefits after completion is seldom performed (Planview 2007). In addition to the fact that evaluation of IS investments "requires multidimensional measures and is a complex tangle of financial, organizational, social, procedural, and technical threads" (Lin et al 2005), the results of those that are performed often show results as low as 25 percent success (PriceWaterhouseCoopers 2003). It has also been pointed out that internally performed benefits realization studies can be made to show any desired outcome (Mello 2001). A final consideration for healthcare relates to the fact that under the current reimbursement process, benefits of IT investment accrue to many beneficiaries, not just to the entity that makes the investments (Vogel 2003).

The discussion surrounding use of any form of impact analysis as a time-consuming and inexact process and that benefits realization studies performed after the fact and by the organization itself are the most inexact has suggested that new metrics beyond the traditional industrial-age measures to focus on cost analysis and savings are needed. Classen et al (2007) describes several approaches for evaluating CPOE systems, including internal organizational studies, vendor studies, CCHIT certification of products, and the Leapfrog Group and National Quality Forum (NQF).

In healthcare, the bottom line is improved quality, cost, and access to care. Quality matters and improved quality does lead to improved cost, even though such improvements cannot be directly quantified. In fact, Mello (2001) suggests that ROI analysis should not be used for projected intangible benefits or broad or necessary strategic initiatives. Whether your organization agrees or not, no EHR impact analysis would be complete without recognizing the nonquantifiable, intangible results of the EHR. The Healthcare Financial Management Association (HFMA) suggests the following six categories of nonquantifiable benefits of an EHR (Kian, et al 1995):

- Data capture and access
- Decision support
- Optimization of clinical practice
- Business management
- Streamlining of patient flow
- Legal/regulatory compliance

An example of data capture and access benefits includes increased productivity due to improved access to patient data. Following is a case in point:

> An EHR system had been implemented 18 months prior to a series of physician interviews about the EHR. When asked about the impact on documentation, most physicians indicated it took longer, a few said it took about the same amount of time as previously, and none indicated it took less time. When asked if physicians went home earlier, later, or the same time, they all indicated earlier or the same time, not volunteering, but agreeing with the interviewer, that there were significant time savings in other areas, such as in not having to track down missing data and not wasting time on the phone clarifying, checking, and correcting.

Decision support is the primary source of quality improvement. This may include decreased complications as a result of improved monitoring and preventive care reminders, reduced malpractice risk for failure to detect inappropriate care or for care omissions, and improved quality of care from giving clinicians information they need to make informed treatment decisions.

Business management benefits contribute to improved ability to negotiate managed care contracts and to improved financial management through the ability to relate clinical status to resource consumption. Streamlining patient flow increases patient satisfaction, improves efficiency in resource use from improved scheduling, and decreases patient no-shows and lost customers, among other things.

Finally, legal and regulatory compliance is enhanced through compliance reminders, enhanced ability to protect patient confidentiality, and decreased interruptions to patient care as a result of appropriate backup and recovery mechanisms.

Any organization's list of intangible benefits to be achieved through an EHR should reflect its strategic goals.

Sources of Funding

A final, though by no means less important, consideration with respect to ROI must be sources of funding. With price tags of $25,000 to $50,000 per physician and potentially millions, if not tens of millions, of dollars for hospitals, EHR projects will clearly take some creative financing. Most projects will require tapping a combination of various sources of funds. Following are some of the sources of capital that a healthcare organization may consider for funding an EHR project (HFMA 2003):

- Organizational reserves is the most obvious source of funds, always used to some extent, and the least desirable source of funding. When provider organizations make investments in affiliated organizations, care must be taken to ensure that all legal ramifications have been dealt with.

- Bank and other financial service company short-term loans are generally available for under $10 million. Larger loans always require some form of collateral, which could result in loss of control of the organization.

- Capital leases are traditionally used for large equipment acquisitions and could be negotiated for major IT investments as well. Some providers use application service provider (ASP) models of financing IT investments, not only as a means of financing, but also as an ongoing means of technical support.

- Vendor discounts and incentives are fairly common and can contribute to lowering the total cost of ownership. They frequently require something in return, where the provider may need to serve as a development partner or spokesperson or follow specific rules for implementation and use.

- A joint venture or partnership extends the notion of development partner with vendor to a tighter relationship or may be a business venture that supports the EHR implementation and sells services to others. Some of these partnerships entail alpha or beta testing of products. Alpha testing is quite risky and usually avoided by healthcare organizations. Serving as a beta test site, however, can be helpful in

lowering cost and ensuring that the system is designed to the organization's specifications. In such a situation, however, the installation may take longer and require
considerable patience until the vendor works out system bugs.

- Health plans and plan sponsors may be willing to negotiate favorable contractual
arrangements based on adoption of EHRs. This is the idea behind The Leapfrog
Group discussed in chapter 15. Many health plans and employers are willing to
provide incentives to those providers who will support disease management activities through enhanced use of IT.

- Private philanthropy/foundations may be a source of some funding for IT investments, although they typically prefer to fund more tangible assets or support educational endeavors, such as fellowships, university chairs, and so on.

- Pharmaceutical companies have often provided assistance to providers who are
willing to conduct clinical trials or supply data relative to product use. However,
these activities must be entered into carefully.

- Public grants are sources of funding depending on the government's current initiatives. Starting in 2004, a number of major federal funding grants for value assessment, demonstration, and implementation of IT infrastructure projects have been
made available, where just a few years earlier virtually no such money was available.
Most such grants require an application process, are competitive, and often require
some form of research study, documentation, or other requirements to secure funding. These also often have matching funds requirements where the organization
must make an equal investment. Finally, many do not support capital investments.

- State legislative initiatives are a final source of funding in some cases. These may
be tied to various state government projects, especially for improving service to the
poor or persons with certain disease classes or for supporting small community and
rural health initiatives.

- Process improvement as a financing mechanism may seem strange, but many hospitals are finding that identifying and improving inefficient processes and building
consensus around the need for change actually goes a long way toward improving
overall efficiency and is a contributing factor to recognizing investments in IT systems as a major component of the capital budget (McLennan 2005; Perry 2004).
Physician practices also benefit from such process improvements. A physician
practice of 10 physicians found $247,500 on unnecessarily complex and redundant
administrative tasks, most of which could be improved even prior to acquiring an
EHR (McKee 2004).

Because of the federal government interest in promoting EHRs, the Medicare Modernization Act of 2003 called for exceptions and safe harbors to the Stark and Anti-Kickback
regulations. The Centers for Medicare and Medicaid Services (CMS) issued exceptions to
the physician self-referral prohibitions (commonly referred to as the Stark Law) for donations of EHR and e-prescribing systems in 2006. Likewise, the Department of Health and

Human Services (HHS) Office of Inspector General (OIG) provided safe harbors to the Anti-Kickback rules. These changes have enabled hospitals to make certain types of donations to physicians for EHR (and e-prescribing) systems. In addition, with the emphasis on HIE organizations, the existing community-wide health network exception that already existed under the Stark Law may be invoked by regional health information organizations (RHIOs) and other HIEs to support acquisition of EHRs.

Conclusion

Many healthcare organizations want to have some idea, up front, of what the EHR system will cost. A pro forma cost–benefit analysis projects costs and savings over a specified period of time. As vendor selection is undertaken and more accurate cost and benefit data can be determined, an economic projection for the value of the investment can be made. Some organizations require a specific return on investment before proceeding with the EHR; others believe the EHR is a strategic investment for which a precise economic benefit cannot be determined but want to have a ballpark estimate for budgeting and establishing benefits expectations. Benefits realization studies are not performed as frequently as they perhaps should be, but they can contribute to both demonstrating value and highlighting areas where improvements are necessary.

In healthcare, the major economic value is derived initially from operational savings that are relatively easy to quantify. Later, qualitative benefits will accrue that are difficult to measure but are much more important. In whatever form it takes, an impact analysis must be done within the context of qualitative benefits.

References and Resources

AHA Solutions, Retrospective Clinical Denials Management, www.aha-solutions.org.

Anthes, G.H. 2003 (Feb. 17). ROI guide: Internal rate of return. *Computerworld*. www.computerworld.com.

Arlotto, P. 2003. An interview with Pam Arlotto, healthcare IT strategist. *Journal of Healthcare Information Management* 17(4):18–19.

Bauer, J.C. 2003. Return on investment: Going beyond traditional analysis. *Journal of Healthcare Information Management* 17(4):4–5.

Chaiken, B.P. 2003. Clinical ROI: Not just costs versus benefits. *Journal of Healthcare Information Management* 17(4):36–41.

Clark, RL, 2006 (Feb. 22). Quoted in HFMA research details barriers to national EHR adoption. HFMA Publications.

Classen, D.C., et al. 2007. Evaluation and certification for computerized provider order entry systems, *Journal of the American Medical Informatics Association*, 14(1): 48–55.

Dunham-Taylor J., and JZ Pinczuk, (2005) *Health Care Financial Management for Nurse Managers*. Jones & Bartlett, p. 96.

Dunn, R. 1999. *Finance Principles for the Health Information Manager*. Chicago: American Health Information Management Association.

Federal Register. 2006 (August 8). Final Rule: Medicare program: Physicians' referrals to the health care entities with which they have financial relationships; Exceptions for certain electronic prescribing and electronic health record arrangements.

Federal Register. 2006 (August 8). Final Rule: Medicare and state health care programs: fraud and abuse; Safe harbor for certain electronic prescribing arrangements under the Anti-Kickback Statute.

Goldstein, D. and P. Groen. 2006 (July 18). Value measurement and return on investment for EHRs. *Virtual Medical Worlds Monthly.*

Grieger, D.L., et al. 2007 (July). A pilot study to document the return on investment for implementing an ambulatory electronic health record at an Academic Medical Center, *Journal of the American College of Surgeons* 205(1), pp. 89–96.

Healthcare Financial Management Association, in partnership with GE Healthcare Financial Services. 2003. *How are Hospitals Financing the Future? Access to Capital in Health Care Today.* Westchester, IL: HFMA.

Health Information Management Systems Society. 2003. EHR and the Return on Investment. www.himss.org/content/file/EHR-ROI.pdf.

Kian, L.A., M.W. Stewart, C. Bagby, and J. Robertson. 1995. (July). Justifying the cost of a computer-based patient record. *Healthcare Financial Management* 49(7): 58–67.

Lin, C., et al. 2005 (August). IS/IT Investment Evaluation and Benefits Realization Issues in Australia. *Journal of Research and Practice in Information Technology* 37(3).

Linder J.A., et al. 2007. Electronic health record use and the quality of ambulatory care in the United States, *Archives of Internal Medicine* 167(13):1400–1405.

McKee, K. 2004 (Nov. 19). 10 ways to work smarter. *Medical Economics* 36–38.

McLennan, D. 2005 (June). Financing investments in health care IT. *ADVANCE for Health Information Executives* 9(6):37–46.

Mello, A. 2001 (Oct. 3). Why ROI Can Sometimes Lie. TechUpdate.

Miller, R.H., 2007. The value of electronic health records incommunity health centers: Policy Implications, Health Affairs 26(1): 206–214.

Perry, B. 2004. Unearthing hidden benefits. *ADVANCE for Health Information Executives* 8(6):63–65.

Planview. Benefits Realization a Key IT Challenge for Fortune 1000 Companies. www.benefitsrealization.blogspot.com/2007/10.

PriceWaterhouseCoopers. 2003. Benefits Realization Online Survey Results. www.pwcglobal.com.

Robbins, B.C., and H.C. Werner. 2003. Financial modeling for the EHR. *ADVANCE for Health Information Executives* 7(12):16–20.

Sarasohn-Kahn, J. 2007 (July 31). EHRs, Media and Statistics: Misinterpreted Results Skew Understanding. *iHealthBeat.*

Solovy, A. 2005 (June 30). Capital catch-22. Hospitals & Health Networks 79(6): 32–40.

Vogel, L.H. 2003. Finding value from IT investments: Exploring the elusive ROI in Healthcare. *Journal of Healthcare Information Management* 17(4):20–28.

Wise, P. 2007 (June 27). Quoted in Return on investment does not drive EHR adoption in hospitals, *EmpowerMed.*

Chapter 12
EHR Selection and Contract Negotiation

As momentum for electronic health records (EHR) grows, the process for selecting a vendor has become increasingly challenging. This is true whether the selection being made is for a comprehensive suite of EHR components for a hospital, an EHR for a physician office, or any of an EHR's individual components or associated bridge technologies.

The EHR marketplace is highly dynamic—with vendors entering and leaving the market all the time, and many vendors selling products as EHRs that are not truly EHRs—at least by the criteria used by the Certification Commission on Health Information Technology (CCHIT). In the past 20 years, it is likely that there have been more than 500 companies that have attempted to sell ambulatory EHRs. In 2006, there were estimated to be about 250 vendors selling ambulatory EHRs, and approximately 80 had been certified by CCHIT. By mid-2008, the number certified against the more strict, 2007 criteria (which then included e-prescribing) was 43, including 19 vendors with products conditionally certified or having been granted a 90-day extension on the 2006 certification. The hospital market is smaller, but not without its own unique challenges. Many hospital vendors "grew up" as "hospital information systems," well equipped to handle administrative, financial, and ancillary departmental needs of hospitals, but largely not focused on clinical capabilities, which is the hallmark of an EHR. CCHIT estimates there are about 24 vendors that might eventually qualify for CCHIT certification of inpatient EHRs. In 2008, 11 vendors had inpatient EHR products that were certified or premarket conditionally certified against the 2007 criteria. The 2007 criteria for inpatient EHRs (which was the first year in which inpatient EHRs were certified) required products to have computerized provider order entry [CPOE] and bar code medication administration record [BC-MAR] capabilities with connectivity to patient and provider demographics and ancillary systems.

Instability in the marketplace and the focus of EHR truly on clinical information processing makes vendor selection challenging. This chapter:

- Summarizes the critical role advance planning plays in vendor selection

- Discusses the build–borrow–buy–blend–rip and replace decision

- Describes the steps commonly taken in selecting a vendor

Key Terms		
Application service provider	Due diligence	Request for proposal
	Interface engine	Rip and replace
Clinical Context Object Workgroup	Request for information	Systems integrators

- Distinguishes between request for information (RFI) and request for proposal (RFP)
- Offers suggestions for managing the vendor selection process
- Describes the critical tasks of due diligence and contract negotiation

Executing EHR Planning

This book emphasizes the importance of planning for the EHR. Although some would want to move into vendor selection quickly, the thoroughness of up-front planning without vendor influence pays tremendous dividends. EHR strategic planning ensures that the organization is clear about its vision for the EHR and that the EHR complements the organization's strategic initiatives and business plan. As mentioned earlier, executive management commitment and support are critical success factors in the EHR project. Developing a migration path to achieve the vision of the EHR establishes a comprehensive plan that reduces the risk of reactive purchasing. Goal setting aids in establishing expectations for full utilization and hence benefits realization. Assessing the processes impacted by the EHR, identifying functional needs, and understanding the data and technology infrastructure help to clarify the functional requirements, establish design parameters, and commit users to change and to achieving specific, measurable return on investment (ROI).

Making the Build–Buy–Borrow–Blend–Rip and Replace Decision

It is critical that planning be accomplished before any vendors are asked for a proposal. However, there is one other important decision to make prior to initiating a vendor selection process that is more oriented to *how* an EHR is going to be acquired, rather than on *what* the EHR is. This decision relates to whether an organization is going to consider self development of a system (that is, "build"), buy—which is actually license—clinical components from its incumbent vendor, acquire a product through an **application service provider** (ASP) arrangement—which is the concept of "borrowing" a product, buying clinical components from another vendor thereby blending these with the administrative/financial components of the incumbent vendor, or largely starting over from scratch with a new vendor replacing most existing applications. The mere fact that there are so many strategies as well as many other factors makes the acquisition strategy a difficult decision.

Build vs. Buy

The build or buy (acquire an EHR from a commercial vendor) decision is a fairly historical decision. In the past, when there were few EHR vendors and products were not comprehensive, some organizations considered building their own EHR. Many of these systems were developed in academic medical centers or with a commercial partner who was interested in developing an EHR product. Indeed, many of these projects were the forerunners to current EHR systems. Now, most organizations recognize that commercial products can meet their needs and that most will far surpass the functionality that could be self-developed. Still, this decision is not totally dead. Some physicians are intrigued with developing their own, "perfect" system, and some hospitals have development teams they do not want to give up.

An organization's decision to build or buy should be based on a careful review of the marketplace because currently it is generally more expensive to undertake self-development. Unless self-development is coupled with vendor partnership that leads to commercialization, a self-developed system also can be a drawback when attempting to integrate with commercial products as the organization grows, merges, or acquires affiliates.

Buy vs. Borrow

To buy (that is, to license a product from a commercial vendor) or "borrow" (using an ASP arrangement) is often an economic decision. Licensing software and either buying or leasing hardware for an EHR is a costly proposition. An EHR requires considerable access to capital as well as considerable ongoing maintenance, upgrades, and enhancements. However, many organizations are considering an ASP model as one way to obtain EHR functionality without the heavy capital outlays and IT staffing that buying an EHR entails.

Essentially, an ASP is an arrangement that involves a customer paying a subscription fee to access a software application and their data that reside on secure computers managed off-site by a vendor. In this model, there is much less upfront capital outlay and fewer IT staff required in-house. In fact, the ASP acquisition strategy may be considered essentially a financing model. The ASP model of acquiring computing power is actually not new; many organizations shared computing services when computers were first being developed. Still popular today, many vendors find that the steady stream of revenue from an ASP arrangement is a good business strategy. (Sometimes these arrangements go by other names, such as remote connectivity option [RCO] or service bureau.) New technologies have greatly enhanced the basic model of leasing access to sophisticated systems.

There are several types of ASPs. One type hosts various applications developed by a number of software vendors from a remote data center and delivers them to its customers over a secure Internet connection or a private network. Another type of ASP manages and supports is own software applications while partnering with telecommunications and data center companies to deliver a complete solution for its customers. Another variation is the vertical service provider (VSP), which focuses on offering industry-specific application hosting services to customers in a particular vertical market, such as healthcare. VSPs may target specific applications such as diagnostics, medical record management, purchasing, claims processing, scheduling, or human resources.

Organizations that choose any of the ASP forms of acquiring an EHR, however, should bear in mind that they still have to acquire the hardware to be used by individual users. Hardware can be purchased or leased. Purchasing hardware allows the organization to take advantage of immediate ownership and the flexibility to do whatever it chooses with the equipment. However, it also creates an immediate asset on the balance sheet, as well as a potential cash flow problem. Leasing minimizes the burden of ownership, typically requires no down payment, and may remove the risk of obsolescence (depending on the length of the lease). Operating leases usually qualify for off-balance sheet treatment for accounting purposes and so will not impact financial ratios and may conserve bank lines of credit for other acquisitions (Zadrozny 2005). It is a good idea to evaluate such options thoroughly from an accounting perspective, as paying over time could end up costing more than buying. In addition to cost factors, the organization needs to be aware that confidentiality issues could arise if appropriate measures are not taken to destroy all data on the equipment prior to returning it to the leasing agent. Moreover, there may be monetary penalties for loss or damage to equipment or for returning it early.

Yet another option to acquiring an EHR is outsourcing. Outsourcing is a contractual relationship with a specialized outside service provider for work traditionally done in-house. In some respects, it is broader than ASP because ASP generally refers to the utilization of computer services whereas outsourcing can include both computer services and various management services. Outsourcing sometimes is equated with the use of offshore services. However, outsourcing does not have to be offshore or even off-premises. It can provide management of services directly at the provider's site.

The advantages and disadvantages to the ASP/outsourcing model are summarized in table 12.1.

As with any set of advantages and disadvantages, careful management of the process can offset disadvantages and capitalize on advantages. Perhaps the most critical element of ASP/outsourcing is a strong service-level agreement (SLA) that establishes the terms of service the ASP/outsourcers will provide.

Table 12.1.   ASP/outsourcing advantages and disadvantages

Advantages	Disadvantages
Lower up-front costs for hardware and installation	Potential higher cost over long term
Software becomes an operating cost versus capital expenditure	Integration issues if ASP/outsourced functions must connect to in-house systems
Fewer data center headaches	Less ability to customize
Access to new and/or better technologies, especially for security	Loss of control/accountability issues

Blend: Best of Breed, Best of Fit, or Best of Suite?

Another consideration with respect to acquiring an EHR is whether to continue with an existing vendor's product line or mix vendor products. This decision occurs because many information systems (ISs) products have been highly proprietary and therefore not interoperable with products from other vendors. This means that when a commitment is made to acquire, for example, a hospital IS (or a practice management system for a physician office) from one vendor, fitting products from other vendors into the mix becomes more difficult.

Best of fit, or single source, is a scenario in which an organization acquires products from primarily one vendor, and that vendor's suite of products are integrated or fit well together because they were developed from the same platform. Best of breed is the opposite situation, where an organization has acquired the "best" products from various vendors. It is then difficult to get the products to share data with one another. Multiple interfaces must be written and managed, and often these are not totally satisfactory. The result is that each individual organization unit may be happy with its chosen product, but as the organization moves toward adding clinical components that rely on the various other systems as a source of data or to which data must be sent, the challenge to exchange such data can be overwhelming (Briggs 2003).

Many healthcare organizations have tended toward best-of-fit scenarios, with only occasional use of another vendor for a very specific application, which usually is a stand-alone application. However, some vendors who offer tightly integrated products (that is, highly proprietary) have not always kept up with the marketplace in the latest EHR technology. In this case, providers have had to think about compromising on functionality with their existing vendor or spending a lot of money on interfacing their other products. Most providers are reluctant to scrap an entire infrastructure, although doing so is not entirely unheard of, especially when the systems are old or have not been regularly upgraded.

In deciding whether to wait out a best-of-fit vendor's EHR strategy or adopt a best-of-breed strategy, the best of suite, or dual core, strategy is another option to consider. Best of suite is essentially a combination of two primary vendors, usually the incumbent vendor providing the financial/administrative functions and another vendor providing the clinical functionality. Some vendors have recognized that they are unable to provide every solution for everyone and have been developing systems to accommodate a more blended approach.

Rip and Replace

The scenario in which an organization decides to switch to an entirely new (single) vendor has been dubbed **rip and replace**. Although this strategy may seem very expensive and most experts recommend against the strategy, a number of organizations are finding that it may be economically feasible in an environment where it is costly to manage potentially hundreds of interfaces or where their existing systems are out of date. A number of hospitals have adopted this strategy recently when they have found that either their incumbent, proprietary vendor with an outmoded technical platform has been struggling to develop clinical systems, or the hospital's acquisition strategy has been best of breed and there is no single vendor on which to build. In general, the best-of-fit strategy is intended to reflect the highest level of integration among components, making it easy to exchange data.

Physician offices and clinics are even more frequently looking to rip and replace as many EHR vendors are tightly integrating practice management system (PMS) functionality with the EHR. Although perhaps not representing quite the upheaval as it would in a hospital setting with many source systems, the rip and replace strategy in a clinic is often guided by the fact that not only is the PMS based on older technology, but it may not have been upgraded recently. Many offices fail to upgrade their systems as upgrades become available, making the cost of a new system often less than the cost of upgrading the system out of cycle and developing an interface.

Some Caveats

The ultimate goal of most organizations as they approach EHR is to achieve interoperability. This is highly desirable, especially as an EHR, by definition, is a system that draws data from multiple sources for its use. Few organizations set as their goal for EHR a best-of-breed environment. As a result, the concepts of interoperability, open source, and Web services architecture are important to bear in mind.

Interoperability

Interoperability refers to the ability of two disparate systems to exchange data seamlessly. In making an acquisition strategy decision, it is important to understand what any given vendor is truly offering for product and thus how likely it will be to achieve interoperability. Components from a single vendor may not always represent best of fit, or true integration and hence interoperability. Some vendors develop almost all their products themselves, from a single technology platform. Even when the technology platform is old, they work well together. If the platform is new and the vendor is as facile at developing clinical components as it is at developing administrative/financial components, the system should be highly interoperable. However, it is the strategy of some vendors not to develop all components themselves, but rather to acquire products from another vendor (or acquire the vendor itself) to round out its suite of products. In this case, the vendor is primarily a "system integrator," not a developer. Although the result is a well-interfaced suite of products that work reasonably well together, the result will never be as satisfactory as when the products are all developed from the same platform. So, when considering vendor A, understand whether A is its own developer, or an integrator of products from B, C, D, etc.

Open Source

Open source is another concept that sometimes trips people up in thinking they will achieve interoperability from such products. Open source refers to software applications in which the code used to create the program is freely available to use, view, and modify, often based on an open source operating system, such as Linux. Sometimes open source software is freely distributed with the intent of getting others to perfect the product; however, not all open source software is necessarily distributed without charge. Physicians, in particular, have sometimes been enamored by the concept of open source applications, not only because they are free or low cost, but because they tend to like to think they can refine them to suit their own needs. Interestingly, the American Academy of Family Physicians (AAFP) describes the open source phenomenon as one where some success has been achieved "where the developers of applications are also the users." In general, however, they note that there has been slow adoption because "the vast majority of users (clinicians) are not software developers (or even so-called power users)" (AAFP 2008).

Some of the interest in open source came about when the federal government decided to make the source code for the EHR software developed by the U.S. Department of Veterans Affairs, VistA, available to the public through the Freedom of Information Act. Although VistA has been taken by a few vendors who have tweaked it and implemented it successfully in a few hospitals and ambulatory care facilities (Medsphere 2008), it remains largely an interesting "project." (Note that this EHR software has nothing to do with Microsoft's Vista operating system.)

Web-based Products

Finally, when one seeks to achieve interoperability, one may think of the Web, and specifically Web services architecture. Although standards and products are moving toward Web Services Architecture (WSA), XML, and other such structures, not many EHR vendors have made much of a move (Oswald 2004). This is largely because the healthcare industry in the U.S. has such a huge investment in legacy systems that are not Web-based. However, progress is being made in standards setting and recognition of XML for document dissemination. There are also other parts of the world that are more embracing. The openEHR Framework, for example, is a specification maintained by the openEHR Foundation, which is an organization predominantly composed of European and Australian researchers who support development and implementation of EHRs based on open specifications. The openEHR Framework is consistent with the new Electronic Health Record Communication Standard (EN 13606) and is being used in parts of the UK NHS Connecting for Health Programme (openEHR 2008).

It should also be noted that "Web-based EHRs" could mean either those based in WSA and distributed as Software as a Service (SaaS) (Traudt and Konary 2005), or any software handled by an ASP (Gordon 2008).

Selecting a Vendor

Whatever decisions are made about building, buying, borrowing, blending, or replacing systems, there is a selection process that must be undertaken. The acquisition strategy is one of many elements to consider. It is also common for care delivery organizations to approach vendor selection with some open mindedness concerning their acquisition strategy. Several vendors offer their products for both traditional leasing ("buy") and ASP. It also may not be until a vendor selection is undertaken that the precise strategy to be used will be formulated.

Controlling the Selection Process

As the organization begins to undertake vendor selection, it should control interactions with vendors to ensure a fair representation of products and to keep marketing hype and accusations of competitive advantage to a minimum. Most organizations require all vendor interactions to go through one designated individual. The vendors who make the first cut should be treated evenly, with equal opportunity to demonstrate their products and interact with the selection team. In addition, the organization should select firm criteria.

The healthcare organization is buying a product or service, not "salesmanship." This is as true for a poor salesperson as for a good one. Some have suggested that the more marketing techniques a salesperson must apply to the product, the less likely the product meets the requirements to sell itself. People can be highly swayed by friendliness, fancy dinners, and promises. Likewise, they can be turned off by surly salespersons who show little interest in the organization, even though their product may be outstanding.

Controlling the selection process is as much about *looking past* the salesperson as it is about *looking at* the product. The vendor's salesperson will *not* be responsible for installation, training, or ongoing support. A good salesperson represents the company as a whole and should be a member of a collaborative team that learns the buyer's needs, understands its business requirements, and offers proactive suggestions. However, the bottom line is that the salesperson's responsibility is sales. He or she will generally not be around when there are implementation problems.

In the EHR marketplace, it is important to recognize that the products are not commodities. Although many good EHR products are on the market and many are certified as meeting the certification criteria, they still differ from each other significantly. A good product for one organization is not necessarily a good product for another. This fact emphasizes the need for thorough planning and a carefully controlled selection process.

Figure 12.1 provides a schematic of a process that most healthcare organizations find helpful in narrowing down the universe of potential EHR vendors. The process really

Figure 12.1.   Vendor selection process

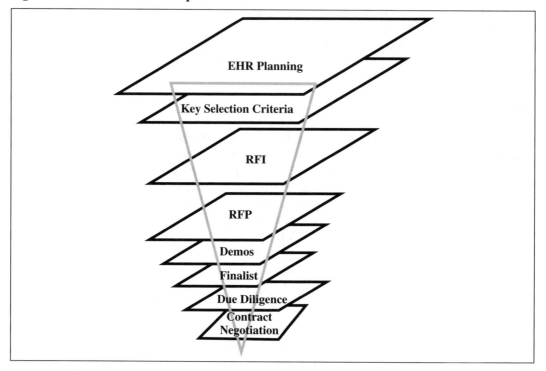

is about using a set of filters to focus the candidate pool on the organization's specific requirements.

Differentiating among Associated Products and Services

Many lists of EHR vendors include a wide variety of products and services, not just EHR products. Many EHR vendors also sell associated products and services. The vendors of associated products and services often include EHR consultants, systems integrators, component producers, and niche or specialty products.

EHR Consultants

EHR consultants provide everything from EHR strategic planning, process redesign, and vendor selection to system integration, implementation, and ASP services or outsourcing support. Any, all, or none of these types of consultants may be appropriate for your project.

Many organizations find that a consultant is extremely helpful in facilitating definition of the EHR vision, goal setting, and overseeing process assessment efforts. A consultant for this aspect of the project should be open-minded, an excellent communicator, and someone who values details but is not mired in minutiae. The organization's users should take ownership of process assessment but will likely need direction and support.

Many organizations also find it useful to have a consultant oversee the vendor selection process. In this case, the consultant should have a broad range of experience and be highly vendor-neutral. Many organizations take as much care in selecting their EHR consultant as they do in selecting the EHR itself. However, many organizations also make the mistake of engaging a consultant who they perceive can carry them through all phases of the project—from visioning through implementation to ongoing support and benefits realization. This is often not the best strategy because a consultant who has sufficient experience in implementing a given product is likely to be highly biased toward that product and generally is not right for the planning stages or the postimplementation benefits realization activities.

Most organizations need to supplement their own staff with persons who can help implement the product. In many cases, the vendor itself supplies these persons. In other cases, the vendor outsources this function. In still other situations, the organization may decide to obtain its own resources or use a mix of vendor and other resources. Too many different companies involved in the project can become a project management nightmare. However, where there are unusual interfaces to be developed, an accelerated time line, or special types of technology, it may be necessary to have multiple companies providing services.

Systems Integrators

Systems integrators are companies, or parts of companies, that specialize in getting disparate vendor products to work together. They may write interface programs or supply an **interface engine,** which is a software tool that manages connections among many disparate systems. Sometimes this is called middleware.

An interface engine supports multiple communications protocols, including (but not exclusively) Health Level 7 (HL7), by mapping data formats between two otherwise incompatible applications. In addition to connectivity, an interface engine supports enhanced security functionality. Within the clinical information context, **Clinical Context Object Workgroup** (CCOW) is a vendor-independent standard developed by HL7 to support clinical application integration. CCOW achieves simultaneous sign-on to multiple clinical applications by using mapping agents that map equivalent identifiers without sharing the same identification information for patients or users (often referred to as single sign-on) (CCOW 2003).

Component Producers

Component producers sell products that support the EHR. Although the EHR relies on all source systems as well as point-of-care data capture for its data, there are a number of tools that manage the data in a variety of ways. Some of these may be data capture tools, such as document-imaging systems and voice recognition systems. Other tools serve to process the data. These might include a clinical decision support system, report writing tools, or data warehousing. The system integration tools mentioned earlier could be considered component products. The CPOE, e-prescribing, and BC-MAR tools are important components of an EHR.

Niche or Specialty Products

Niche or specialty products provide EHR systems that are primarily designed for one type of clinical specialty. For example, the field of behavioral health services is quite different from that of general medical and surgical services. Certain vendors support EHRs exclusively for behavioral health services. Many specialty-based EHR products have been designed for physician office specialties, such as for cardiologists, nephrologists, and others.

Narrowing the Universe of Vendors

No healthcare organization has the resources to evaluate hundreds of vendors to find one that will be the best fit. Some organizations narrow the universe of vendors by developing a short list of key selection criteria and then issuing a **request for information** (RFI) to some 10 to 20 vendors (at most) in an effort to focus on perhaps four or five to evaluate seriously. Many organizations are eliminating this step in favor of reviewing Web demos and attending trade shows. When the field is narrowed to a manageable number, the organization issues a **request for proposal** (RFP) to obtain more detailed information.

Key Selection Criteria

Organizations should draw from their planning activities to establish a set of initial vendor-screening criteria. Questions to ask include:

- Does the vendor share the organization's *vision* for the EHR?

- Does the vendor's product provide the key *functionality* needed to achieve the organization's vision?

- Does the vendor utilize the desired *technology*?

- Does the vendor qualify under the organization's *acquisition* policies, including CCHIT certification?

- Can the vendor support the organization's desired *implementation* strategy?

- What is the vendor's track record for *operations and maintenance* support?

- What is the vendor's understanding of the *implications* of implementing an EHR system?

Request for Information (RFI)

An RFI is basically a means to accumulate marketing literature. Because most vendors provide much of this information on their Web sites, RFIs currently are not as often used as in the past.

When an RFI is used, having an external advisor send it out on the organization's behalf (without identifying the organization) can be helpful for the organization to understand the marketplace without being inundated with vendors attempting to make sales calls. Generally, an RFI is limited to a two- or three-page set of questions on the following areas:

- *Company background:* Obtain information on the vendor's size and financial stability

- *Product information:* Obtain the product name, primary market, technical platform, and overview of product capabilities that will be matched with key functionality criteria

- *Market information:* Ask the vendor to identify its major competitors and explain how the vendor differs from them

- *Installed base and clients:* Identify the number of EHR products the vendor has sold, is currently implementing, and has fully installed

- *Special criteria:* Collect information on any unique features or functions the vendor has established as critical

Figure 12.2 is a vendor comparison map that can be used to plot the responses to the RFI. This tool helps narrow down a large list of vendors.

The vendor comparison map can accommodate any limited number of key criteria an organization desires. The figure illustrates the following example:

A physician office has identified four major criteria to consider in making the initial cut. As an ambulatory care organization, its primary focus is outpatient workflow. Thus, it wants a vendor that can supply a full product suite in case the organization wants to replace its outdated practice management system. It also anticipates increased managed care contracting and thus wants to be able to move into that operation with the same vendor. Although wanting new technology, the organization is unwilling to risk accepting a new market entrant but, rather, prefers to buy from a stable vendor. Some 16 vendors (labeled A through P for illustrative purposes) were considered likely candidates and plotted on a vendor comparison map. The vendors in the upper-right quadrant are the most suitable for the organization to evaluate further. In this case, five vendors will receive RFPs.

In making the initial selection of vendors to whom to send RFPs, external advisors can offer neutral and unbiased advice, generally based on their broader familiarity with

Figure 12.2.   Vendor comparison map

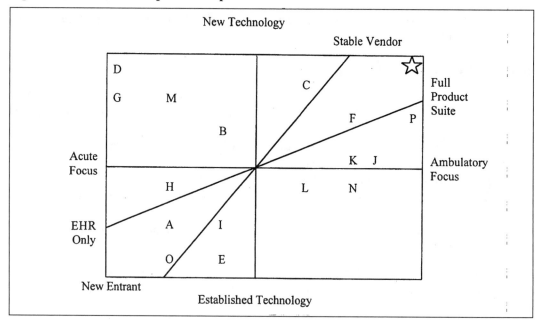

the marketplace. In some cases, organizations may find that some of their staff members, especially those serving on the EHR steering committee and even some representatives of facilities within an integrated delivery system, may already have experience with one or more EHR products. Their experience may be as a direct user or the result of having seen product demonstrations at trade shows. However, sometimes these individuals can have a vested interest in the selection of a particular vendor.

Request for Proposal (RFP)

An RFP is a formal document sent to vendors inviting them to submit bids for the organization's EHR project. The number of vendors to whom an RFP should be sent generally should be fairly small, such as to the four or five that seem to best fit the organization's overall criteria after they have studied the marketplace. The number of RFPs sent may depend on whether the healthcare organization is public or private. Public organizations often have requirements for getting RFPs to any eligible vendor and hence may send them to many more than four or five.

Some industry observers suggest that RFPs no longer serve their intended purpose because they often lack substance. However, a well-constructed RFP serves two important purposes. First, it solidifies the planning information and organizational requirements into a single document. In a way, it is the culmination of the organization's strategic EHR planning. There is value in bringing this information together for the EHR steering committee and the organization as a whole. Second, when developed and managed correctly, the RFP provides valuable insights into the vendor's operations and products and tends to level the playing field in terms of asking all the vendors the same questions. Additionally, it can serve as a source document for the contract that provides the license to use the vendor's software.

It requires skill to write an RFP that results in more than a set of checkmarks in a yes column on a form. The intent of the RFP should be to elicit a description of how the vendor believes its product solves the healthcare organization's specific problems and meets its requirements.

The RFP usually has some fairly standard components, including the following:

- *Organizational profile:* The first section describes the healthcare organization, including its basic demographics, mission and goals, vision for the EHR, current information infrastructure, and specific constraints (such as its particular time line). This section also contains the organization's instructions for responding (for example, to whom the bid should be sent, how many copies will be sent, and how vendor questions will be handled).

- *Vendor information:* This section, which may be placed next or last in the proposal, asks the vendor for a description of its demographics. The description should include the vendor's size and longevity (years in business, revenues, profitability, number of employees), product research and development history and plans, types of installations (number, size, status), corporate composition (organizational makeup, employee qualifications and tenure, country in which most work is performed), references, user group information (leader, size, frequency of meetings), and contract history (any defaults, pending lawsuits, Internal Revenue Service [IRS] status).

- *Functional specifications:* In this section, the organization requests a description of functional capability, such as the process flows the product supports, and compares these against its redesigned processes. Alternatively, the organization may develop a script describing a scenario, or use case, based on its redesigned processes and ask the vendor how its product would perform the inherent functions. This approach can be useful for avoiding yes and no responses.

- *Operational requirements:* This section should elicit information on the EHR product's data architecture, analytical processes supported, necessary interfaces, reliability and security features, system capacity, expansion capabilities, response time, downtime, and other issues associated with system maintenance.

- *Technical requirements:* In this section, the vendor should propose the appropriate technical architecture to meet the organization's EHR functional specifications and operational requirements, delineating the specific hardware, networking, and software requirements. Many organizations are asking vendors to describe both minimum and optimum requirements, as some vendors have only supplied minimum requirements that have not worked well after implementation.

- *Application support:* The vendor uses this section to propose an implementation schedule and to describe data conversion, acceptance-testing, training, and documentation, as well as the ongoing support, maintenance, and upgrades it will supply.

- *Licensing and contractual details:* In this section, the vendor is asked to supply its specific bid for one-time and recurring costs based on the organization's requirements. This section also should include a request for the vendor's standard contract, financing arrangements, proposed relationships with hardware vendors, and warranty information. This section should include clauses that protect the healthcare organization in the event the vendor goes out of business.

    Many organizations request that the pricing information be provided in a separate section of the response. Doing so removes the influence of cost from other critical evaluation factors. Pricing models and proclivity to discount vary so much among vendors that it is often easier for a financial specialist to attempt to normalize these for comparison purposes before the EHR steering or selection committee reviews them.

- *Evaluation criteria:* Some organizations add their evaluation criteria to the RFP so that the vendor knows up front the most important elements of the evaluation. This would indicate how the organization weighs various factors. For instance, evaluation criteria may identify that cost is weighed at 50 percent of the organization's decision-making criteria or that it is acceptable for the vendor to outsource interface development, but not maintenance.

Organizations and external advisors may have standard RFP formats or alternatives that they prefer to use.

Managing the Vendor Selection Process

Managing the RFP issuance, receipt, and evaluation is as important as preparing its content. RFPs should be sent to all vendors on the organization's short list at the same time, and all vendors should be given the same amount of time to respond. If a vendor requests an extension, it should be granted only for extenuating circumstances and only before any other vendor has submitted a response. All vendors then should be notified immediately that they have an equal extension period. A request for an extension may be viewed as a red flag for potential problems, although with the current surge in momentum for acquiring an EHR, such a request is becoming more commonplace and should not necessarily deter consideration of the vendor. Alternatively, if a vendor does not respond at all to an RFP, it may be that it recognizes that its product is not a "right fit" for the organization or simply has to make choices based on its own capacity. If an organization is interested in such a vendor, it may contact the vendor to find out why a proposal was not received and decide whether to accept one late if the vendor becomes interested in responding.

Bergeron (1999) suggests that issuance of the RFP instantly establishes a "competitive feeding frenzy." The EHR steering committee should discuss the potential (inevitability) of this occurring and plan for it directly. Some organizations try to keep potential vendors' identities confidential; others include the potential vendors' names in the RFP. A middle ground is perhaps more common: The short list is not revealed, but respondents are not kept secret (which is virtually impossible anyway). Most organizations do not accept proposals from vendors other than the ones to whom RFPs have been directed. If an exception is made, the EHR steering committee should vote on it and give the vendor no extra time, unless the committee deems the omission to be an oversight on the part of the organization. This should not occur when sufficient planning and careful construction of the selection criteria have taken place.

Some organizations hold a bidders' conference to respond to questions about the RFP. In this situation, the RFPs include the specific date, time, and location for the conference. Any vendor may attend and ask questions. Thus, all vendors hear all questions and obtain the same answers, keeping the playing field even. Unfortunately, most vendors either do not attend or attend only to learn what other vendors are asking.

When no bidders' conference is scheduled, the organization should decide whether it will respond to questions, who will respond, and how. Notifying vendors that questions must be put in writing and that the questions and answers will be shared with all vendors receiving the RFP can serve the same purpose as a bidders' conference. How tightly the bidding process is controlled is up to the organization.

Many organizations are starting to use vendor selection codes of conduct to advise and remind the members of their steering committee and others of the practices to which they want to adhere. This helps achieve an objective and fair vendor selection process.

Evaluating the RFP

A first step in RFP evaluation may be to assess the vendor's overall response: Was it received early or on time? Did the vendor ask appropriate questions or simply questions to gain competitive advantage? Did the vendor follow the organization's instructions on how to respond? The answers to these and other such questions can be revealing. The organization also may want to learn why certain vendors did not respond.

After obtaining some initial impressions, the organization should do an in-depth analysis of the responses and how they compare to the selection criteria. Because a comprehensive EHR is a big project, some organizations find it useful to allocate sections of it to different subject teams for in-depth evaluation. The teams then report back to the group as a whole. Many organizations use some form of scoring methodology to evaluate the proposal against the criteria and a formal group process technique to ensure everyone's input.

A Likert scale may be used to do a quantitative analysis on the results of the RFP. Figure 12.3 provides an example of a Likert scale, which compares 6 vendors (A through F) against 10 weighted selection criteria. The figure illustrates the following example:

> A hospital has prioritized 10 criteria. It has assigned a simple numeric weight to each criterion, ranging from 1 (least important) to 10 (most important). (It is possible to use a different scale and assign different weights to each criterion. For example, a scale of 1 to 5 may be used. The first two criteria may be considered most important and both weighted as 5, the next three may be weighted as 3, and the remaining 5 weighted as 2.)
>
> To calculate each vendor's score, the sum of each criterion's weight is multiplied by the vendor's rating on that criterion. (In figure 12.3, vendor A earned 1.5 on the first criterion weighted 10, thus the 10 x 1.5 equals 15; it earned 2.0 on the second criterion weighted 9, the 9 x 2.0 equals 18; and so on. These are then totaled. In this case, vendor A earned a total of 100.5 points.)
>
> In the final analysis, vendors F and E have the most potential for this organization because they are 60 points ahead of the next group of vendors consisting of D, B, and C.

Figure 12.3.   Vendor comparison on Likert scale

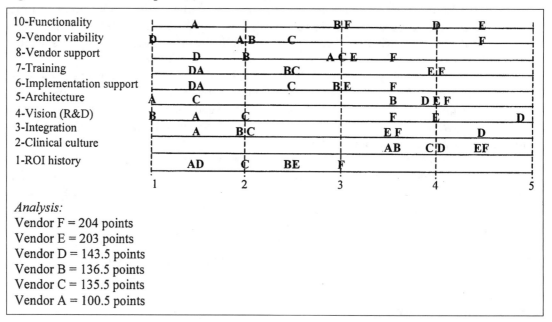

Analysis:
Vendor F = 204 points
Vendor E = 203 points
Vendor D = 143.5 points
Vendor B = 136.5 points
Vendor C = 135.5 points
Vendor A = 100.5 points

At the conclusion of this evaluation, one vendor may rise to the top or several vendors may warrant further, in-depth review. At this stage, it is important to rule out any vendors who are subpar.

One thing few organizations discuss but might consider at this stage is the concept of good customership. Customers often chide vendors for their sales tactics and "vaporware," and yet vendors often expend considerable resources in responding to RFPs, conducting demonstrations, and performing other legitimate sales activities. Although these expenses are factored into the price of the product, frivolous demands should be avoided. When the organization is not serious about a particular vendor after reviewing the RFP, it should eliminate the vendor as politely as possible and extend appreciation for the vendor's response.

Due Diligence to Determine the Vendor Finalist(s)

The next set of steps are often referred to as **due diligence**, or a formal process of investigation to ensure that the product is as stated in the RFP and is truly right for the organization. Due diligence is an analysis of the product via demonstrations, site visits, reference checks, and corporate visits. This process should culminate in identifying the vendor with whom to begin contract negotiation. Although care should be taken not to rush and to ensure a thorough due diligence, this is also the time when "analysis paralysis" can set in and needs to be managed. It can be helpful to remember that acquiring an EHR is not just about the product, but that people, policy, and process play a tremendous role in how successful one can be with an EHR.

Product Demonstrations

Most organizations invite the vendors who have passed the initial RFP phase to conduct a demonstration of their EHR products on-site. Demonstrations are valuable for several reasons, even in cases where the organization has viewed demonstrations previously. First, the demonstration acquaints as many of the potential users as possible with the product to make everyone feel a part of the process and to obtain everyone's feedback. Potentially hundreds of persons may view a demonstration, and so a feedback mechanism should be devised to focus on the highlights. A second reason to conduct a demonstration is to evaluate products side by side. Finally, the demonstration illustrates the vendor's understanding of the organization's specific requirements. The requirements should be reflected in how the vendor conducts the post-RFP demonstration; earlier demonstrations probably would have been generic.

As with the RFP, one option for the organization is to prepare a script the vendor must follow during demonstrations to highlight the key processes the organization wants to observe. Although vendors will not be able to completely customize a product to match the script, through the use of PowerPoint and Visual Basic programming language, they should at least be able to simulate processes to meet the organization's requirements. This is an excellent test of whether the vendor fully understands the organization's situation. If the vendor cannot meet a specific requirement and indicates this fact during the demonstration, its honesty is certainly a point in its favor as long as the requirement was not a major factor.

However, it is important to be aware that just as vendors are easily able to create a simulation, they also can create an illusion. (After all, that is how they create vaporware. However, it is appropriate to remember that from the vendor's perspective, what organizations consider vaporware may be considered a prototype to evaluate response to product ideas.) The EHR product being demonstrated in response to the RFP should be based on the current, real release of the product, and any attempt to do otherwise should disqualify the vendor.

A demonstration may be conducted in several segments. One segment is for many users who will spend just 5 or 10 minutes at the demonstration to get a sense of the look and feel of the product. A small, but important, use of the product should be scripted for such a purpose. Another segment might be a 1- or 2-hour demonstration of a more comprehensive scenario for members of the steering committee. In this segment, committee members should challenge the vendor and encourage the vendor to ask questions. The steering committee should include users of all types, including physicians, other clinicians, and administrative professionals. This ensures that all aspects of the EHR are evaluated thoroughly. A demonstration also may be planned for the organization's technical team to evaluate the interfaces, see the source code, understand modification procedures, and so on.

Vendors should be given adequate time to set up their equipment and test their software and network connections. Some organizations try to have all the vendors demonstrate at the same time, but in separate locations. When this is not feasible, conducting the demonstrations as close together in time as possible is important for comparison purposes. As soon after the demonstrations as possible, evaluations should be collected and the selection committee debriefed.

Site Visits

Organizations often visit vendor client sites that are similar to their own. The purpose of the visits is to assess the vendor's product in action. Site visits offer an opportunity to learn about the installation process and obtain feedback from direct users. They also can be valuable for learning other "lessons" from the client, even apart from their relationship to the product. Even though most vendors arrange site visits at their "best" sites (and often compensate the organization for their time in hosting the site visit), there are still valuable lessons to be learned. (The buying organization should pay for the trip and not accept the vendor's offer to do so.)

The site visit team should include a representative group composed of clinician users, information management representatives, and others. Typically, this is a core group of the larger steering committee. It is preferable to have the same group go on all visits. Generally, one or two visits per vendor are made, and often visits are made to the clients of the two candidates that lead the field after the demonstrations.

It is advisable to establish an agenda for the site visit. The vendor may be present during introductions, but the rest of the site visit must be done without the vendor present. Team members should not hesitate to speak to people other than those scheduled (and potentially primed by the vendor). It is useful to observe as many people as possible who are not on the formal agenda. (Insofar as possible, these individuals should be typical users.) Even so, because the site needs its vendor to survive, people working at the site rarely give the vendor bad marks. In addition, questions will need to be crafted carefully so that the responses reveal important insights about the vendor's level of service and support without offending the vendor's representatives. Another reason to proceed cautiously is that vendors may have outsourced staff to the site; thus, it is possible that some of the IS staff, trainers, and others at the site may actually be employees of the vendor.

At the conclusion of each site visit, participants should be debriefed immediately before they forget their impressions or confuse their reactions with those they had at other site visits.

Checking References

At the same time that site visits are being conducted, reference calls should be made to as many of the vendor's other clients as possible. The organization has the right to ask for a complete list of the vendor's clients, and any vendor who does not provide a list at this point should be suspected of having something to hide. Some vendors may ask you to sign a contract not to contact clients other than those they identify. This, obviously, is not something desirable.

As for site visits, an agenda should be established for conducting reference calls to ensure that no key questions are forgotten. A conference call or a series of calls to talk with equivalent users, technical staff, and administrators might be a useful tactic. Moreover, conversations with the leaders of the vendor's user group and reviews of agendas and meeting attendance lists can be helpful in supplementing reference checks.

Conducting Corporate Visits

If after site visits and reference checks it is still difficult to narrow the field to one vendor, a few other activities may be undertaken. One such activity is a corporate visit. Representatives from the healthcare organization, such as the CEO, CFO, and medical director, meet with their counterparts at the vendor's company. The CIO may meet with the vendor's chief technology officer (CTO)

Corporate visits are particularly helpful as vendors start to merge and acquire other companies. The culture of the vendor can make a difference in how well you may interact with them in the future, the trust you place in their promises, and so on.

Creating the Implementation Plan

Another activity that is useful in making the finalist selection is to request that the vendor's technical staff conduct a walk-through of the healthcare organization. This activity would help ensure that the vendors fully understand the technical infrastructure that exists and any customization that may be required. The walk-through should result in a detailed implementation plan and firm up any potential change in the initial cost estimates provided in the RFP.

Most organizations phase in EHR projects because EHR projects are so large and impose significant change. Some organizations may want to conduct a pilot program even before they consider phasing in a full implementation. Because the difference between conducting a pilot program and phasing in implementation can have a significant impact on contract negotiations, it is important to understand the purposes of both options.

A pilot program is a limited implementation of a proposed change for a selected group, after which the organization decides whether it will proceed with the rest of the project. A phased implementation is a confirmed project carried out in small segments over a period of time until all groups are implemented. Sometimes organizations can save money by having the vendor do the first few phases and then having the organization complete the rest. Phased implementation helps manage the impact of change on the organization whereas a pilot program is part of the decision-making process.

Healthcare organizations may decide to conduct pilot EHR programs for any number of reasons, including, among others, to determine the project's potential ROI, to compare the features of competing products, to determine the product's fit with the organization, to validate new hardware or software, to buy time to gain user acceptance, or to determine the organization's readiness for an EHR system. Often the underlying reason for conducting a pilot program, however, is some other factor, including fear of change, difficulty in managing change, insufficient funding, and uncertainty about whether any EHR will fulfill its potential. All of these factors are poor reasons to do a pilot; in such environments, pilots are likely to fail.

Another consideration is that for a pilot program to be successful, the vendor must install most of the product so that the organization can evaluate its interfaces and users can obtain the full value of data collection from source systems. Vendors recognize the issues presented by pilots and often steer clear of them. Unless a vendor is a new market entrant and needs a foot in the door, most vendors offer phasing and some have begun to offer risk-sharing contracts instead of pilots. A vendor that accepts a pilot contract will necessarily have to price the project higher than a phased project to overcome the risk. Sometimes the difference can be recouped by accepting the full product within a designated period of time (Amatayakul and Cohen 1999).

When an EHR project is phased in, consideration should be given to whether a direct cutover or parallel conversion will be used. The direct cutover has the advantage of not having to maintain two systems, but it requires considerable up-front preparation, including uploading data for active patients either before the cutover or as each patient is scheduled. Parallel conversion is more comfortable because the organization knows that everything is backed up, but it sometimes extends reliance on paper systems into perpetuity.

Often the nature of the organization (inpatient or outpatient, size, number of locations) and the extent of data already automated determine the form of conversion. Straight cutovers and parallel conversions are rarely done for an entire EHR implementation except in a small environment.

Making the Final Decision

Ultimately, the organization must narrow the field to a single vendor of choice, which is the vendor in which the organization is most interested. Usually, the steering committee is responsible for recommending the finalist, although the decision is best made with input from all participants.

No product will meet all the organization's requirements exactly. Customization is possible, but adapting the organization's requirements to adjust to a close match keeps costs down. Moreover, customization can have a long-term impact on the organization's ability to implement system upgrades successfully.

Even at this point in the project, the tendency may still exist to hold on to old, familiar ways. Vendors may even encourage an organization to buy a product that most closely matches its current processes (is there any wonder that ROI opportunity is low for such products). Many who will be new users of such systems will tend to look for products that appear easy to use—even though they may not be sophisticated and could end up frustrating users as they become more comfortable with the EHR. It is important for an organization to facilitate a true understanding of its EHR vision and goals in those who will make the selection decision or recommendation.

Price should be the last factor considered in finalist selection. Many factors influence the pricing of EHR products. Hard-line negotiation seldom proves beneficial over the long term. At this point, prices should not be significantly different across the vendor finalists unless the products are significantly different. If the products are significantly different, the decision is often one of price vs. functionality. When balancing functionality and price, the organization must consider its migration strategy carefully. It may be appropriate to phase in functionality, and good vendors should be able to show how this can be done. Alternatively, being penny-wise and pound-foolish can result in problems down the road, as the following scenario illustrates:

> A large group practice bought a comprehensive EHR system and expected to achieve significant cost savings through clinical decision support. Unable to fund workstations for every examining room, the practice decided to provide interim functionality through printouts and to have physicians use workstations centralized at the nurses' stations. Even though queues rarely formed at the workstations, physicians found the practice inconvenient and got their nurses to enter their data. Not only did this defeat the opportunity to benefit from clinical decision support at the point of care, but it also reduced the expected benefit to nursing personnel. The bottom line was that the physicians were essentially unhappy with the system. Although an investment in more workstations would have paid for itself, the physicians would not agree to the expenditure, seeing the entire system as being less than successful and beneficial only from an operational, not a clinical, view.

The following example illustrates a successful implementation:

An integrated delivery system (IDS) with many small- and medium-sized physician practice affiliates scattered across nearly an entire state needed a way to improve communications. Physician practices varied greatly, from not having an EHR to having fairly sophisticated systems. The IDS considered investing in the purchase of a single system for all affiliates. At the time, the cost was prohibitive, but supporting a Web-enabled system to exchange data and to begin feeding a repository was a significant advantage to all practices. Such a system also would accomplish a common look and feel among the hospitals and the practices. When practices wanted more functionality or upgrades for their current systems, they migrated to a common vendor.

Performing Final Due Diligence and Negotiating the Contract

The final steps before signing on the dotted line are final due diligence to investigate the vendor of choice and contract negotiation.

Final Due Diligence

Demonstrations, site visits, reference checks, and even corporate site visits are all parts of due diligence. However, these activities focus primarily on the product. For a major investment such as an EHR, the healthcare organization also needs to assess the vendor's viability and how well it believes it can work with the company.

Credit checks on the company and its officers may be performed, especially if the vendor is not well established. Depending on whether the company is public, some information may be easier to obtain than other information. Still, considering the size of the investment the healthcare organization is making, even a nonpublic company should disclose reasonable financial information at this point. The market status of other products in the vendor's product line is also a good indicator of its financial status and ability to meet its contractual obligations (Grams 1998).

Contract Negotiation

The following discussion is not a substitute for legal advice but provides some tried-and-true suggestions for effective contract negotiation.

Before beginning the actual contract negotiation, one other element to consider is whether to negotiate with one or two vendors. Some consultants suggest that the wisest approach is to narrow the field to two vendors and negotiate with the primary candidate first, leaving the second choice available in the event contract negotiations break down. Again, good customership is advised. If the process of contract negotiation is expected to be fairly rapid, a second vendor may be able to be managed. But there are many variables in contract negotiation and a second vendor kept waiting for a very long time may become frustrated and not provide the best second choice. If the negotiation fails with the first vendor, the organization may opt to begin the process again instead of returning to the second vendor (Cohen 2004).

Contract negotiation with a vendor begins with folding in a copy of the original RFP and the vendor's response into the vendor's standard contract. It also should include a thorough review of exactly what is being acquired. This may seem unnecessary after the comprehensive selection process just performed. Making sure what the vendor is actually providing in terms of software licenses, hardware, and services, however, may be somewhat nebulous in the final analysis. For example, will the vendor provide and install the hardware (or will the organization do one or both)? How many hours of training are included? Does the license agreement include only the EHR provided by the company, or does it also include licenses to third-party software necessary to support coding (for example, the license to use CPT from the AMA), the drug knowledge base, and even the database design (Sterling 2005). The final implementation plan also should be included in the contract. By themselves, the vendor's response to the RFP and the implementation plan are not legally binding documents.

Contracts should include a milestone-based payment schedule based on issues such as installation period, customer use, satisfaction, and projected savings. Compensation adjustments for product delivery delays and nonperformance should be specified. Maintenance contracts should include a clause that correlates problems with appropriate response times.

The Healthcare Financial Management Association (HFMA) has compiled a guide to IT contract negotiation that identifies ten critical components. These are included in table 12.2.

In addition to these critical components, some organizations look to protect themselves in the event the vendor goes out of business or is acquired by another vendor. Terms of the contract should include the fact that the product will be kept up to date for a specified number of years as long as the maintenance agreement fees are paid. This also should obligate any company acquiring the vendor to these terms. To protect against the vendor going out of business, some organizations require the vendor to put the source code and data schema for the product into an escrow account, making it available to a programmer the organization may acquire to assist in keeping the product current, at least until a new selection process can be undertaken. Some vendors require a separate fee for this process (O'Connor 2005; Uretz 2005).

Consideration also might be given to asking the vendor to supply evidence that the data retained in the EHR system can be converted to another platform if necessary. Some companies have been developed to perform just such services. If you use an ASP, the contract should also address that the data will be returned to the organization. Negotiating an ASP versus straight licensure contract has a number of different elements, including disposition and protection of data, as well as even more attention on service level. The extent to which you want to incorporate such protections in the contract depends on the risk profile of the organization and the perceived stability of the vendor in the marketplace (Amatayakul and Lazarus 2005).

Conclusion

Although the EHR project is not just about vendor selection, vendor selection is its most obvious activity. Planning is critical to successful vendor selection. The organization that understands its environment, information needs, functional requirements, and ability to

Table 12.2.   Critical contract negotiation components

Component	Description
1. Product definition and contract structure	• Define the system components covered by the contract; include response to the RFP to ensure comprehensive functionality description • Determine whether software license agreement, maintenance provisions (including service-level agreement), and installation agreement are included in one contract or separate contracts
2. Scope of license	• Recommends a fully paid, perpetual, royalty-free, nonexclusive, nontransferable license for use by, or on behalf of, affiliates, as specified • Reviews a vendor's standard set of restrictions on licenses and negotiates incremental pricing, if necessary
3. Pricing structure	• One-time costs • Ongoing maintenance, including response to federal regulations • Operational changes
4. Implementation	• Includes specific work plan for implementation • Includes provisions for breach of agreement
5. Key personnel	• Qualifications • Replacement provisions • Third parties • Selection rights for key staff
6. Acceptance testing and payment terms	• Define testing stages (unit testing, integration testing, interface/network testing, stress testing, and live testing) • Define acceptance at each stage • Provide for correction of errors • Provide for resting and remedies
7. Performance warranties	• Response time • Uptime • Batch processing throughput assurance
8. Limitations on liability	• Ensure mutuality of liability • Insurances
9. Change in vendor control and product obsolescence	• Defines triggering events • Identifies remedies if a triggering event occurs • Identifies exclusions for limitation of liability
10. Dispute resolution and exit strategies	• Process • Mediation or binding arbitration • Exit clauses that outline right to deliverables and interim payment

Source: Adapted from HFMA 2004.

effect change will have a much easier time articulating its needs to potential vendors and helping users adapt to the system. Such planning reflects an organization that is well run and carries over into managing the selection process and the installation. Every element of planning has an impact on the selection and installation process.

Specific vendor selection is essentially the application of filters to the universe of vendors. The filters are formed through the organization's advanced planning and should be applied through unbiased facilitation.

The conclusion of the vendor selection process is successful contract negotiation, which also is the start of implementation and ongoing maintenance.

References and Resources

Altis. 1999–2004. Assessing an Interface Engine. www.altisinc.com/IE/assess.html.

Amatayakul, M., and M. Cohen. 1999 (May 1). Conducting a successful EHR pilot. *TEPR 1999 Conference Proceedings.* Orlando, FL: Medical Records Institute.

Amatayakul, M., and S.S. Lazarus. 2005. *Electronic Health Records: Transforming Your Medical Practice.* Denver: Medical Group Management Association, 169–173.

American Academy of Family Physician's Center for Health Information Technology. 2008. What is open source software?

Bates, G.W. 2001 (Feb.). Transitioning to an electronic medical record: the essential elements to consider when choosing a system. *Group Practice Journal* 50(2):38–40.

Bergeron, B. 1999. A keystone in your change-agent strategy: the RFP. *ADVANCE for Health Information Executives* 3(3):65–70.

Briggs, B. 2003 (June). The main event: Best-of-breed vs. single-source. *Health Data Management,* 41–48.

Certification Commission on Health Information Technology. 2008. www.cchit.org.

Clinical Context Object Workgroup. 1999–2003. www.hl7.org.

CIO Executive Summaries. 2002. Service-Level Agreement. www.cio.com/summaries/outsourcing/sla.

Cohen, M. 2004 (May 19). Negotiating successful CPR/EMR contracts. *TEPR 2004 Conference Proceedings.* Fort Lauderdale, FL: Medical Records Institute.

Gillespie, G. 2003 (June). Doing your homework: Execs should analyze vendors' financial statement before they sign on the dotted line. *Health Data Management,* 56–64.

Gordon, L. 2008 (June 4). Are you thinking of using a web-based EHR? www.emrblog.com.

Grams, R.R. 1998. Shopping in the health care information systems market. *ADVANCE for Health Information Executives* 2(7):37–40.

Hagland, M. 2003 (June). Choosing a vendor. *Healthcare Informatics,* 87–88.

Healthcare Financial Management Association. 2004. *Dotting the i's and Crossing the t's: Ensuring the Best IT Contract* (promotional material). Westchester, IL: HFMA.

Hjort, B. 2000. Surviving and thriving during contract negotiations. *Journal of AHIMA* 71(7):73.

Medsphere. 2008. Press Release: Medsphere Implementation at West Virginia Hospital Confirms Suitability of OpenVista Solution Across Continuum of Care. June 10, 2008.

Miranda, D. 1998. What works in point-of-care data collection systems. *ADVANCE for Health Information Executives* 2(4):37–40.

Monahan, T. 2001 (Feb.). Nine hot trends. *Healthcare Informatics* 18(2):54–56.

Morse, D. 2003. White paper: Looking outside: Using external capital sources to overcome budget constraints. HCT Project, GE Healthcare Financial Services. www.hctproject.com/white.asp.

O'Connor, K.J. 2005 (winter). Everything you always wanted to know about software escrow agreements—and then some! *Journal of Healthcare Information Management* 19(1):10–12.

OpenEHR. 2008 (May 17). http://www.openehr.org/home.html.

Oswald, M. 2004. The Future of Clinical Integration, MSHUG, World of Health Congress.

Schooler, R., and T. Dotson. 2003. Rolling out the CIS. *ADVANCE for Health Information Executives* 7(10):51–58.

Sheridan, C. 2001. Do you need an ASP ASAP? *Journal of AHIMA* 72(8):38–42.

Sterling, R. 2005 (July 8). 6 EMR Contract Terms that Avoid Big Headaches Later. Presentation at the Electronic Medical Records for Physician Practices conference, Washington, DC.

Traudt, E. and A. Konary (June 2005). *2005 Software as a Service Taxonomy and Research Guide.* www.idc.com.

Uretz, M. 2005. How to Survive Your EHR Contract. www.ehrgroup.com.

Zadrozny, B. 2005. Joining the HIT revolution: Should you buy or lease the tools you need? *Healthcare Informatics* 22(2):97.

Chapter 13
EHR System Implementation and Ongoing Maintenance

The implementation process begins after the contract is signed. Some suggest that this is when the real work begins. Many organizations are unprepared for the enormity of the task. Implementing an EHR is many times more complex than implementing a departmental system or even other cross-departmental applications. However, if the steps outlined in the previous chapters have been carried out as part of planning for the EHR, much of the implementation process should be to carry out the plans. Some experts in EHR implementation also suggest that neither planning nor implementation is ever finished. This is consistent with the philosophy of a migration path. Yet, implementing any one or more of the components of the migration path reflects a defined project and should be treated as a milestone that needs to be reached and celebrated. This chapter:

- Emphasizes the importance of project planning and management

- Describes infrastructure preparedness issues and reinforces the need for process redesign and change management

- Lists examples of items required for system build

- Defines testing stages and preconversion activities

- Provides training and support strategies

- Describes ongoing EHR activities

Project Planning and Management

As described in chapter 4, strategic planning for an EHR includes alignment of organizational goals and EHR initiatives, executive management support, medical staff and other user involvement, and project resources. Project resources explicitly include adoption of project management standards, definition of the project life cycle, skills and job description for a project manager, and project management techniques.

Key Terms

Acceptance testing   Clinical pathways   Roll-out strategy

Chart conversion   Configuration   Turnover strategy
                         management

Also critical to effective project planning and management are establishing an appropriate organizational structure for the implementation and gaining participation of key stakeholders. Some organizations dissolve their EHR steering committee after vendor selection has occurred and use, instead, dedicated staff to perform the implementation function. Other organizations organize a new implementation committee or domain teams to assist dedicated staff with the implementation functions. The scope of the EHR project and nature of the organization determine the approach, although most organizations find that a user stakeholder committee or other form of input is essential for implementation.

Part of the reason for dissolving the steering committee is literally because members are tired or because different skill sets are needed. A cautionary note was suggested, however, when describing the five stages of group development. The importance of the adjourning stage should not be minimized. In fact, it may be appropriate for steering committee members to identify their preference for staying on as implementation committee members. They might even be asked to qualify themselves for this new role. Organizations find transitioning members useful and, where necessary, can find adjunct roles for those whose skills do not translate directly to implementation.

All the project management techniques of building a project plan, facilitating meetings, and managing change are critical to the implementation phase of the EHR project. Two levels of planning are often useful. The first is an overall approach; the second encompasses specific tasks, dependencies, milestones, resources, and budget.

Overall Approach

As part of its various planning activities (functional needs, data and technology assessments, and the vendor selection process), the organization should have determined the overall scope of change the EHR will have on the organization. This likely reflects where the organization is with its migration path. The scope of change should help determine the project's roll-out and turnover strategies and the level of effort required by all concerned. Complementary to roll-out and turnover strategies is chart and data conversion.

Roll-Out Strategy

Roll-out strategy describes whether an organization will phase-in or follow a "big bang" approach to rolling out an EHR or its components. Because an EHR implementation typically is a huge undertaking, most organizations implement an EHR using a phased roll-out strategy. (See table 13.1.) However, the phasing may vary, and may be constructed in a multilevel, matrix-like approach.

Table 13.1. Summary of Roll-Out and Turnover Strategies

Type of Roll-Out Strategy	Consider using if Healthcare Organization Is:
Phased ■ Implementation of an EHR component, or functions of a component, in one or a few organizational units at a time ■ Plan exists to follow on with full roll-out in same manner	• Multispecialty clinic • Medium- to large-sized clinic or hospital • Multi-site facility • Implementing a complex EHR
Big Bang ■ Implementation of all aspects of an EHR component (or entire EHR in an ambulatory setting) in all organizational units virtually simultaneously	• Single specialty clinic • Small clinic or very small hospital • Other size/type clinic or hospital with considerable staff resources and vendor support
Pilot ■ Application of straight turnover or parallel processing in one or a few organizational units ■ Determination whether to proceed to full roll-out or not is made after some period of use ■ (Often not acceptable to vendors because level of effort needed to represent product fairly is too great)	• Implementing a product new to market • New to computerization • Medium to large size • One with previous bad experience with EHR
Type of Turnover Strategy	**Consider using if Healthcare Organization Is:**
Straight Turnover ■ Paper processes cease shortly after go-live ■ Close monitoring and cycle checking ensure system works as planned	• Most EHR environments
Parallel processing ■ Paper processes continue until system works as planned ■ Requires diligence in keeping both paper and electronic systems complete, accurate, and timely	• Select processes, such as patient accounting • Some BC-MAR applications (with poor results) • Organizations new to computerization in general • Implementing a product new to market

It is virtually a necessity to phase in an EHR via components, such as listed in chapter 1. However, many organizations also phase in implementation of each component, such as by nursing stations, departments, physician specialties, sites, and so on. Sometimes the phasing depends on the module being implemented and the interest of the users. For example, a computerized provider order entry (CPOE) might be implemented first on a medical-surgical inpatient unit because this is where it might have the greatest impact; a document-imaging system might begin in the emergency department (ED) because the ED has fewer forms to deal with; or an outpatient EHR may be implemented in the physician champion's clinic first because he or she might be more experienced and willing to work through bugs. Careful consideration should be given to the size of the organizational unit (not too big or too small), balancing the level of interest of the users (not the curmudgeons and not the cyberdocs), the complexity of the unit (that influences the degree of customization needed), and so on.

Another element of the phasing might relate to the functions performed by the component being implemented. If conducive to breaking down component by specific functions, it is also possible to have users adopt only one or a set of functions at a time. For example, some organizations get everyone up to speed on rudimentary processes and then phase in more specific processes. This can be both advantageous and disadvantageous, and often depends on what module is being implemented. For example, if bar code medication administration record (BC-MAR) is being implemented first through electronically generated MAR forms and then through a full bar coding process, the phasing can be helpful to acquaint nurses with computer systems and achieve patient safety benefits while potentially upgrading the pharmacy system, acquiring medication supply systems, adding bar code processing, and so on. Alternatively, some hospitals have tried implementing CPOE only for medication orders or for orders without a full complement of clinical decision support. Neither of these is acceptable to physicians, who either find it time-consuming to have to enter orders in both electronic and manual modes or who consider order entry without clinical decision support merely a clerical duty. In clinics, physicians may decide to first use the EHR only to retrieve laboratory results and documents from the hospital, then to perform e-prescribing, and finally move to documenting via templates.

In addition to phasing in by organizational unit and/or function, it should be determined whether the organization will require all users (within the organizational units targeted for implementation) to use the system or permit only those interested. In general, this applies to physicians, although a few organizations have permitted some nursing units to opt out of adoption. In one large clinic, for example, the physicians decided to permit only those interested to use the EHR and others to continue to use paper records, but they would be charged a paper processing fee. (Thankfully, few physicians opted for paper records initially, and even they quickly realized that not only were they losing money, but they also were having to learn the system anyway to manage their partners' patients. The need to process paper records in parallel with electronic records was phased out within a year.) In another example, a hospital decided to exclude its behavioral health unit because the general EHR was not suitable for such documentation and there were concerns about confidentiality.

Most healthcare organizations prefer to allow for some pacing, but desire ultimate adoption by all. Maintaining a hybrid environment is costly and can be a patient safety issue. In any hybrid record situation, it may never be completely clear where the latest information is actually available. Unfortunately, because of the need to implement an EHR in components and phases in most hospitals, the hybrid record situation is all too often the norm. This is less common in a physician office, because even though there may be phasing, the phasing can be accomplished more quickly.

Because of concerns about hybrid records, or even simply gaining full adoption, some organizations have tried and successfully accomplished implementing at least the major components of an EHR in a big bang approach. This also may be called rapid implementation. To do so, however, there must be extremely careful planning up front, virtually 100 percent commitment by all users, and an enormous amount of support during go-live (Badger et al 2005). Some physician offices are also considering the big bang approach, both to reduce the overhead of maintaining both paper and electronic systems and to ensure that every physician is on board. Typically such roll-outs are more successful in smaller practices.

Sometimes pilot testing also is referred to as a roll-out strategy. Pilot testing usually means that an information system will be tested with one group of users, and if they do not like it, use of the system will be discontinued. Because the EHR is such an enormous undertaking, it generally is not feasible to do a true pilot test. Even though many organizations will call their first go-live phase a pilot, it is not a true pilot unless the intent is to evaluate its continuance. Most first phases are conducted to work out bugs in both the software and processes, not to decide to scrap the entire project (although some larger organizations have come close and some small clinics or physician offices have actually done this).

Turnover Strategy

Two other considerations need to be considered with respect to the overall implementation approach. **Turnover strategy** refers to whether the paper system will cease on go-live, or whether it will be run parallel for some period of time after go-live.

- Straight turnover refers to having everyone in the designated group go live at one time, with paper processes ceasing virtually immediately after go-live. This is the most typical form of turnover for EHRs because most organizations find that any reliance on former paper processing not only ends up being too time-consuming but also sends a message that the system is not to be trusted. Although this may seem to be a risky strategy, it frequently is found that staff really cannot perform both paper and electronic processes accurately, completely, or on a timely basis. Furthermore, a straight turnover does not apply that quality checks are forsaken. Some interim paper processing may be necessary for a few days, and part of the go-live support should be to ensure the electronic processes are performed correctly and completely. However, staff should quickly move to the new environment, because not to do so will be a patient safety risk and a risk for not realizing your expected return on investment (RIO).

- Parallel processing is a turnover strategy where the organization continues processing in manual form as well as electronic form. The intent is to validate the electronic processing against the manual processing, such as at the end of a day, week, or month. Most organizations find this too time-consuming and error prone. For instance, in one hospital, nurses wanted to run parallel processing when implementing BC-MAR. The result was that some nurses used the BC-MAR primarily, often forgetting to document also on paper, while other nurses did the opposite. The staff checking the accuracy of the system thought there were major problems, until it was recognized that this was an implementation problem, not a system problem. Some form of parallel processing, such as using worksheets until certain the EHR has processed the documentation, may be necessary during the initial stages of go-live, but this is not what is typically meant by parallel processing, where every action is duplicated.

Conversion Strategy

Another component of the overall implementation that is closely related to roll-out and turnover strategies is conversion strategy, sometimes also referred to as pre-load strategy. This refers to how much of the existing paper records (**chart conversion**) or data in other electronic systems (data conversion) will be moved to the EHR prior to or during go-live. (Data conversion is discussed later in this chapter.)

For the acute care processes in hospitals, chart conversion may actually be somewhat less of an issue than for clinics or the ambulatory areas of a hospital. Most hospitals apply a straight turnover approach to chart conversion, where the new system is used on go-live and users must rely on paper records (which may or may not be scanned) for past admission information. This is generally an acceptable approach because any given admission is more often a unique episode of care. Virtually every admission includes a comprehensive history and physical (H&P) examination that is used as the basis for care. Past records can be useful, but generally data from them that are not included in the new H&P (such as current medications and allergies) are not needed in clinical decision support systems. However, if the hospital has a high readmission rate, it may be necessary to consider some of the chart conversion strategies identified for the ambulatory environment.

More often, the issue for a hospital is the hybrid record, where only parts of the EHR are available for use and some parts of the current chart must be on paper. For example, a hospital may have had a digital dictation system (for the H&P, radiology, and some other diagnostic studies results) and a laboratory results reporting system for some time. It then may add a CPOE system and a BC-MAR system, but progress notes and nursing graphics may continue to be handwritten. Unless the hospital prints everything out, a hybrid record is the result. Where a hospital declares its electronic components of the chart to be the official legal source (see appendix C.2 for AHIMA's practice briefs on the legal health record), it usually finds the need to include reminders in the paper chart that certain documents or data are accessible only electronically. Unfortunately, such a system can still lead to confusion, especially where not all users are willing to use both the electronic and paper chart components. (For example, those physicians not interested in EHRs may request that the electronic content be printed. If the physician writes notes on printed charts, it then may become "original health record" content that needs to be filed into the paper chart, potentially resulting in more than one version of information. If other physicians or clinicians rely on the fact that the electronic source is the "official source," the annotation may be missed, presenting a potential patient safety issue. Still other physicians may prefer to access the electronic system and ignore paper content.)

In a clinic or other ambulatory environment, reliance on previous visit information is often more essential than in a hospital because an episode of care can last for several visits. Furthermore, the time spent with a patient during any given visit is usually not long enough to re-create, to create again an entire medical history for the new EHR. As such, the chart conversion strategy requires careful consideration of what data from the charts need to be converted, how, and when.

Some organizations choose to backfill all content of active charts for 6 months or 1 year using document imaging, abstraction, or a combination of both. A timing issue can arise in this situation, where a chart may be converted too early and a visit occurs prior to EHR go-live, in which case the visit must be remembered to be converted. Other issues, of course, entail whether only an image of the past information is sufficient or whether some of the information is desired to be in discrete form and ready to be used in clinical decision support. It is for this reason that many clinics consider adopting both scanning and abstracting for chart conversion. Whoever performs the abstracting, however, must be knowledgeable about clinical processes, medical terminology, and drug names. In fact, some clinics are finding that the physicians can abstract a small amount of data more efficiently and accurately than having staff perform this function. Table 13.2 compares paper chart conversion strategies.

Time Frame for Implementation

Another part of the overall planning approach is the time frame for implementing each phase. The vendor should be able to offer estimates of the time it will take to get any given organizational unit up "live" on the system. The organization then needs to decide the level of effort it is willing to commit so that an actual estimate is determined. It is generally recommended that the first organizational unit that is phased in be used to obtain a solid

Table 13.2.   Chart conversion strategies

Technique	Advantages	Disadvantages
Continue pulling paper chart	• Makes available entire chart • Often acceptable for hospitals, especially those with a relatively low readmission rate	• Requires paper charts to be available for many years after EHR go-live • May result in a hybrid record if some clinicians will not use EHR for current care
Scan paper charts of active patients	• Makes entire content of paper chart available electronically • Acceptable process for both acute and ambulatory care • Allows destruction of paper chart, unless only parts of paper chart are scanned	• Does not provide discrete data for processing in clinical decision support, so for some period of time, an electronically hybrid record results • Cost/benefit issues of degree of indexing must be addressed
Abstract data from paper charts of active patients	• Makes data available for electronic processing of reminders and alerts • Some vendors are supporting templates that capture key data and distribute them to appropriate place in EHR	• Error prone if performed by nonphysician • Time consuming if performed by physician • Rarely used by hospitals; increasingly used by clinics
Use a combination of above	• Achieves all benefits relating to access • Most often used for a short period of time in which chart is pulled for any additional scanning or abstracting	• May be confusing if not consistently applied • Probably most costly to implement due to variations in instructions

Table 13.3. Installation vs. implementation

Installation	Implementation
Assemble hardware components	Review contract and develop detailed implementation plan (see chapter 13)
	Implement communication plan (see figure 14.1)
Connect devices	Establish issues management system (Figure 14.2)
Run hardware setup	Prepare site, such as data center enhancements, user area shelving, and so on (see chapter 10)
Lay network cable	Procure hardware, accept delivery, inventory, and tag
Install network devices, including wireless access points	Install (see left)
Test network connectivity	Design process improvement changes (see chapter 7)
Load application software	Build data dictionaries, tables, rules logic, file designs, screen layouts, data quality edits, report designs, repository structures (see chapters 8 and 9)
	Design technical controls, including security access controls (see chapter 10)
	Configuration management (see figure 14.3)
	Test (see table 14.4)
	Train (see table 14.5)
	Document policies and procedures
	Check/rehearse
	Go-live
	Evaluate
	Celebrate/correct course
	Transition to full adoption
	Acceptance testing

estimate of the time it takes to install, train, and obtain adoption. Subsequent units should take less time, but the organization may decide to give every unit the same time or to step up the process where some units are implemented in parallel. Again, the level of staff availability and experience and the scope of the project are the determining factors.

Specific Tasks

When overall phasing and time frames are established, detailed tasks should be plotted on a project plan. This is perhaps where the distinction between installation and implementation is most apparent. Installation refers to merely setting up and plugging in hardware, and loading software onto the computer. Implementation includes installation and much more. Key differences between installation and implementation are illustrated in table 13.3.

Figure 13.1. Issues log and sample entry

#	Issue	Source	Date ID	Reference	Escalation	Resolution	Date Tested	Sign Off
33	Screen does not display error correction	Mary	3/2	M3.S4.D2	No	Source code correction (vendor)	3/10	J.P.

Copyright © 2008, Margret\A Consulting, LLC. Reprinted with permission.

Because the tasks, people involved, budget, and myriad other details need to be tracked, an EHR project plan could well include thousands of tasks. Again, many vendors use detailed project plan templates when working with healthcare organizations. As previously noted, such plans should be a part of the contractual agreement when acquiring the system. However, it should be the task of the organization's project manager to manage the organization's own project plan. This plan should carry forward the key milestones of the vendor's plan as well as include the myriad tasks for which the organization itself is responsible. The project manager should be directly involved in harmonizing the plans and reviewing and signing off on task completion, monitoring task dependencies, ensuring milestones are met, and leveling resources.

Issues Management

Because of the number of tasks and their complexity and dependencies, it is important to have an issues management program (also called problem management or exception management). An issues management program serves to receive and document issues and track them to their resolution. Figure 13.1 shows a sample issues log.

Again, it is the project manager's task to receive issue reports, log them, identify the resources needed to take corrective action, and document resolution. He or she must understand the scope of issues that need to be tracked as well as the nature of issues that need to be escalated to a higher authority. For example, a week's delay in obtaining extra printers is not as critical as a report from the system integrator that an interface will require several hundred additional hours of work. The project manager probably can find a work-around for the shortage of printers but will need to report the issue of the interface to the CIO, board, or other authority. Certainly, any issue that would have a material bearing on the project's timeliness, budget, or desired outcome is one that needs to be escalated.

Infrastructure Preparedness

When the project plan has been established, there are many preparatory tasks. Some of these address the equipment and physical plant of the organization; others address people and processes.

Hardware Infrastructure

Among the first tasks on the project plan will likely be to prepare the organization's infrastructure for the EHR system. This may entail purchasing and installing hardware, upgrading the network, and even making changes in the physical plant. For example, some organizations must do extensive cabling or even expand or rebuild their data center. There often are issues associated with workstation location, ability to use computers on wheels (COWs), patient kiosks, printers, and so on. If a large-scale scanning program or chart abstraction process for chart conversion will be conducted, there may be considerable extra space needed for staging charts, high-speed scanners, and so on. This often entails a completely separate area apart from the file area, and often a courier process to move charts from the file area to the scanning operation and then to a temporary archive location. Additional storage devices and sometimes off-site disaster recovery sites must be added. Many organizations establish a test system separate from their production system for testing and training. This may entail acquiring additional space and hardware, as well as a "war room" where system build can occur and a separate training room. Many of these tasks must be performed before software is installed; some are ongoing.

Hardware purchasing and delivery also are two important tasks. It may be appropriate to purchase all human–computer interfaces (HCIs) at one time and have them either delivered in batches or all delivered at the same time and store the ones not immediately needed. These are just a few of the many details the project manager must include in the project plan and about which decisions must be made. HCI acquisition and delivery may seem to be a straightforward task, but the difference in price to be realized by buying in quantity and having the capacity to store a large number of PCs makes the task more complex than it initially appears to be.

Process Infrastructure

Other infrastructure preparation issues include process assessment and redesign (if not performed earlier). The earlier in the planning these can be performed the better, as many processes can be improved in their manual form that will aid in implementing the EHR. A good example of this is the use of **clinical pathways**, order sets, and evidence-based medicine (EBM). Although these tools are not new, not every clinician has actually used them or documented against them. In a paper environment, such tools for some clinicians were often treated as general "guidance" rather than required processes. Clinicians frequently did not give much consideration to the standardization of terminology such use would require. They were certainly not held accountable for their use as there was virtually no means to document their use. Reviewing what clinical tools exist, understanding and agreeing to use of the standard terminology they include, developing new tools or modifying existing ones as needed, and starting to use them more fully can be initiated in the paper environment prior to full EHR implementation.

Identifying and obtaining agreement on all form of standards may be something to prepare for in advance of actual software installation. For example, some vendors offer a proprietary vocabulary or the option to adopt a standard vocabulary. Although this is probably at least partially decided prior to contract negotiation, reviewing the vocabulary and deciding specifically how it will be used may be necessary at this point. Perhaps only a limited portion of standard vocabulary will be adopted. The vendor may provide options for a number of nursing vocabularies. It may be necessary to perform some mapping from the vendor's vocabulary, or even standard vocabulary, to standard data sets prior to software installation. Performing as many of these types of tasks prior to system build, the next major task, helps it go smoothly (and keeps costs in line with budget).

Certainly, policies, procedures, training materials, and user manuals can be developed, or at least initiated, in advance. Again, many vendors have templates for some of these, but they all need review and adaptation to the organization's culture or unique characteristics. Clinicians responsible for using clinical guidelines, templates, macros or smart text, structured data-entry screens, and decision support rules need to be involved in reviewing, developing, and acquiring these components. For example, if a vendor offers the organization a choice of drug knowledge sources, the organization will need to make a selection. If one of the choices included in the vendor's product is different from the drug knowledge source the clinicians are familiar with, it would be appropriate for the clinicians to come up to speed on the different choice. Another example is the "favorites" list of medications, problems, or other frequently generated data. In some cases, the EHR can "learn" what a clinician's favorites are by frequency of use. However, many organizations take proactive steps to ensure that each clinician's favorites are already built into the system prior to go-live.

People Preparation

As part of infrastructure preparedness, preparing people for the level of change should begin in earnest as soon as the implementation is initiated. The project manager should have a defined communication strategy and plan. Figure 13.2 shows a sample communication plan. Some options include creating a newsletter that explains what is going on with the EHR implementation, putting a general status report on the organization's intranet, or even starting a list serve of frequently asked questions. Some one-on-one communication with key individuals who need to be convinced also is in order. Anything that will help the clinical transformation and ease the minds of staff is essential.

Reassuring staff is significant. In fact, staff reticence and uncertainty can make implementation difficult, impact productivity, cause an increase in errors, and have other negative effects on the organization. Sometimes it is not even clear that these issues are arising. The smart project manager must anticipate them.

For example, one organization implementing CPOE found that the pharmacists were more concerned than the physicians about the system's impact. The pharmacists thought that with the level of decision support embedded in CPOE, they would no longer be needed or at least significantly fewer of them would be needed. In this case, the opposite was actually true, especially with The Joint Commission's emphasis on medication reconciliation (2006). Before it was recognized that pharmacists were concerned about losing their jobs, however, evidence of the issue was seen, instead, in various positioning strategies, such as requesting new positions and creating more complex processes to perform their tasks.

Such a scenario can play out in virtually every professional field, from other clinical staff such as laboratory technicians, dietitians, nurses, and therapists to coders, transcriptionists, business office staff, schedulers, and even information technology (IT) staff.

Figure 13.2.   Sample communication plan

Key Messages	To (All staff, BOD, EHR Team, MDs, Patients)	From (Med Dir, Admin, EHR Team, MDIS, Proj Mgr)	Medium (E-mail blast, hot line, intranet, media kit, meeting, newsletter, personal comm., Pol & Proc, Poster, Report, Script, Web site)	Date(s) or Milestones
EHR Planning				
EHR Education				
Computer Skills				
EHR Migration Path				
Stakeholder engagement				
Benefits/Value				
Selection Process				
Code of Conduct				
Process Improvement				
Expectations				
ROI				
Contract Signing				
Implementation Plan				
Chart Conversion Strategy				
EHR Testing				
EHR Training				
Suggestions				
Celebration				
Adoption Rate				
Patient Satisfaction				
Physician Satisfaction				
Staff Satisfaction				
Quality Measures				

However, most organizations believe that the productivity improvements anticipated with EHR systems will lead to more direct patient care time, customer service time, accuracy, or even revenue generation rather than the diminution of staff. For example, a clinic converting to an EHR and anticipating the discontinuance of transcription decided to sell transcription services to other providers until transcription could be phased out through attrition. Such planning is essential, and its communication even more critical.

People preparation also may be as simple as some early PC training for users unfamiliar with basic Windows functions or how to use a navigational device. This type of training has nothing to do with the EHR application itself but can help these individuals become comfortable with learning how to use the EHR when the EHR training actually takes place. Moreover, early PC training can contribute to easing people's minds about the impending changes. Of course, these new skills must continue to be used so new policies on communications, for instance, may need to be adopted. For example, a facility may require that everyone obtain his or her schedule from the computer, all meeting announcements only be posted electronically, and all performance reviews be done online.

Communication about the new EHR also is important with patients. For example, many vendors provide big signs that describe the organization as undergoing "EHR construction" and a short pamphlet explaining what an EHR is, how it changes their provider's access to information, and how it will benefit them. One organization undergoing EHR implementation perhaps said it best: "You cannot over-communicate!"

System Build

Actual system build is the process in which the software is configured with all the various data dictionaries, table development, rules logic, data and code set mapping, file designs, screen layouts, data quality edits, report designs, repository structures, and technical controls, including security access controls and error correction routines.

Need for System Build

EHR systems vary in their degree of customizability, but all have some system build issues. Some vendor products have a very low degree of flexibility; others can be almost totally customizable. Part of the vendor selection process is to determine the degree to which the organization needs and wants to customize its system. Some organizations make a conscious effort to reduce the level of customization simply because they think standards are a good thing. Other organizations want to accommodate every conceivable nuance and may have the resources to do so. Most organizations are somewhere in the middle, recognizing that the system needs to accommodate many of their unique aspects while still improving processes through standardization.

System build includes the most detailed of tasks and is often the most labor-intensive step in the overall implementation process. It is the most fundamental step to making the EHR system work. However, it should be noted that, although a basic system platform should be established initially, some aspects of system build can, will, and should go on for many years. A prime example of this is in the area of clinical decision support. Most organizations are finding it necessary to have just the "right" amount of decision support on go-live, and then building it up as users become accustomed to the system. (Finding what is the "right" amount for an organization can be difficult to determine and is still usually a matter of trial and error.) For example, one organization chose to implement what it described as a "boatload" of alerts and reminders only to have the clinicians up in arms about the hassle of dealing with them all. After a relatively short period of time with all the vendor-supplied alerts and reminders having been implemented, the organization removed all of them and then slowly reapplied them as they came to be identified as needed.

Configuration Management

An important part of system build is **configuration management**, or change control. As changes are made to customize the system to the organization's specifications, a record should be kept of them. This is especially important in a clinical environment, where a single change, such as in the valid values of a data element or whether a data element is required or optional, can directly impact clinical decision support. The term *metadata* was defined earlier in this book as data about data. Configuration management should be linked to the metadata in the system's data dictionary in a data dictionary change control log, such as the one shown in figure 13.3.

Figure 13.3.   Data dictionary change control log

Data Element Characteristic	Original	Change	Change Requested by:	Change Approved by:	Change Performed by:	Change Tested by:	Final Change Date:
Name of entry							
Table							
Physical name							
Synonym(s)							
Definition							
Reference							
Source of data							
Derivations							
Valid values							
Conditionality							
Default							
Lexicon							
Relationship							
Access restrictions							
Process rules							

Copyright © 2008, Margret\A Consulting, LLC. Reprinted with permission.

After go-live, changes will continue to be made to the configuration of the screens, reports, decision support rules, and other processes. Because a change to any one part of the system potentially impacts many other parts, it is essential to thoroughly understand the information flow and data model that the change request impacts. Such changes are generally made at the request of an individual or group. The organization should have a policy concerning who may make a change, how it should be documented and authorized, and what priority it will be given. Many organizations require that all changes be made using a formal change request process, which would include a master change control log and request forms.

Testing

Testing is a critical step that is sometimes overlooked or shortchanged, especially in smaller organizations. In fact, some vendors (especially those selling to physician offices) assume because they have previously implemented their product in numerous other client organizations that further testing is not necessary, or that testing will take place during end user training. However, it should be clear from the previous discussion on system build that every implementation is different and needs to be tested. Many tasks are associated with testing.

Establishing a Test Environment

The first task is to establish a test environment (sometimes called a development environment). Because testing will continue throughout the implementation process, it is important that it not disrupt the production environment. In addition, fixes, upgrades, and modifications will be needed routinely in the future and also should be tested in a manner that does not slow down, or cause errors to occur in, the actual system used on a day-to-day basis. At a minimum, the test environment should include separate hardware and installation of software. Ideally, it would include test data. Many vendors provide test data, but many organizations prefer to develop their own test data to ensure that all conceivable issues are tested.

Some vendors and organizations recommend using actual data (though not "live" data) for testing. This can be a good strategy because it is sometimes difficult to create test data from scratch that cover every type of data to be encountered, but it raises the issue of whether the data should be deidentified. In response to a frequently asked question, the Web site maintained by the Department of Health and Human Services (HHS) Office of Civil Rights, which oversees HIPAA privacy rule compliance, offers that such test data do not have to be deidentified because their use is part of the organization's operations. Still, many organizations prefer not to take the chance that the actual data will include a current employee, relative or friend of an employee, or community VIP and will at least change the names of the actual patients.

Developing a Test Plan and Schedule

Once a test environment is established, a test plan and schedule should be developed to include the necessary tests. Tests that typically should be performed are described in table 13.4. It is noted that the names of the testing types are not standardized, so their description should guide the project manager to ensure that all appropriate testing is performed.

Table 13.4.   Types of system testing

Test	Description
Unit and function testing	Testing of individual modules or applications. This is the most basic test to ensure that each separate component works as expected. This test would look at screen design to ensure that all the tables load properly, reports are generated correctly, and so on.
System testing	Tests how well modules or applications work together. It also looks at work flow within a department or other organization unit and across units. If data are to flow from one department to another and do not, this is a problem.
Integrated system testing, or interface testing	Testing of systems that had to be interfaced to ensure the proper exchange of data.
Performance and stress, or load, testing	Testing of system performance, including response time, with volumes of data as anticipated in a live setting; and testing of performance that simulates peak volumes.

Copyright © 2008, Margret\A Consulting, LLC. Reprinted with permission.

Test Scenarios and Testing

Test data are required to conduct the various levels of testing. However, without a scenario, or story, that sets the data in context and describes expected inputs, processes, and outputs, testing is not as thorough as it could be. Many organizations utilize use cases that describe the sequence of actions a system should take with respect to a specific task or function. Use case development was described in chapter 8 with respect to defining EHR functional requirements.

Users or domain experts must develop the clinical use cases and also should be the ones to conduct their testing. It is only clinicians who can explain the nature of a thought process desired to be aided by the EHR and hence to ensure that a system has been built properly. Engaging users to not only write but also conduct the tests helps their peer group develop trust in the system. In many situations, anyone responsible for conducting an EHR system test is required to sign off that the system performed the test to specifications. An issue log, or separate testing log, should be maintained to ensure that all test failures are corrected. Figure 13.4 uses a variation of use case modeling (Larmon 2002) to describe (part of) a scenario that might be used for testing a CPOE system. Although not every conceivable drug ordered via a CPOE system needs to be tested, a small number of typical, complex, and unusual scenarios from each clinical specialty should be constructed and tested.

Obviously, if any one or more of the above tests reveal problems, the problems need to be fixed by the vendor and contract language should cover the vendor's obligation to do so.

Acceptance testing is a term often used to in EHR implementation to describe the point at which the organization signs off that the implementation is working as expected. This is somewhat different than acceptance testing in typical software development, where it is the completion of use case testing that triggers acceptance. The EHR vendor and organization should agree on the criteria with which an implementation is accepted; but for an

Figure 13.4.   Portion of sample use case model for CPOE system test

Provider	System
Primary Success Scenario: Receive appropriate D-D, D-L, D-A, D-W, and D-Dose	CPOE with interface from ADT, Problem List, Medication List, Allergy Documentation, Laboratory, Pharmacy, and Referral systems
Secondary Success Scenario: Retrieve list of patients who may be pregnant, become pregnant, or nursing to advise them of birth defect warning	Data mining capability
Basic Flow: 1. Provider enters order for Paxil 2. D-D contraindication alert if patient taking MAOIs or thioridazine 3. D-L alert if patient has severe renal or hepatic impairment 4. D-A alert if patient has a hypersensitivity to paraxetine (active ingredient in Paxil) or any inactive ingredients 5. D-W (obtain psych consult reminder)if patient is at risk for suicide 6. D-dose recalculation for starting dose in pediatric patients	1. System finds structured product label (SPL) information from drug knowledge base 2. System compares D-D contraindications from SPL to active medication list 3. System compares most recent creatinine clearance with SPL warning of <30 mL/min 4. System compares ingredients in Paxil to drug allergy information on SPL 5. System checks patient problem list for suicide risk 6. System recalculates starting dose for patients under specified age, height, and weight
Extensions (or alternative flows): 2-a: Alert with respect to MAOIs or thioridazine fires 1. Cancels order 2. Requests to see detailed SPL 3. Selects alternative antidepressant 4. Overrides alert and retains for Paxil 2-b: Override presents list of potential rationales required for order to be accepted 1. Selects rationale 2. Cancels order	1. System deletes order for Paxil 2. System supplies content of SPL 3. System performs checks as above on alternative order 4. System accept override request and supplies rationale requirement per organizational policy
Secondary Flow: 1. Request system to search for all patients for whom Paxil was ordered AND who are women between 12 and 50 years old. . . 2. Produce mailing labels of all patients on report	

Copyright © 2008, Margret\A Consulting, LLC. Reprinted with permission.

EHR, acceptance typically occurs at least 30 to 60 days, or longer, after go-live. This is because not every conceivable scenario can be anticipated in advance. Some issues often go unidentified until the system is working in the production environment for some period of time. Some vendors plan to retain their staff in an organization until the formal sign-off on acceptance has occurred; others will have staff return later to review the system's performance with organizational representatives. At a minimum, for an organization to sign off on acceptance, it should ensure that all issues have been satisfactorily resolved, that users are adopting the system as expected and their satisfaction is acceptable, and they have completed one "cycle" of processing on their own without issues. Such a cycle should ensure that all charges have been captured, regular reports can be run, and that information needed for subsequent care is available.

Performance warranties also may be considered part of acceptance testing. In many cases, vendors make claims about productivity or performance capabilities and will go "at risk" for these performance criteria. However, they will not do this unless the organization has appropriate metrics, baseline data, and documentary evidence of improvement, or lack thereof. If the vendor is unwilling to go at risk, the organization may still wish to conduct its own benefits realization studies to take corrective action internally where needed (and to celebrate success).

Training

Training is an aspect of implementation that occurs at various points in the process, targeted at different individuals, and for different purposes. Training of varying intensity, methodology, and purpose occur periodically and strategically throughout the implementation process. Table 13.5 lists the various types of training that should be incorporated throughout the entire EHR systems development life cycle (SDLC).

Unfortunately, it is common for organizations to have used up their EHR budget prior to the time they get to instruction or support for end users, or even earlier for skills building. Skimping in these areas results in users who are not properly trained and either do not make maximal use of the system or are reluctant to use it. The overall result is that the system's anticipated benefits are not realized. Executive management is then (and rightly so) in the position of wondering where its ROI is.

Some vendors are as much at fault for minimal training as organizations are because they portray their systems as easy to use and intuitive to learn. However, busy professionals need hands-on training and reinforcement to ensure that what may appear intuitive to an IS technician or EHR developer is truly something discernable. Although much training will have to occur after testing just prior to go-live, and continue after go-live, as much training as possible should be done early on.

Training Approach and Modalities

Many organizations follow a train-the-trainer approach for user training. When trained staff members have completed the initial training, they become trainers for other staff members. Of course, use of the train-the-trainer approach varies with the size of the organization and who is being trained.

Table 13.5. EHR training throughout the SDLC

Type of Training	Target Audience/Modality	Key Message(s)
Introduction	• Everyone in the organization • Short sound bites at meetings, in newsletters, and so on	• An EHR is an essential technology for patient safety, quality of care, and user satisfaction • An EHR is a complex system with which the organization will migrate to and with all users involved
Education	• Initially steering committee, executive management, and other decision makers • Ultimately all developers and super users • Seminars and briefings that introduce theoretical and practical knowledge targeted to specific audience	• An EHR introduces a clinical transformation • An EHR is a system of systems designed for knowledge management • An EHR requires thorough planning and highly detailed and specific implementation, testing, and training
Briefings	Project sponsors • Project managers (organization and vendor) • Dashboards, regular meetings to keep key individuals up to date	• Current progress, issues, and successes with EHR implementation
Skills building	• Super users in person classroom/online training to build process mapping competencies, screen layout design competencies, and so on • End users on computer navigation using classroom or personal training tools, then on EHR functionality in various forms of communications, including demos	• An EHR is a tool that aids clinician decision making • Data entry should be performed by the individual closest to the source of the data, including the patient where possible • An EHR requires competency in navigating a computer
Instruction	• Super users on vendor-specific requirements, usually at vendor training seminar or onsite hands-on • End users to perform specific functions using train-the-trainer, training workstations, instruction manuals, "cheat sheets," and automated help function	• How this EHR works, may be customized, should be trained on • How this EHR works and tasks performed
Support	• End users provided stand-by assistance for navigating screens or any other assistance during go-live	• Achieve comfort using the EHR to gain full adoption
Retraining/ Refresher training/ coaching	• Super users to relearn or refresh for later upgrades often via online or seminar • End users who have created work-arounds to use of system in meeting • End users who are not fully adopted by one-on-one training	• Ongoing monitoring of system use and continue to support system as it evolves • Achieve comfort using the EHR to achieve benefits

In addition, different training modalities should be considered. In general, some "classroom" training is required, with on-the-job support also provided. However, the classroom training could be intranet based and taken at home or help screen-based, where users are more on their own. Although different types of users may have different preferences, a 1- to 2-hour course on the basics is a minimum essential for a comprehensive EHR system. Most organizations reduce the clinicians' patient load during the training period and for the first few weeks after go-live. Additionally, organizations should make trainers available to provide almost instantaneous assistance and many have their trainers wear distinctive clothing, such as red jackets, for this purpose.

The first group of users to go live often ends up serving as both partial system designers and testers because glitches almost inevitably occur. The more the system can be tested in advance, the better off the live process will be and the more likely the users will be to adapt to the new system. Another issue with the first group of users is that they also sometimes become trainers. New users often turn to the first group of users for help, especially when the number of trained trainers available is insufficient for subsequent implementations. There is some risk in this approach. First, it is time-consuming for the initial group of users, who by now should be in full production mode. Second, the initial users may have developed bad habits because they had to learn intuitively or did not learn correctly the first time. (This also points to the need not only for initial training, but also for monitoring to ensure that ongoing use is appropriate.)

Theoretically, by the time the second group of users goes live, system problems will have been worked out and only operational problems will need to be addressed. In actual practice, the more data flowing through the system, the more likely it is that unforeseen system problems will still occur, although they should be less frequent.

Human Resource/Labor Relations Issues

Various human resource/labor relations issues are associated with training that should be planned for in advance. One issue in a union shop is the extent to which the job changes. Early collaboration with union representatives can forestall many problems with union staff. Another issue for all types of organizations is how and when training will occur—during the workday, in overtime, or on personal time. Will users be required to achieve a certain level of competency that is tested and certified? Users are often given new access and authentication mechanisms that may be accompanied by signing a confidentiality agreement. For physicians, incentives or compensation may need to be considered.

Another issue is the subsequent role of staff members who worked on the EHR project. On an individual level, most physician champions move into an informatics role, supporting ongoing knowledge development. Nurse trainers may assume technical support roles or provide informatics support for nursing care. Nurse educators continuously monitor and update materials made available to the healthcare organization's consumers. Health information management (HIM) professionals can serve as excellent monitors of ongoing EHR use, evaluate emerging technology, conduct benefits realization studies, and contribute to ongoing process improvement, operations analysis and redesign, and workflow changes. Other roles for a variety of persons include database maintenance, data quality monitoring, outcomes management, consumer informatics (merging consumer education with individual health data), information security, knowledge management, and user relations.

Pre-Live Data Conversion and Other Activities Prior to Go-Live

The final phases of testing, conversion, and training are often performed in overlapping time frames. Obviously, training must occur early for those users who will help build out the system and perform tests, but end user training can and should wait until closer to go-live.

Data Conversion

Pre-live conversion generally includes data conversion. Data conversion is the preparation of data, files, and program loading to the production environment. Data conversion is often required when data is currently maintained in one system and needs to be moved to another, new system. For example, if part of an electronic medication administration record (EMAR) implementation requires a new pharmacy system, data currently in the pharmacy system will need to be converted to the new system. Decisions about how and when data conversion will take place will have been made earlier in the process, but actual data conversion would occur at this point.

Go-live Rehearsal

A go-live rehearsal may be performed, especially for EHR systems where there will be straight turnover and a cutoff of paper chart retrieval except in emergencies. Every stakeholder should be involved in this process.

Support

Finally, the day of go-live should be one in which "all hands are on board." Many organizations will attempt to identify a "light" day, such as a weekend day, night shift, or other time when fewer patients are expected and the minimum number of users are required. If a light day cannot be identified, the organization might create one by not scheduling as many patients or by closing part of a unit and shifting patients to another unit. Whatever strategy is adopted, a full complement of support personnel should be available to provide assistance. For a major EHR implementation, a full complement of vendor support staff also should be made available. If the EHR is being implemented in a small physician office and vendor support staff will not be on site, there should be assurances that vendor support will be available via telephone.

Murphy's Law that "If anything can go wrong, it will" should be anticipated on go-live. To avoid mishaps, preparedness is crucial.

EHR Adoption

Although go-live signifies the time when the end user starts to use the system, this should not be considered the end of the EHR implementation activities but, rather, the start of the adoption phase of implementation. The RAND Corporation makes a distinction between a system being installed vs. a system being adopted. It notes that "an organization may invest in a system and expose clinicians to it, but adoption requires acceptance and use of the system on a regular basis" (Fonkych and Taylor 2005, 18). The Center for Information Technology Leadership (C!TL) also makes this observation, reporting on a study demonstrating that 32 percent of hospitals indicated they had a CPOE system, yet only 13.7 percent required its use by physicians (Johnston 2003). Similar variations in reporting EHR adoption rates in general, and discrepancies between installation and adoption, are reported for clinic settings as well.

Monitoring System Usage

Many organizations monitor system use by new users so that they can assess the level of adoption. This is a good step to begin the process of determining adoption rates; however, other strategies also are appropriate.

Conducting Satisfaction Surveys

Conducting a user satisfaction survey is a visible way for the organization to recognize the importance of adoption and to obtain some consistent feedback. Two or three short satisfaction surveys might be used to gauge adoption, especially because interventional efforts may be taken after each one.

Especially for ambulatory care environments, conducting a patient satisfaction survey also can be a powerful tool. Many are finding that patients value having online access to their medical records and that physicians are significantly more likely than patients to anticipate concerns about EHR (Ross, et al 2005). Such a dichotomy may actually help physicians overcome concerns that their patients do not like them using the EHR.

Emphasizing Celebration

Celebration may be considered a form of communication, change management, or other element associated with EHR leadership. Regardless of its categorization, the value of celebration cannot be overemphasized. Celebration does not have to be loud and raucous. It can be tasteful and in keeping with the culture of the organization, but it needs to be a way of life for organizations that see as many stresses as healthcare organizations do. Ideally, celebration should occur at strategic milestones throughout the project's implementation phases. Timing celebrations with achievement of milestones also allows recognition that progress is being made and the implementation is not an endless journey but rather a series of steps. Individuals, departments, and others should be recognized for their contributions. Celebration in the form of recognition engages users and honestly affords appreciation for much extra effort. Celebration is an opportunity not only to recognize, but also to obtain informal feedback.

Conducting a Benefits Realization Study

Formal benefits realization studies are not easy to do and require benchmark data to be valid. However, they can reassure users (and executive management) that the system is having an impact and is worth bearing with any interim issues.

Creating a Customer Service Attitude

Another important strategy to help gain adoption is to create a customer service attitude within your organization. This may be easier said than done, but there are many ways to take small steps toward this goal. For example, holding a pizza lunch or donut breakfast once a week by the IT staff, executive management team, medical director of information systems, or others initially after go-live is an opportunity to obtain feedback in a nonthreatening way. Remember, individuals struggling to use the system may think that their jobs are at risk, may be embarrassed in front of their peers, or may have other perceptions that need to be debunked. Furthermore, if they are struggling or not using the system at all for some reason, that absolutely must be addressed. All support staff, help desk personnel, supervisors, and others need to understand the importance of a customer service attitude when a system such as the EHR is being implemented. The level of change and potential risk in the system is one that many find stressful.

Conducting Walk-throughs

A final way to promote better adoption is to conduct walk-throughs of the various areas that have gone live, not just once shortly after go-live to thank everyone (which should also be done), but several weeks or months after go-live, and periodically after that. It may be surprising to learn what is really happening as opposed to what you think is happening. Additionally, this is a terrific way for staff to realize that leaders are genuinely interested in the EHR and its continued success. Despite the best of intentions, good customer service, and other efforts, it is conceivable that individuals who should be fully using the system are still using work-arounds, putting up with slow response time, or are simply not sure what an icon on the screen means.

Walk-throughs should be conducted by a variety of staff and should become a routine means of gaining feedback. Done en masse and only once or twice can imply an investigation with the potential for blame.

EHR System Documentation

A final element of EHR implementation is documentation. Documentation concerning the project itself has been described for virtually every step along the way. This is critical for management of the project. However, documentation of the system itself—the user manuals, practice guidelines that support templates, decision support rules, and other system documentation—is critical for ongoing maintenance.

In addition to system documentation, policies and procedures that reflect the directives relative to use of the EHR in various processes also are important to document. Many organizations do not have policies with respect to system use, relying instead on general policies for professional credentialing, compliance, privacy and security, human resources, and other issues. However, EHRs bring enhanced opportunities in the privacy and security area, as well as in other policy-related matters. These should be codified as revisions to existing policies and procedures or added to the existing set of policies. For example, under HIPAA, individuals have the right to request restrictions on use and disclosure of protected health information (PHI). Many healthcare organizations must turn such requests down in the paper realm because they are impossible to manage. With an EHR, some restrictions may be more feasible, and at least policies should be reviewed and revised, if applicable. Moreover, the EHR brings new ethical dilemmas to the fore. For example, should a rationale be required to be documented when a decision support rule fires an alert? There is currently a considerable difference of opinion (Rollins 2005), but each organization should address its preferences in policy. Other policies may center on tighter access controls, disaster recovery planning, release of information, and acceptance of content from a personal health record (PHR).

Ongoing Strategies

Most healthcare organizations claim that no EHR system is ever fully implemented. Initial installation may be over, but modifications, enhancements, and upgrades are virtually ongoing. Some of the decision making concerning level of customization and benefits realization, for instance, requires as much facilitation and finesse as the initial selection process.

Many lessons will be learned throughout the implementation process. Whether formally tracked and documented or simply recognized and dealt with, the lessons learned should be anticipated and accepted. It may be the culture of some organizations that lessons learned are seen as failures and blame is quickly placed. This is not a healthy position and should be avoided. In fact, it would be wise to discuss this issue in one of the early steering committee meetings and reinforce it in training sessions. Although EHRs are not completely immature products, they are still new and often more comprehensive than any other change the organization has dealt with in the past. Undoubtedly, lessons will need to be learned; ideally, organizations will be willing to write articles and contribute case studies so that others can benefit from the lessons they have learned.

Finally, the EHR is not only implemented in phases but also in a migration path that will continue to be enhanced with new technology, new knowledge sources, and new ideas. Generally, it is understood and accepted that vendor upgrades need to be applied, new regulatory initiatives must be incorporated, and routine system maintenance must occur. In addition, it can be expected that when the EHR is on its migration path, users will see the path enhanced continuously.

Conclusion

Although any discussion of implementation strategies makes installation, testing, training, and go-live sound rather straightforward, expecting the unexpected should be the norm. Both patience and ongoing monitoring are key ingredients to a successful implementation that transforms the healthcare organization's clinical process and achieves its desired benefits.

References and Resources

Badger Sl, et al. 2005. Rapid Implementation of an Electronic Health Record in an Academic Setting, *Journal of Health Information Management* 19(2) 34–40.

Fonkych, K., and R. Taylor. 2005. The State and Pattern of Health Information Technology Adoption. The RAND Corporation. www.rand.org.

Friedman, D., et al. 2003. White paper: Change management: An integral component of clinical transformation. HCT Project Cap Gemini Ernst & Young. www.hctproject.com/white.asp.

Healthcare Financial Management Association. 2004. Promotional material: Dotting the i's and Crossing the t's: Ensuring the Best IT Contract. Westchester, IL: HFMA.

Hitti, M. 2005 (Sept. 27). Paxil's birth defects warning strengthened. WebMD Medical News. www.webmd.com/content/article/112/110504.htm.

Johnston, D., et al. 2003. The value of computerized provider order entry in ambulatory settings. Wellesley, MA: Center for Information Technology Leadership. www.citl.org/research/ACPOE_Executive_Preview.pdf.

Joint Commission. 2006 (Jan. 25). Using medication reconciliation to prevent errors. Sentinel Event Alert 35.

Larmon, C. 2002. *Applying UML and Patterns: An Introduction to Objected-Oriented Analysis and Design and the Unified Process*, 2nd ed. Upper Saddle River, NJ: Pearson Prentice Hall, p. 53.

Rollins, Gina. 2005. The prompt, the alert, and the legal record: Documenting clinical decision support systems. *Journal of AHIMA* 76(2):24–28.

Ross, S.E., et al. 2005. Expectations of patients and physicians regarding patient-accessible medical records. *Journal of Medical Internet Research* 7(2):article e13.

RxList. n.d. Paroxetine Hydrochloride (Paxil). www.rxlist.com.

Schooler, R., and T. Dotson 2003. Rolling out the CIS. A*DVANCE for Health Information Executives* 7(10):51–58.

Walizer, D. 2004. Post-implementation support. *ADVANCE for Health Information Executives* 8(1):22–23.

Chapter 14
EHR Bridge Technologies

Whether starting on a migration path to an EHR, filling in the gaps where EHR components are missing, or supporting cross-enterprise communications, bridge technologies for EHR have an important place in healthcare organizations. The two most common bridge technologies are often considered to be electronic document management systems and clinical messaging. This chapter:

- Describes how bridge technologies fit into the overall EHR migration path

- Discusses issues associated with hybrid records

- Defines electronic document and content management (ED/CM) systems and how they support chart access and work flow within and beyond the health information management (HIM) department

- Describes the technology options, issues, and functionality for an ED/CM

- Provides tips and a case study (on the CD) for the planning and implementation of an ED/CM

- Describes clinical messaging and how it supports enterprise interoperability

Bridge Technologies as an IT Strategy

At AHIMA's National Convention in 2006, Reino and Hyde described the challenges hospital face with the hybrid record and observed that "as we move toward the electronic health record (EHR) . . . we are faced with an array of challenges—challenges that normally stem from an industry that does not always like change. Changes are required to take a highly individualized world and make it standardized in some fashion. Changes surround workers who have not grown up with technology as a requirement and now have to face it on a daily basis." In 2003, AHIMA's e-HIM work group described the fact that most

Key Terms

Bridge technologies	Content management systems	Enterprise report management
Clinical		
Clinical Document Architecture	Electronic signature authentication	Hybrid record
		Workflow management systems

healthcare organizations "continue to be plagued by paper-based health information . . . using a hybrid medical record: partially computer-generated and partially paper-based." And that "wherever organizations lie on the EHR evolutionary timeline, they are learning that the technologies of electronic document management are a necessity." This remains true today, and for both hospitals and physician offices, although in different ways.

Needs for Hospitals

For hospitals, the multiplicity of source systems, even when following a best-of-fit IT strategy, combined with lack of applications for some types of documentation makes it difficult to meet even the first part of the EHR definition: *collect data from multiple sources*. The result almost certainly is a **hybrid record** that follows one of three patterns:

- Some parts on paper only and some parts electronic only

- Some parts on paper only, some parts electronic, but ultimately printed to paper

- Some parts on paper only and some parts electronic only, but are routinely requested to be printed out during patient care episode

Although any of these patterns may provide the content for a legal health record, the fact that there are multiple places to look for the complete content of the legal health record make such a hybrid structure a challenge to use. A survey of current practices suggests hospitals have an almost equal chance of being in one of these three states; the first is difficult to achieve because it almost always turns into the last (Amatayakul and Cohen 2005). The second situation may actually be one that is migrating into a totally paperless record through scanning remaining documents into an electronic document management system (EDMS) or coupling scanning and content management into an electronic document and content management (ED/CM) system, also called enterprise content and records management (ECRM) system. (Distinctions between EDMS and ED/CM, or ECRM, are described later in this chapter.)

The theory behind such systems is that despite the increasing demand for clinical applications that collect and process discrete data for clinical decision support, such as in computerized provider order entry (CPOE), bar code medication administration record (BC-MAR), and point-of-care (POC) charting systems, there still is the need to present

Figure 14.1.   Nature and Use of Information Content

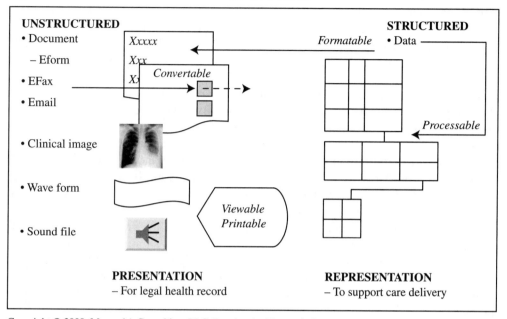

information in a manner that is consistent with the human culture of use, both for organizational users and to present a record in court if called on to do so. The desire, then, is to have a single location from where all content may be easily retrieved. An ED/CM system enables the electronic storage of scanned documents, other unstructured digital content, and structured data that have been formatted into "print files" to be maintained together in one electronic record system.

Strong (2008) notes "ECRM is the strategy, technology, and processes for managing information assets facilitated by information technology. . . It addresses issues related to technology, process improvement, legal and regulatory requirements, and cultural and behavioral change." Figure 14.1 illustrates the nature and use of information content that resides within a care delivery organization. Although any structured data can be formatted and processed into viewable or printable information (theoretically), such data typically reside in a data repository from which multiple views and formats can be derived. To settle legal disputes, the transaction presentation, not representation, is required for business records (Kohn 2006). Although it is not impossible to generate such a transaction presentation at the time a record would be called into evidence, there are many other processes that care delivery organization staff prefer to perform using such a format.

It is noted that the generation of printable information *theoretically* should be able to be performed by an EHR system. This note is made because some of the early CPOE, BC-MAR, and POC charting systems were not designed to do so, or did so in a manner that was not typical of the paper-based health record presentation format. For example, several vendors' CPOE systems were originally designed only to print orders as lists specific to the elements of the order's destination. In other words, a single order for labs, medications, special diet, and nursing services was generated as separate lists of all labs, all medications, all diet requests, and all nursing services for the given patient. (These vendors have subsequently revised their systems to print orders by order set, although it was a "hard sell" to achieve this, and there is no telling how the software for other, new applications may be written.)

In addition to the lack of applications or all documentation requirements of health records, many vendors for hospital EHRs have not fully developed a robust data repository and applications to support its integration of data for use at the point of care. It is one thing to have systems that support a specific function, such as laboratory information management or nursing admission assessment, but quite another to be able to pull discrete data from each of these into a robust database that supports yet another caregiver in achieving, for example, an accurate medication list supported by laboratory data that might contraindicate ordering a given drug or require recalibrating a dose of a given drug. Vendors working in this direction may begin by providing an integrated view of the different data but have not necessarily created the ability for the system to interact fully with the data from the different sources. Such systems are highly complex to develop, and until recently there has not been much willingness to pay for them. Hence, organizations have largely been left to their own devices to integrate the data into a legal health record presentation format.

Another issue for hospitals is not only the lack of product functionality, but also the lack of support for their use. The Center for Information Technology Leadership (C!TL) makes this observation, reporting on a study demonstrating that 32 percent of hospitals indicated they had a CPOE system, but only 13.7 percent required its use by physicians (C!TL 2003). These numbers currently are largely unchanged, as Modern Healthcare found that 49 percent of hospitals indicated they had a CPOE system in 2006; although adoption rates from the Leapfrog Group, which measures CPOE use for its incentive program, reported even lower results at 6.7 percent in 2006; and HIMSS Analytics data reveal CPOE adoption at 3.0 percent for 2006. (Differences may be attributable to many factors, including whether the hospital considers adoption to be 100 percent utilization or the ability to pass 75 percent of all orders through its system—the Leapfrog Group's criteria, or includes clinical protocols, which is the definition used by HIMSS Analytics.)

As a result of these issues, yet with strong need for access to data and better management of information, hospitals are faced with structuring a migration path that fills the gaps between the disparate systems. In some cases, these gaps are felt acutely by clinicians and the push is to focus more on EHR. Even then, however, **bridge technologies** are needed to fill gaps where there is no information system support. In some cases, these are messaging systems where views to data are provided. In many cases, however, the solution is an EDMS or ECRM system, at least to make chart content accessible for follow-up and subsequent admissions. In other cases, the gaps for hospitals continue to be more of a concern for administrative functions, hence the focus on EDMS as a means to pull existing record content together and make it more accessible for coding, billing, quality, and so on.

Needs for Physician Offices

For physician offices, EHR products tend to be more inclusive and often convert structured data into narrative format routinely, and therefore are more able to produce a representation of the legal health record. Virtually all aspects of clinical information flow and documentation within an office can be addressed by the EHR. Furthermore, other than a practice management system (PMS) and perhaps a lab system, physician offices tend not to have many other systems. Moreover, EHR vendors are integrating PMS and EHR more tightly. As a result, there are fewer "gaps" in physician offices.

However, gaps do occur in physician offices in two main areas. One major gap area is between the hospital and the office. In fact, physicians often feel this gap more acutely and prior to the need in their own office for more robust systems. In this case, **clinical messaging** is an appropriate bridge strategy (and may well be an ongoing strategy). Clinical messaging is a service that provides a secure, electronic infrastructure to automate the delivery of health data to any site where clinical patient care decisions are made (Henning 2008). The other major gap area is in chart conversion. When a patient is readmitted to a hospital, the admission may or may not be related to the reason for a previous admission. There may be a significant period of time between one admission and another, where having previous admission information is not absolutely time-sensitive (Stiell et al 2003). Having discrete data from a previous admission brought forward for use in a current admission, then, is not always as important as information from previous visits in a physician office.

Most physician offices need their patients' problem list, medication list, record of immunizations, recent labs, and so on for each visit across an episode of care. When an EHR is acquired, this information needs to be brought forward to the EHR. This process of chart conversion may be accomplished in several ways to include abstraction, scanning of documents, or simply pulling previous records for a period of time. Many offices find that scanning documents is an efficient and effective way to get access to data, even if it is not interactive within the EHR.

Managing the Hybrid Record

AHIMA's practice brief titled "The Complete Medical Record in a Hybrid EHR Environment" defines a hybrid record as "a system with functional components that (1) include both paper and electronic documents and (2) use both manual and electronic processes" (AHIMA e-HIM Work Group on Hybrid Records 2003). (See appendix C.3 on the enclosed CD.) The practice brief notes that not only is managing health information in this hybrid environment challenging, but, in fact, some risk may be associated with a hybrid record for patient quality of care.

Impact of the Hybrid Record on the HIM Department

From the perspective of the HIM department, there are authoring and printing issues, access and disclosure issues, and other operational impacts of hybrid records on the department. Figure 14.2 supplies strategic practice guidelines for HIM functions in a hybrid environment.

Figure 14.2.   Strategic practice guidelines for traditional and emerging HIM operational functions

#	HIM Operational Function	Operational Considerations	Strategic Practice Guidelines
1	Transcription/ Coding Staffing	In-house, home-based, outsourced, or offshore	• Familiarize and synchronize with your organization's strategic plan • Become knowledgeable about system integration capabilities, limitations, and opportunities of both source and interfacing information systems • Ensure availability and operationalization of quality control features and reporting capabilities of all source and interfacing systems (for example, for Part ID quality controls) • Ensure compliance with any and all privacy, confidentiality, and security laws (for example, state, federal, or organization specific) • Ensure organization has carefully planned its off-site EHR content prior to operationalizing any off-site coding or transcription functions (for example, have major clinical documentation needed by coders, such as MD progress notes, available online to coders before implementing off-site coding)
2	Transcription Delivery Media	Fax, tape, disk, paper, electronic (for example, batch mode, uploading, integrity maintenance)	• Standardize delivery media to minimize paper and/or duplicate delivery modalities • Ensure device availability (for example, remote access) and notification to recipients of delivered electronic documents • Ensure proper privacy and security controls are in place regardless of media
3	Electronic Signature	Transcription and other critical EHR documentation	• Review and consider e-signature processing capabilities, limitations, opportunities (see separate Practice Brief on e-signature) • Clearly understand minimal operational workflow requirements for processing e-signatures when working with information systems and vendor representatives

(continued)

Figure 14.2.   (Continued)

#	HIM Operational Function	Operational Considerations	Strategic Practice Guidelines
4	Release of information (ROI)	Customer service when ROI function off-site or remote. Electronic transfers rather than paper printing	• Consider expansion of HIM responsibilities for ROI functions into decentralized areas including off-site clinics, if not already responsible • Consider how to continue to meet standards/laws if ROI function is decentralized (for example, disclosure laws with respect to ETOH/ HIV/ mental health; have HIM continue to handle all requests for amendments coming through ROI) • Consider whether HIM will continue to maintain oversight or be subject matter resource to those managing ROI • Ensure EHR plans incorporate ROI workflow capabilities both on site and remotely (for example, disclosure tracking and auditing capabilities) • Consider electronic rules/alerts on ROI requirements to allow for expanded delegation of ROI operational capabilities and responsibilities
5	Record Processing	Completion, abstracting, assembly, indexing	• Establish business rules for online EHR viewing based on individual's role and completion status of online document (for example, ROI only sees "complete" online records) • Ensure EHR system capabilities to monitor/track record completion (for example, online alerts to individual clinicians, aggregated management screens/reports for HIM) • Regardless of where organization is along EHR transition continuum, management of record completion business processes will still be needed • As the need to print and assemble paper-based records diminishes, HIM management will need to transfer and/or retrain staff to other operational areas (for example, assemblers => preppers/ scanners where imaging has been deployed) • Where EHR being printed, develop standardized assembly order based on the user's needs (for example, different EHR views may necessitate different assembly orders [lawyers, patients, and so on]) • Work with EHR vendor toward use of expert rules for automated abstracting, where possible
6	EHR Data Back Loading	Data quality/integrity	• Ensure a precleanup prior to any back loading (including back scanning) to an EHR

(continued)

Figure 14.2. (Continued)

#	HIM Operational Function	Operational Considerations	Strategic Practice Guidelines
9	Data Integration Issues	System merges, conversion issues, and multiple EHR systems in a given environment	• For multifacility and/or multidepartmental EHR system integrations, ensure appropriate quality control mechanisms are in place to ensure data integrity (for example, enterprisewide master patient index [MPI] encounters or episodes as part of the overall IT conversion process) • HIM should play a strong role in all quality control planning and implementation activities (for example, audit reporting/monitoring)
10	Retention/ Destruction Issues	State and federal mandates, legal counsel recommendations, and system limitations and needs	• Conduct a compliance review to ensure current policies are up to date with all state and federal laws on retention and destruction • Where the legal medical record is defined as a hybrid environment, ensure that your retention and destruction policies include those components of the legal medical record that are stored in non-paper-based media (for example, remote/local servers, tapes, film, fiche) • Ensure that EHR systems have the ability to retain and destroy health information in accordance with your facility's legal medical record definition (for example, fetal monitor data)
11	Definitions/ Glossary of Terms	Varying definitions of original, legal, complete, or hard-copy record; business rules; other definitions as we proceed through process	Define what a "complete" medical record is in paper-based vs. EHR environment (for example, transcribed outpatient clinic notes)

Source: AHIMA 2003a.

Impact of the Hybrid Record of Patient Quality of Care and Documentation

Patient quality of care issues can arise in a hybrid environment because such an environment essentially creates two sources for potentially the same information. For example, if the expectation is to review laboratory results online, but some physicians want them printed out, the result is two forms of the same data. This may not cause a problem if the paper copy is used only for review of the results and then discarded; however, if the paper copy is used for annotation in any way, it is possible that the next clinician looking for the laboratory results online may be unaware of the printed version with annotation and take action that would have benefited from review of the annotation.

Alternatively, not finding a laboratory result printed and placed in the paper chart might result in the false assumption that the results are not back or somehow the test was never performed. A second order might be placed for the test, potentially putting the patient at risk because of either the nature of the test or a delay in taking action on the results, which would certainly result in an unnecessary cost to the system. Unfortunately, if hospitals are having difficulty gaining adoption for CPOE, as suggested by the C!TL results cited above, use of two sources of information about the patient, one of which being something clinicians prefer not to do, will be a difficult sell.

Some hospitals have attempted to solve the problem of where to look for information by including a table of contents at the front of the chart. As more electronic systems are added over time as sources of chart content, the table of contents will guide chart review based on what systems were available when.

In addition to patient quality of care issues, potential documentation issues are associated with a hybrid environment. Questions may arise concerning how results review is to be documented. Will this increase the burden on the clinician in having to annotate in the paper chart that results were reviewed? Can an assumption be made that they were reviewed based on subsequent action alone? To some extent, these questions raise the bar from the standard of documentation in the paper record, where the assumption is, in fact, that if the results are in the chart, they must have been reviewed for there to be a subsequent note or order. The assumption in this case is relatively safe. When the results are available only online, there will not be any reconciliation between an audit trail and the paper chart, especially when someone else may have printed the results and the clinician discarded them after review because of a hospital policy that they not be added to the paper record. (Discarding the printout adds its own burden to the already burgeoning load of secure destruction.)

EDMS

Clearly, the goal of most healthcare organizations is to reduce the burden of having a hybrid record or eliminating it altogether. As a result, many hospitals are moving to EDMS to support their EHR effort. AHIMA's practice brief titled "Electronic Document Management as a Component of the Electronic Health Record" (AHIMA e-HIM Work Group on Electronic Document Management 2003a) describes six key functions for EDMS:

1. Document capture

2. Document indexing, bar coding, character and form recognition, and forms design

3. Document retrieval, viewing, and distribution

4. Document management

5. Automated forms processing

6. Electronic signature, document annotation, and editing

(See appendix C.4 on the enclosed CD.)

Document Capture

Document capture is the function most typically thought of when introducing EDMS. Although a variety of technologies may be used to capture documents, scanning and electronic transactions are the most common.

Document scanning, or imaging, creates an image of a document that is retrievable from multiple workstations. Although it provides access to documents, the scanning process can be quite burdensome for the organization. Most healthcare organizations want to be able to at least index the documents scanned for easier retrieval, so part of planning for document scanning is determining how and when such indexing operations will be performed. (See the next section.) As a result, many healthcare organizations look first to determine what documents already in digital form are able to be electronically fed (often still referred to as computer output to laser disk (COLD) fed) into the EDMS.

Documents that originate as digital dictation, transcriptions, print files from other systems (for example, lab), digital pictures, faxes, or e-mail can be COLD fed into a repository. The result is that hopefully a smaller amount of the chart documents need to be scanned. Of course, care must be taken to clearly establish a procedure so that documents that are COLD fed into the repository but also printed out during the care process do not end up also being scanned.

Document Indexing, Bar Coding, Character and Form Recognition, and Forms Design

To enhance retrieval of scanned documents, some form of indexing needs to take place in order to organize the documents for easy retrieval. Ideally, each form that is scanned or otherwise created should have a bar code or some other forms recognition feature, or features, associated with it. Bar coding is an entire science in itself, with at least two primary types of bar code standards available for use.

Most EDMSs support the Code 39 bar code standard, also called the linear bar code. This is an alphanumeric, self-checking, variable-length code that has been standardized by the Health Industry Bar Code Council (HIBCC). It also is the standard the Food and Drug Administration (FDA) requires for use on drug products and biologicals.

Another bar code standard, Code 128, also called a two-dimensional bar code, can encode more complex information. It is produced by the Uniform Code Council (UCC). Hospitals may use either or both Code 39 and Code 128 bar code on patient wristbands. The FDA has indicated that, although the linear bar code must be used to encode the National Drug Code (NDC) of the drug or biological, it is acceptable to add information via the two-dimensional bar code or other means (for example, radio frequency identification [RFID]).

The reason the issue of multiple standards for bar coding and RFID is raised in a discussion of EDMS is that questions have been raised about how desirable it may be for EDMS bar coding to be interoperable with other forms of bar coding for use in the healthcare organization. For now, it seems the linear bar code is the basic standard and will be used at a minimum.

In addition to bar codes on medical record documents, other optical character recognition (OCR) and forms recognition characteristics may be available to enhance the accuracy of indexing features on forms. Careful consideration should be given to understanding bar code specifications, bar code content, and issues related to bar code placement and any OCR on the forms prepared for use in medical records.

Healthcare organizations that approach EDMS should plan ahead to incorporate bar codes on their forms or be faced with using an interim solution for indexing, such as bar-coded separator sheets to distinguish between different types of documents in the chart (for example, all progress notes, all vital signs, and so on).

Document Retrieval, Viewing, and Distribution

The ability to retrieve documents from an EDMS is determined by the underlying technology used to store the documents. In some cases, documents from an EDMS are only available through a separate application on the desktop or potentially through the organization's intranet. The ability to search for a specific document or even content within a document then will depend on the level of indexing incorporated onto the form (that is, the content of the bar code and any use of OCR).

If the organization has an EHR with a clinical data repository (CDR), it is possible that there will be enhanced ability to call up a document as other components of the EHR are viewed. Again, depending on the CDR's level of indexing and sophistication, documents may be retrieved from a list of document types or may even be pushed to a particular view. The presence of a document or other image (for example, from a picture archiving and communication system [PACS]) on a given view may be indicated via an icon.

Viewing, printing, faxing, and attaching documents to e-mails all are capabilities the healthcare organization needs to address in its EDMS.

Document Management

Document management is an important function of EDMS. Although documents can be scanned, indexed, and retrieved, the abilities to conduct version control, access control, audit trails, content management, report management, and workflow are also distinct advantages of EDMS.

Version Control
Version control is a particularly critical component of EDMS when an EDMS is used as a key component of the EHR (as opposed to a means to archive inactive charts). Depending on when documents are scanned or COLD fed into the EDMS, it is very likely that some documents will not have been completed and authenticated and will need to be printed out, completed/signed, and rescanned. In some cases, EDMS is used for automated forms processing (discussed later in this chapter), in which case there is an even likelier chance of multiple versions. What is done with the former version is an important matter of healthcare organization policy and should be determined in conjunction with the clinicians who will use the record as well as with legal counsel.

Access Controls and Audit Trails
Just as in any electronic environment, an EDMS requires access privileges to be authorized, established, and enforced; a record of accesses is needed as a means to audit. Document management technology should provide such access controls and audit trails.

Content Management

In the broadest sense, **content management systems** refer to the ability to deliver document/content life cycle management, collaboration, search and navigation, Web access, workflow, knowledge management, and business process automation. At the core of a content management system is a repository for capturing, managing, and storing information from workgroups, folders, documents, discussions, memos, links, and other objectives. Content life cycle management includes check-in/check-out (access), version control, audit trails, and document-level security for all kinds of document file types, including word-processing documents, Web pages, and images. In many businesses, *enterprise content management* (ECM) refers to the ability to manage data collected on Web forms for customer relationship management. AIIM, formerly the Association for Information and Image Management, provides a cross-industry, global resource for ECM as well as being an ANSI-accredited standards development organization, producing standards for micrographics, advanced data storage systems, electronic imaging, document management technologies, EMDS, metadata, interoperable ECM (iECM), and PDF archiving, engineering, and universal accessibility (Amadeus n.d.).

In healthcare organizations, ECM typically has a somewhat more narrow focus on the management of content, although as more information is available in a variety of digital formats, the more expansive ED/CM, ECRM, becomes more commonplace. Certainly, EDMS is no longer just scanned documents, but includes documents that are electronically (COLD) fed, content retrieved through email or efax, sound files, and clinical images and wave forms from PACS.

Report Management

Enterprise report management (ERM) is the term typically used across industries to refer to technologies and formatting behind bringing electronic files into an EDMS. Healthcare organizations tend to use *COLD* to describe the ability to automatically move a dictated and transcribed document (or other document generated as a print file from an application, such as a laboratory information system) into the EDMS without printing or otherwise handling a paper version of the document. Because magnetic disks are often more commonly used than laser disks, the term "electronic feed" is simply used instead of COLD.

In order to COLD feed documents into an EDMS, an interface is required. For healthcare, this interface usually requires an HL7 message (although other transport solutions, such ASC X12, are feasible). HL7's **Clinical Document Architecture** (CDA) is a document markup standard that specifies the structure and semantics of a clinical document (its metadata) for the purpose of this exchange. CDA documents are encoded in eXtensible Markup Language (XML). Figure 14.3 provides an example of the major components of a CDA document.

Workflow

Many EDMS add a workflow component to their functionality. This enables documents to be proactively directed to where work needs to be performed. For example, some logic may indicate that as soon as key documents have been scanned, the record is ready for coding and would send an alert to a workstation in the HIM department (or wherever such work may be performed, including to a remote coder).

Figure 14.3.   Major components of a CDA document

```
<ClinicalDocument>
     . . .  CDA Header . . .
     <structuredBody>
          <section>
                    <text>(a.k.a. "narrative block")</text>
                    <observation> . . . </observation>
          . . .
          </section>
     </structuredBody>
</ClinicalDocument>
```

A number of terms are associated with workflow and its management (Andrew and Bruegel 2003). *Workflow* refers to the sequence of tasks that need to be performed within a process. *Workflow management* is the planning, organizing, directing, and controlling of the workflow. **Workflow management systems** store workflow definitions as a collection of tasks, resources, and conditional logic. They then retrieve workflow information from the database to guide work as transactions pass through the organization (Retsema 2003).

Workflow technology helps to organize, automate, and improve processes by dividing them into component tasks, specifying who performs each task, identifying the business rules for performing the tasks, describing the potential outputs, and indicating who performs the next step in the process. Based on these factors, workflow technology:

- Assembles the information needed to perform each task

- Provides guidance for performing each task according to the correct and consistent business rules

- Routes the task, along with the information needed to perform it, to the appropriate person

- Potentially speeds up a process by dividing it into tasks or parts, coordinating the work of multiple people on the various parts, and reassembling the parts to complete the original process

HL7 defines workflow management functions as those intended to "support work flow functions including both the management and setup of work queues, personnel and system interfaces, as well as the implementation functions that use workflow-related business rules to direct the flow of work assignments" (Andrew and Bruegel 2005).

A survey of EHR vendors reported by Andrew and Bruegel in 2005 revealed that some 60 percent to 80 percent of respondents indicated that they had workflow functionality, although just less than 50 percent indicated they had a "workflow engine." Andrew and Bruegel define a *workflow engine* as a system that takes care of the management of workflow, including task assignment generation, resource allocation, activity performance, case preparation and modification, launching applications, and the recording of logistical information.

Suffice it to say, workflow management technology is an important adjunct to EDMS as well as EHR.

Automated Forms Processing

An article in *AIIM E-Doc Magazine* compares and contrasts document image capture and forms automation. AIIM describes both as involving scanning and use of image-processing capabilities to enhance or evaluate a document image. In both cases, indexing and other data are extracted from the scanned image.

The main difference between the two applications has to do with the way each one treats imaged data. With document capture, imaged data are entered (manually, through bar codes, or via OCR) with reference to one or a small number of index fields. With forms automation, most or all of the imaged data on each form are intelligently recognized and extracted using intelligent character recognition (ICR). The result of an image capture application is a document image. The result of automated forms processing typically is the extracted data. In fact, AIIM suggests that the form image is thrown out after the data are successfully extracted (Gingrande 2005).

Electronic Signature, Document Annotation, and Editing

Another key component of EDMS included in workflow technology is the ability to electronically sign, add notes to, and edit documents.

It should be noted that the signature referred to here is the electronic form of signature, which is neither the digitized form nor the digital signature. In **electronic signature authentication** (ESA), a standard log-on and password, biometric, and/or token authentication mechanism is used.

Alternatively, a digitized signature conforms to the minimum requirements set for in the Electronic Signatures in Global and National Commerce Act (ESIGN) of 2000, which is any "electronic sound, symbol, or process attached to or logically associated with an electronic record and executed or adopted by a person with the intent to sign the record electronically." Despite the much heralded legislation, there have been no subsequent federal regulations to further enable its use. However, it was based on the Uniform Electronic Transactions Act (UETA). This is a model act adopted by the National Conference of Commissioners on Uniform State Laws (NCCUSL) in 1999 that gives electronic signatures and records the same validity and enforceability as manual signatures and paper-based transactions. It has been adopted by 46 states, including several states that explicitly refer to individually identifiable health information. States that have not adopted this particular uniform act have statutes pertaining to electronic transactions (NCSL 2008). The most frequently used digitized form of signature under ESIGN is the signature pad, which captures an image of a person's signature and is used in the retail industry. (Also refer to chapter 3.)

Readers may also recall from chapter 10 that a digital signature uses encryption to authenticate and provide nonrepudiation services. There currently are no federal laws requiring use of the digital form of signature for healthcare.

Functionality for EDMS

EDMS is often spearheaded in a hospital by the HIM department because of its many benefits to record assembly, forms management, late report filing, transcription, coding, chart completion, release of information, and external reporting.

Other areas that have benefited significantly from the workflow components of EDMS include patient financial services and billing and quality. Radiology finds EDMS a useful way to manage the documents often stored in pockets of film jackets after a PACS is implemented. Emergency departments (EDs) often seek to manage ED reports via EDMS because they are so frequently accessed within a short period of time after an ED visit. Non-care delivery departments also benefit from EDMS, including human resources, procurement, and legal.

As a care delivery organization proceeds to utilize EDMS, it should do so not only within the context of its EHR migration path, but by evaluating the entire organization's information assets. It is not uncommon to find hospitals, particularly, with multiple, different EDMS systems that are not interoperable. Although it may not appear to be necessary for a human resources department to have a system that integrates with the EHR, there may be economies of scale reasons to at least utilize the same EDMS technology platform. Ultimately, there may be reasons to integrate some documents, such as for nurse staffing or inventory management.

Planning for EDMS

Taking EDMS beyond the HIM and other financial, administrative, or clinical department arena, hospitals are finding significant benefits. Although careful planning is required, an enterprisewide EDMS can rapidly put a hospital in position to achieve a paperless environment. (See appendix D.1 on the enclosed CD.)

Clinical Messaging

It has been noted that another bridge technology in preparation for and supplementary to EHR is clinical messaging. Defined as the secure transmission of clinical information between organizations and across the continuum of care, many hospitals are opening portals for physicians and patients, and many physician offices are using clinical messaging in several forms for communication with hospitals and other providers with whom they refer patients. Clinical messaging is described more fully in chapter 16.

Conclusion

Unfortunately, hospitals often face a bigger challenge to implement EHRs than other types of facilities. Legacy systems abound and they are difficult to integrate, especially if they are different vendors' products. Vendors generally do not supply a single, all-encompassing EHR module for hospitals, but rather multiple modules. Hospitals have many sources of data and more unique processes necessitating a modular and migratory approach. Even in cases where all modules are acquired at once from the same vendor, and the modules are implemented during a short time span, each component tends to be focused on a specific process. As a result, many hospitals have chosen a migration path that starts with an EDMS. If this is done in the context of moving forward with additional modules, it is an excellent strategy. There is some risk, however, that an EDMS that is largely a document imaging systems meets an immediate need, the organization could be lulled into thinking that further progress toward a more comprehensive system is not imperative. This approach also does not fully provide for context-sensitive, evidence-based clinical decision support at the point of care or in real time.

References and Resources

AHIMA e-HIM Work Group on Electronic Document Management as a Component of EHR. 2003a (Oct.). Practice brief: Electronic document management as a component of EHR. *Journal of AHIMA*. http://library.ahima.org/xpedio/groups/public/documents/ahima/bok1_021594.hcsp?dDocName=bok1_021594.

AHIMA e-HIM Work Group on Health Information in a Hybrid Records. 2003b (Oct.). Practice Brief: The complete medical record in a hybrid EHR environment. *Journal of AHIMA*. http://library.ahima.org/xpedio/groups/public/documents/ahima/bok1_022142.hcsp?dDocName=bok1_022142

AIIM Standards Committee. (2007). AIIM Recommended Practice (ARP1-2007), Analysis, Selection, and Implementation Guidelines Associated with Electronic Document Management Systems (EDMS). www.aiim.org/standards.

Amadeus. n.d. Electronic Content Management. www.amadeussolutions.com/english/practice/bp_ecm.htm.

Amatayakul, M.A., and M.R. Cohen. 2005 (April 28). HC Pro AudioConference Polling Question: Managing hybrid records.

Andrew, W.F., and R.B. Bruegel. 2005. 2005. EHR workflow management review and survey results. *ADVANCE for Health Information Executives* 9(2):34–50.

Andrew, W.F., and R.B. Bruegel. 2003. Workflow management and the CPR. *ADVANCE for Health Information Executives* 7(2):49–53.

Berman, P. 2004. Enterprise image management. *ADVANCE for Health Information Executives* 8(2):87–89.

Brock, C., J. Vasko, and B. Fugitt. Business Case: Electronic Records/Electronic Document Management System, Federal Information and Records Managers Council. www.pages.zdnet.com/firmweb/federal_records/id41.html.

Center for Information Technology Leadership. 2003. The value of computerized provider order entry in ambulatory settings. *Executive Preview*. www.citl.org.

Conn, J.2007 (March 19). CPOE Adoption Slowly Gaining Ground: Survey. *Modern Healthcare*.

Dolin, R.H., et al. 2006. HL7 Clinical Document Architecture, Release 2. *Journal of the American Medical Informatics Association* 13(1):30–38.

Fox, LA and PT Sheridan. 2005 (July 18). From the Trenches: EHR Strategies and the Role of Health Information Management, Advance for Health Information Professionals.

Friedman, B. 2005. The state of document management. *Journal of AHIMA* 76(4):30–33.

Gingrande, A. 2005 (Jan./Feb.). Automated forms processing. *AIIM E-Doc Magazine*. www.edocmagazine.com/article_new.asp?ID=29431.

Grzbowski, D. 2006 (Feb.). Reconcile COLD-feed systems interfaces. *Electronic Health Records Briefing*, suppl. Marblehead, MA: HCPro.

Halamka, J. 2006. Early experiences with positive patient identification. *Journal of Healthcare Information Management* 20(1):25–27.

Health Industry Bar Code (HIBC) Provider Applications Standard, ANSI/HIBC 1–1996.

Henning C. 2008 (July). Clinical Results Delivery Service, Redwood MedNet.

HIMSS Analytics, EMR Adoption Model, 2007. http://www.himssanalytics.org/docs/EMRAM.pdf.

iHealthBeat, 2007 (March 20). CPOE Adoption Remains Low, Slowly Increasing.

Kohn, Deborah. (2006), Informatics in Healthcare in *Health Information Management*, 2nd ed., eds. LaTour K., and S. Eichenwald-Maki, Chicago. American Health Information Management Association, p. 55.

McMillan, J.E. 2005 (Dec.). How digital rights management (DRM) technology will change the way courts work. In *Future Trends in State Courts*. Williamsburg, VA: National Center for State Courts.

Myjer, D., and R. Madamba. 2002. Implementing a document imaging system *Journal of AHIMA* 73(9):44ff.

National Conference of State Legislatures (NCSL), Uniform Electronic Transactions Act. 2008. www.ncsl.org/programs/lis/CIP/ueta-statues.htm.

Reino L and C. Hyde, 2006 (Oct.). From Paper to Electronic, and In Between: The challenges hospitals face with the hybrid record, AHIMAs 78th National Convention and Exhibit Proceedings.

Reitsema, J.D. 2003 (Feb. 1). Evaluating clinical workflow management systems. *ADVANCE for Health Information Executives* 7(2):54–55.

Rhodes, H., and M. Dougherty. 2003. Practice Brief: Document Imaging as a bridge to the EHR. *Journal of American Health Information Management Association* 74(6):56A–G.

Robins, Kaplan, Miller. and Ciresi, LLP. 2000 (July 26). Electronic Signatures in Global and National Commerce Act (ESING). FAQs and Resource Links. www.rkmc.com/Electronic_Signatures_in_Global_and_National_Commerce_Act_ESIGN_FAQs_and_Resource_Links.htm.

Stiell A., et al. 2003 Prevalence of Information Gaps in the Emergency Department and the Effect on Patient Outcomes. *Canadian Medical Association Journal* 169(10).

Strong, K.V. 2008. Enterprise Content and Records Management. *Journal of AHIMA* 80(2): 38–42.

Wieczorek, M.M. 2004. Taking electronic document management beyond the HIM department. *Journal of AHIMA* 75(1):32–36.

Chapter 15
Acute Care EHR Applications

When an acute care hospital establishes a goal of achieving an electronic health record (EHR), the hospital is essentially acquiring many elements that contribute to achieving the functions of its definition of EHR. This is unlike ambulatory care environments where an EHR is more likely to be many functions packaged together. Hence, a hospital really does not acquire "an EHR" but, rather, compiles the applications that lead to an EHR.

In achieving an EHR, a hospital builds on existing source systems by acquiring additional components, not all of which have to be, or probably can be, implemented all at once. The process to get to the point of achieving the organization's vision of an EHR requires carefully addressing the applications, technology, and operational elements along the migration path it has laid out for itself.

Planning, infrastructure preparation, selection, and implementation topics have been covered in previous chapters of this book. This chapter describes the specific clinical applications that typically make up the components of an EHR for a hospital. This chapter:

- Emphasizes the importance of a critically constructed migration path that supports the hospital's journey to an EHR

- Identifies alternatives that help achieve the collection of data from multiple sources that support an EHR

- Describes the importance of the presentation layer for data retrieval and documentation

- Supplies information about point-of-care (POC) charting applications that address quality and productivity improvement

- Provides an overview of medication management applications (for example, computerized provider order entry [CPOE] and bar code medication administration record [BC-MAR]) that address patient safety

- Addresses the inclusion of clinical decision support in a comprehensive EHR

- Recognizes various other components that have clinical as well as financial and administrative, operational, or educational impact for the organization

Key Terms

Benchmarking

Closed loop medication
    management

Defaults

Free text

Graphical user
    interface

Icon

Medication
    reconciliation

Navigational support

Order communication

Presentation layer

Speech recognition

EHR Migration Path for Hospitals

Virtually every hospital today has a set of information systems. As previously described, hospitals typically start with financial/administrative systems (for example, patient accounting [P/A]; registration-admission, discharge, transfer [R-ADT]; master person index [MPI]) and then add departmental operational systems (for example, laboratory, radiology, pharmacy, health information management, surgery, intensive care, emergency department). Although many of these departmental operational systems produce clinical data (such as laboratory results, x-ray reports, and so on), the systems are primarily designed to support the operations of the department. For example, a laboratory information system receives an order for a laboratory test—or if there is no order communication system, staff in the laboratory enter information from a laboratory requisition form. The system then produces a specimen collection list, labels for specimen collection vials, and other tools that support specimen management. Once the specimen is collected, it is processed by a device that may be connected to the laboratory information system, both to generate results and also to manage quality control and other issues. Like other operational systems, the laboratory information system also manages laboratory staffing, inventory of supplies, and other processes. The goal for the EHR is to tap these operational systems for their clinical information, enhance their ability to perform their operational functions with information entered by clinicians, and integrate all this information with clinical decision support to improve patient safety and quality of care.

Impact of IT Acquisition Strategies on EHR

The information technology (IT) acquisition strategies hospitals have deployed, especially for operational systems, have varied. Some hospitals have acquired the best systems for the respective functions, resulting in a best-of-breed strategy where different systems come from different vendors. Other hospitals have preferred to acquire as many of their financial, administrative, and operational systems as possible from a single vendor, following the best-of-fit strategy. These are sometimes referred to as hospital information systems (HIS). As hospitals are now approaching the EHR, the best-of-breed strategy makes it difficult to integrate the data needed for the EHR functions from all the various different source systems. Alternatively, those with a best-of-fit strategy may find that their vendor, who provided a solid offering for financial/administrative applications, may be weaker in clinical applications. This is not to be disparaging of those vendors, but only to point out that a best-of-fit strategy is designed to provide the lowest common denominator in order to keep costs low. Hospitals using these vendor products have not wanted to spend more to gain a much higher level of sophistication.

Although some hospitals are starting to follow a rip and replace strategy where they have literally replaced most of their old systems with a suite of products from a single vendor, unfortunately, many organizations are unwilling or unable to make such an investment. Many hospitals cannot make the business case for such expenditure, or fear that the impact on staff will be too great.

As a result, many hospitals are struggling to define the right migration path that would achieve the clinical support desired from an EHR within the confines of its legacy systems or at least within a logical and realistic approach of new acquisition. Just as was identified in the chapter describing the EHR migration path, no one size fits all. What may be right for one hospital may not work for another hospital. Chapter 14 identifies bridge strategies being used by many hospitals to achieve better access to information in paper or digital form. As hospitals want to move up the value curve and introduce clinical decision support, documentation of discrete data and point-of-care charting will be necessary.

Factors to Consider

As hospitals approach more sophisticated clinical information systems to support the EHR, they have many factors to consider. For example, some hospitals believe that it will be difficult to get their physicians to use CPOE and thus plan to implement it as the last application toward the EHR. Others believe a CPOE system needs to be among the first clinical applications implemented because of patient safety concerns. There may be a dilemma as to whether to have nurses adopt a BC-MAR system prior to CPOE as a means to provide support to physicians after they start using CPOE or whether CPOE is a more critically needed system. Sometimes it is the physicians who want a system like the one they are beginning to acquire in their offices and often are disappointed in the capabilities of the hospital clinical systems.

Such dilemmas are not unique to applications; they also apply to the technical infrastructure. Some believe a clinical data repository is an essential tool on which to build the EHR; others find sufficient integration continuing with a best-of-fit approach. For some hospitals, replacement of some of the operational systems and enhancing the technical infrastructure is believed to be essential to support the new clinical systems. Other hospitals, however, roll out new applications as quickly as possible, backfilling with technical enhancements only in response to complaints about slow response time or lack of functionality. For example, where laboratory results may have been able to be retrieved and viewed for some time in the hospital, the laboratory system may only be generating a print file for such viewing. It may only be after a CPOE system is acquired that it is realized that the laboratory's output will not support drug–laboratory contraindication checking or dose calculation. The hospital then may be faced with deciding among foregoing the drug–laboratory checking, attempting to have an interface written from the laboratory to the CPOE application, or replacing the laboratory system. Some hospitals have not chosen any of these options, with the result that the CPOE is not fully functional, the interface is expensive to write and maintain and the laboratory data limited, or the replacement is yet another cost and implementation project.

Figure 15.1.   EHR value curve

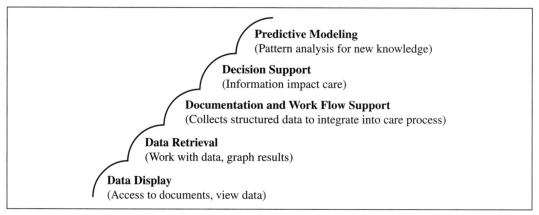

Predictive Modeling
(Pattern analysis for new knowledge)

Decision Support
(Information impact care)

Documentation and Work Flow Support
(Collects structured data to integrate into care process)

Data Retrieval
(Work with data, graph results)

Data Display
(Access to documents, view data)

A hospital should understand that the functions of an EHR, when taken together, are generally going to reflect a value curve. As additional functionality is added, the value returned to the users and to the overall efficiency and effectiveness of providing healthcare increases. This also follows the data–information–knowledge continuum, as it is merely data that are available at the start of the value curve with information and, ultimately, knowledge achieved further along the curve. Figure 15.1 shows a summary of such a value curve. As discussed in earlier chapters, each hospital may select functionality from different points along the value curve to adopt in its migration path. The Institute of Medicine (IOM) EHR Core Functionality, the HL7 EHR System Functional Descriptors, and the requirements of the Certification Commission on Health Information Technology (CCHIT) all build on each other and serve as resources in identifying functionality for implementation suitable for different care settings over a continuum of time.

Critical Analysis of Migration Path

What most hospitals are finding is that educating the organization on EHR concepts, defining specific goals, laying out a migration path wherein relationships among all components of EHR and health information technology in general are identified, and then managing both the acquisition of the elements on the path and the expectations of what the various components along the path will actually achieve are critical steps in realizing EHR benefits.

It cannot be emphasized enough that an EHR for a hospital requires a critical appraisal of what a hospital currently has, what it wants for the future, and what alternatives exist and which among them make the most sense. This must include not only the applications but the technology and operational issues. If a hospital does not have sufficient fail-over capability, bandwidth, or wireless connectivity, user frustration with any system can set in rapidly. Provisions must be made for contingency planning and storage of considerably more data. Plans need to be made to manage the hybrid record situation, and policies are needed to define the legal health record. Engaging clinician stakeholders early in the process gives them an appreciation for what the hospital is facing and can help the hospital make better decisions. A systematic process of mapping current processes to ensure that all control points are retained and new ones added is essential to ensure that these clinical systems do not create errors inadvertently where they were intended to avoid errors. Instituting milestones and checkpoints for completion of an implementation and adoption avoids moving on to another project before a prior one is completely working. Continual monitoring of how clinical systems are used, that they are up to date, that they provide the appropriate level of decision support for their users, that inappropriate workarounds have not been created or new workarounds created because of system glitches that have gone unaddressed, and that they have not inadvertently introduced unintended consequences is essential.

The discussion that follows of various hospital EHR and HIT applications is not intended to reflect a specific sequence of events or imply that there is one right migration path. The sequence of discussion is merely the result of the fact that a book must present information in a sequential rather than a random manner.

Integrated Collection and Use of Data

A hallmark of the EHR is that data from multiple sources can interact together. This means that there must be a way for these data to be placed into a single data repository or to come together at the time data are required for use.

Integration through a Repository

In general, most EHR developers view the centralization of data into a single repository as the most beneficial means of integrating data. Any data needed to support the EHR generated by various source systems would be placed into this repository. When in the repository, database structures can be established to support its interaction with the user.

A repository that collects data from multiple sources and operates with clinical decision support software also generally has the ability to store images of documents, diagnostic images, and other information in digital form such as dictation, e-mail, and e-faxes. This information then would be retrievable through the same presentation layer, perhaps via an **icon** or file structure.

Alternatives to a Repository

Not every vendor that supports HIS has developed a repository structure that is sufficiently robust to integrate both discrete data and images or to work with robust clinical decision support software. As a result, hospitals now have to make tough decisions: Do they wait for their incumbent HIS vendor to develop more functionality? Do they buy from another clinical information system vendor and hope their various source systems can be sufficiently interfaced to be able to contribute data to the new vendor's repository? Do they buy a generic repository and build their own database structures and presentation layer, also expecting to interface their existing source systems? Do they attempt to have clinicians use the various source systems independently, perhaps with an integrated sign on process (single sign on [SSO]) or other middleware that makes the applications look more alike, gaining the benefit of access to the data but still relying on personal cognitive processes rather than robust clinical decision support software to make clinical decisions?

In a way, the dilemma hospitals currently face is something of a chicken-and-egg question, especially in light of clinician adoption concerns. Some hospitals think a slow migration path where only one or two functions are supported first eases clinicians into adoption. Or the hospital attempts to save money by piecing together a system, resulting in what sometimes is described as being a kludgy system. In either case, clinicians may find these situations incomplete and burdensome, and not of sufficient value to bother adopting. Alternatively, because there has been such concern about clinician resistance to systems, some hospitals are reluctant to make huge investments in new systems or attempt a "big bang" rollout strategy where clinician adoption is uncertain. As a result of an increasing number of physicians acquiring EHRs for their own offices, hospitals are starting to find a turnabout in such concerns. In fact, in some environments, it is the physicians who are at the forefront of promoting more sophisticated hospital EHRs. Although this still may not be the norm, hospitals would do well to work closely with their medical staffs and to utilize early physician adopters as champions for hospitalwide projects.

Presentation Layer for Use of Data

It should be obvious that merely pulling data together into a repository is only one aspect of using such integrated data. A **presentation layer** is software that provides screen layout, data capture, and retrieval functionality, and operates on the repository to help users select data from the repository, enter data into it, and be provided with clinical decision support. The presentation layer affords each party to a process—physician, pharmacist, nurse, or other clinician—screens tailored to their needs, with the ability to gain additional knowledge and document specific actions taken.

In fact, data retrieval and documentation strategies may be the key elements of obtaining clinician adoption. Behavioral issues associated with clinician use of the EHR have been discussed extensively. However, how different types of clinicians in different settings interact with the EHR to retrieve and document data directly impacts the type of EHR workstation(s) and screen design necessary for adoption.

Data Retrieval Strategies

To appreciate workstation and screen design features necessary to gain clinician adoption of EHR, it is useful to first appreciate how clinicians currently use information. The model shown in figure 15.2 was introduced more than 20 years ago to describe clinical decision making in general and was based on a model created 10 years earlier for basic information processing (Elson, Faughnan, and Connelly 1997). Its relevance to current data retrieval and documentation strategies design is astounding. It shows that because of system constraints in external memory (primarily paper-based records, but also knowledge sources such as literature and consultants), there is increased reliance on the clinician's long-term memory. And because human memory has significant failings, it is important to build a

Figure 15.2.   Model of impact of system constraints on clinical decision making

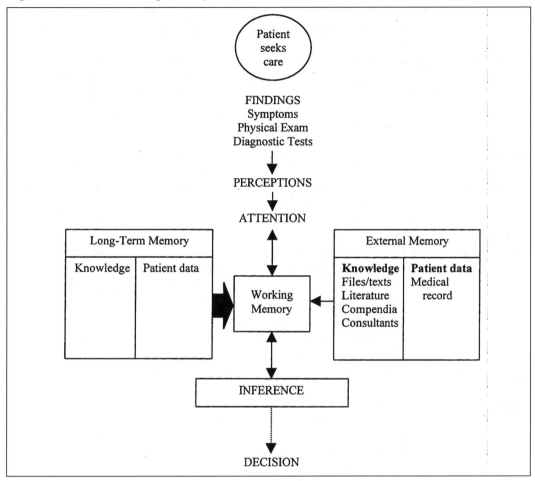

system that will enhance access to external memory for improved decision making. Key to that is an intuitive workstation that can be integrated into clinical workflow.

In using "external memory" support, clinicians can:

- Scan data rapidly to obtain a quick overview and understanding of a new patient

- Retrieve data to refamiliarize themselves with a former patient's history

- Search data for specific facts relative to a current patient

- Review a range of data to solve a problem relative to a current patient

Each of these processes is further accompanied by several levels of text processing, ranging from reading all the words in a paragraph to skipping a paragraph altogether. Even within paper-based documents, graphic, textual, and positional features of the data, logically related and controlled, are essential for orientation, navigation, and effective limitation of search space. With this in mind, is it any wonder that clinicians complain about having to page through too many screens or having a limited amount of data on one screen in a computer system?

There are many considerations relative to data retrieval and the functionality sought in developing functional specifications for an EHR system. These include screen density, size of device, search capability, positioning of content and navigational support, consistency of design and flexibility, graphics, and use of color and icons. Moreover, attention must be paid to matching these characteristics to the applications they serve (*ADVANCE* 2005a).

Screen Density

The Regenstrief Institute for Health Care is a privately endowed healthcare research organization founded in 1969 by the inventor of the modern-day washing machine. Samuel Regenstrief believed that the techniques of systems engineering, industrial engineering, computer sciences, and statistics could improve the delivery and cost of healthcare. He also believed that the healthcare process was chaotic and destined to become more so unless new approaches could be found. Physicians at the Institute, led by Dr. Clement McDonald, are faculty at the Indiana University School of Medicine and work closely with Wishard Memorial Hospital in Indianapolis (McDonald and Tierney 1998). Not only have they created a working EHR system over the past few decades, but they also have studied virtually every aspect of how physicians use data. For example, they can tell the degree of eye movement a physician applies to one of the retrieval strategies described earlier.

McDonald first demonstrated the usefulness of reminders in direct clinical care. He has noted that reminders help clinicians do what they know is correct but for a variety of reasons occasionally fail to do. Physicians simply have too many details to attend to and sometimes can overlook important tasks unless they are reminded to do them.

Members of the Regenstrief Institute have published extensively, especially on the impact that EHR systems can have on the quality and cost of healthcare. They have reached an important conclusion relative to data retrieval and workstation design: the denser the screen, the better it is for data retrieval purposes.

Size of Device

Size of device is a consideration closely related to screen density. Many clinicians want to be more mobile with their computing and are considering migrating to smaller and smaller, and hence more portable, devices. However, what was previously designed for a large monitor may not work on a smaller device and lower-resolution display screen. (The size of a screen is often referred to as the screen's real estate.) In fact, where EHR systems are being designed for use at both PC workstations and handheld device workstations, consideration must be given to how data can be displayed effectively on both and whether the data will look the same.

Smaller screens generally make it more difficult to rapidly scan large volumes of data to obtain a quick overview and understanding of a new patient or to refamiliarize oneself with a former patient's history. However, creative ways are being found to overcome these issues. Figure 15.3 provides a sample patient summary screen. Although this was intended to display on a full-sized monitor, the view of the monthly calendar with "busy" days in boldface is very similar to views used by PDAs. Scanning through a patient-specific calen-

Figure 15.3.   Sample patient summary screen

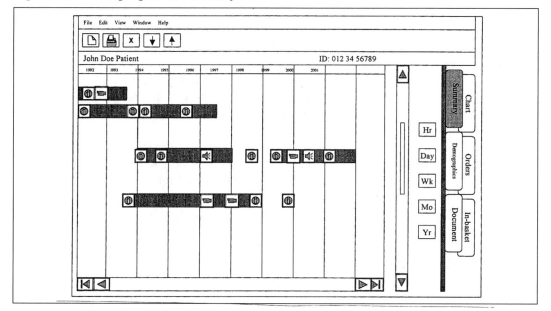

dar that identifies the number of times the patient has been seen can provide the same sense as the thickness of the paper record.

Because the size of the screen has such a large impact on usability, many hospitals are using mobile carts with notebook computers mounted onto them (computers on wheels [COWs]) or specially built kiosks just outside patient rooms that use wireless capability to connect to the hospital's network. Mobile carts can be equipped with bar code scanners and may contain a storage area for blood pressure cuffs or other equipment; some have even been outfitted with small medication dispensing devices (Dullea 2005).

Search Capability

Search capability and the number of levels to drill down are important considerations for all data retrieval strategies. However, they are especially critical for small screen viewing of specific facts relative to a current patient or a range of data to solve a problem relative to a current patient. The EHR needs to have the ability to permit highly structured queries to be made from one screen. Current experience browsing the Web should alert anyone that the more layers one needs to go through to get to data, the more likely one is to get lost. This is equally true for EHRs. In fact, it is one of the reasons why browser-based, advanced search capability technology is becoming popular for EHR systems.

Content Positioning and Navigational Support

Content positioning and navigational support are critical to helping clinicians retrieve data. **Navigational support** with respect to the display screen refers to the ability to move from one screen to another, to drill down to retrieve further detail about something, to access knowledge bases, or to request a graph or other form of display. Navigation is made easy with pull-down menus, buttons, radio dials, and slide bars, all of which can be performed with a mouse or other navigational device. Navigational devices include keyboard, mouse, touch pad, trackball, track point, touch screen, and, to some extent, handwriting recognition and voice commands using **speech recognition**.

Although there are no standard forms designs in paper record systems, there are limited ways to construct a form and to help clinicians navigate through the chart. For example, patient-identifying information typically is put at the top left or top right of each form. Sheets are colored or have color bars on them. There may be tabs, especially for inpatient charts at the nursing station.

Likewise, there are no standards for EHR system display designs, but there generally are more options. Some EHR vendors have attempted to make the EHR look like a paper record, with tabs and colors. Other vendors design screens to look like Microsoft Windows or use still other designs. To some extent, the position of content and navigational support is a matter of personal preference. However, the extent to which such designs can be standardized helps clinicians who may have to use multiple applications, or even multiple EHRs (such as physicians who may have their own office EHR plus have privileges at two different hospitals, each with different EHR systems).

An early step in migrating to an EHR should be to take a forms inventory, reduce redundancy in present forms, evaluate how necessary redundancy in today's forms can be reduced further with an EHR, and plan how the presentation of the legal health record will be achieved in the electronic environment (Quinsey 2007). Many hospitals believe they have to replicate their present paper environment precisely in the electronic environment. Careful planning, however, can streamline even this presentation. For instance, nurses have observed that there are as many as a dozen forms to complete at the time of an admission—often taking 60 to 90 minutes to complete, and with considerable repetition of data entry on each. An electronic documentation system would enable the repetitive data to be prepopulated on each form, also ensuring their accuracy. However, the hospital should be asking, is it necessary to retain all dozen forms? Because access to the data is now available across the hospital, the need for different forms to go to different destinations is no longer necessary. It may be more important to address what specific views are needed and ensure that each view can be captured for the legal health record.

Consistency of Design and Flexibility

Consistency of design and flexibility may seem to be opposing considerations, but both have an important relationship to data retrieval. Although no one has control over the design of different vendor products, within a given system the placement of data and navigational devices ought to be consistent. Screens should essentially all have the same look and feel to make it easier and quicker for both scanning the information and physically navigating through it. However, as noted above, some of this is a matter of personal preference. Therefore, an ideal feature might be to have the flexibility to create unique user designs.

Some experts suggest that flexibility is critical to clinician adoption; others suggest that it may actually hinder adoption because it is not always possible to design a system to exact specifications. Further, they argue that the sooner clinicians learn to be flexible rather than demanding flexibility in the EHR products, the better off they will be. As with most debates, the truth is probably somewhere in the middle.

Graphics

Graphics is one of the especially unique features of retrieving data from an EHR system. Current **graphical user interface** (GUI) technology permits not only straight text and the ability to import images, but also the ability to actually convert text to graphics. The Microsoft Windows operating system also permits many views of different data displayed at one time. Hence, drug dosages and laboratory results can be plotted on a graph while the clinician is viewing an x-ray image and seeing a textual reminder. Graphics can be zoomed in and out for better viewing.

Color and Icons

The use of color and icons is another important consideration when speaking of data retrieval and functionality. For example, many men are color-blind, so relying totally on color to guide navigation may not work in a provider setting where many of the clinicians are male. In addition, different types of display screens display color differently. A lovely shade of green on one screen may look putrid on another. Color can be effective, but it should be accompanied by some other form of indicator.

Icons are popular indicators, and some can be made to flash when they represent an alarm or special form of alert. They can be popular in guiding a clinician through a list. For example, in figure 15.3, icons were used in the sample patient summary time lines to indicate the type of information. A circle with an "i" in it referred to text information. The icon displaying sound referred to the fact that the user could listen to dictation. The camera icon represented an image that could be viewed. Most icons are relatively self-explanatory. Many are spinoffs from road signs. However, some designers can become creative and their icons may not be universally understood.

Data Retrieval for Administrative Functions

Data retrieval for administrative functions is yet another important consideration. In some systems, what is viewable from the screen cannot always be printed in its entirety or is either shifted or reduced in size. Some systems are creating a printer-friendly functionality that creates an appropriately sized printout, or at least enables such a print file to be created and archived should such a printout ever be needed.

Another issue involves the ability to remove identifying information beyond the patient's name and medical record number in order to create deidentified data or a limited data set as may be required by the Health Insurance Portability and Accountability Act (HIPAA). A few systems have gone as far as to be able to remove certain identifying characteristics of the patient for administrative use within the organization (for example, for coding, transcription, or quality improvement). Although this is beyond what is absolutely required by HIPAA because HIPAA does permit use for "operations," the practice goes a long way toward contributing to extra confidentiality measures, especially as some of these functions may be outsourced. This also might be appreciated when a provider treats many of its employees.

Results Notification

Results notification is a frequent function found in EHR systems. One form of results notification is to identify when there are new results not previously retrieved or when a result is out of range or abnormal. This notification may come in various forms. Some presentation layers place a special icon beside the patient's name or result on the display. Others may even set off a clinician's pager.

Documentation Strategies

In addition to the strategies described for data retrieval, data capture for documentation must consider the various forms of data entry and creation, including free-text entry, structured data entry from pick lists or pull-down menus, template-based entry, and natural language processing.

Free Text
Free text is the entry of narrative data, primarily via keyboarding, although dictation, voice recognition, and handwriting recognition are possible. Dictation uses a third party to transcribe the data; hence, there will always be a delay factor in seeing the results.

Speech recognition was once thought to be the panacea for clinician data capture, but there have always been concerns about its accuracy. Its accuracy is improving, but it is still not 100 percent. Most clinicians find that voice recognition is suitable in certain circumstances and not in others. For example, it is excellent in situations where a lot of repetitive data must be entered in a relatively "private" setting. Radiologists and pathologists find voice recognition particularly useful. However, even for physicians who have no objection to having a workstation in an examining room or who currently dictate their notes while in the examining room, it may be awkward to conduct voice recognition while simultaneously speaking with the patient and having to watch the screen to make corrections.

An important issue with voice and handwriting recognition is that, unless the situation is such that there is time for a "correctionist" to review the results, the author must be constantly alert to the system not correctly interpreting the handwriting or speech. Correcting errors can be distracting and possibly more time-consuming than keyboarding. Where data are not highly repetitive and where clinicians may use any number of devices so that no one device gets "trained" on the specific individual's voice pattern, error rates can be as high as from 5 percent to 20 percent. Often errors occur more frequently in common words and phrases than in medical terminology on which the device has been "factory trained." This can be particularly frustrating. In general, most clinicians now regard voice recognition as one option to be considered in certain circumstances.

Data Entry from Pick Lists or Pull-Down Menus
Structured data entry from pick lists or pull-down menus is an important data capture technique. Most EHR systems use a combination of such structured data entry and free text. When using structured data entry, it is important that the data options be clearly defined, comprehensive, and up to date. Ideally, the data should be drawn from a controlled vocabulary and encoded by the EHR system for use in processing. Even if not, however, structured data are essential to ultimately drive clinical decision support.

Structured data entry should be easier and quicker to use than keyboarding, even for experienced typists. To achieve this level of facility with structured data entry, however, the user must go through a learning curve and the system must be well designed, where underlying logic drives the menu options. For example, if a structured data-entry physical examination is being recorded for a female, physical examination components relating only to males should not be presented. To be most effective, structured data entry should be highly tailored to the type of patient. This requires considerable work up front, especially when the setting includes unusual specialties. This is one reason why many physicians prefer to buy EHRs related to their specialty: they come with many premade structured data-entry menus.

Another consideration in structured data entry relates to **defaults**. Structured data entry should be designed so that rules are strictly followed relative to the absence of a response. It is not good documentation to have the default to an unanswered selection be "normal." If there is no response to an item, there should be a prompt to obtain a response for critical items or the default should be "not recorded." Systems designed to prompt for a required response, however, should permit the user to proceed, but the entry should be marked incomplete until a response is generated.

A final feature related to structured data entry is the ability to derive narrative from structured data. For example, after a physician responds to each item on a structured physical examination, some systems embed the responses into a narrative that makes the final output look as though it was dictated or keyed in. For example, if one element is "chief complaint" and the response is "shortness of breath," the EHR system could create this statement: "The patient complains of shortness of breath."

Template-based Entry

Template-based entry is something of a cross between free text and structured data entry. Because many notes follow a repeated structure and include similar types of data, templates may be developed wherein the clinician need only add variable data. Macros that provide phrases or sentences to complete the variable portions of templates can further speed the use of automated templates.

Another form of data capture using a type of template is "cut and paste," or data reuse. In this case, a clinician literally copies an entry from a previous note or a different patient and pastes it into the new entry. Although data reuse can be an effective data capture tool, strong caution must be applied to ensure that the note is entirely applicable for the new entry. Any reference to a different patient or a different time can nullify an entry and cause the entire record to be suspect. Clinicians should not only be careful, but also understand from a technical standpoint what the implications are of cutting and pasting (actually copying and pasting). It is possible that in so doing, more (or less) than the intended data are moved to the new record. Because this process is designed to speed data entry, in haste, the clinician may not be aware of the additional or missing data, resulting in misrepresenting the case and potentially resulting in submitting a fraudulent claim for reimbursement (Dimick 2008). Because the functionality is so prevalent in EHR products, it is essential that every organization evaluate how it might be used and develop solid application rules to ensure accurate use (Amatayakul and Brandt 2003). Many suggest that the functionality not be permitted. Although this may be desirable, the key to not permitting such functionality is not making it available. If such a function is available, policy alone is generally insufficient to impact action.

An example of a data capture screen that includes both pull-down menus for structured data and the results of macros is displayed in figure 15.4.

Natural Language Processing

Deriving structure from unstructured text refers to natural language processing (NLP). This is one of the biggest remaining challenges currently faced by computer scientists today. NLP is a technical process in which highly sophisticated computer programs "read" strings

Figure 15.4.   Example of structured data-entry template with macros

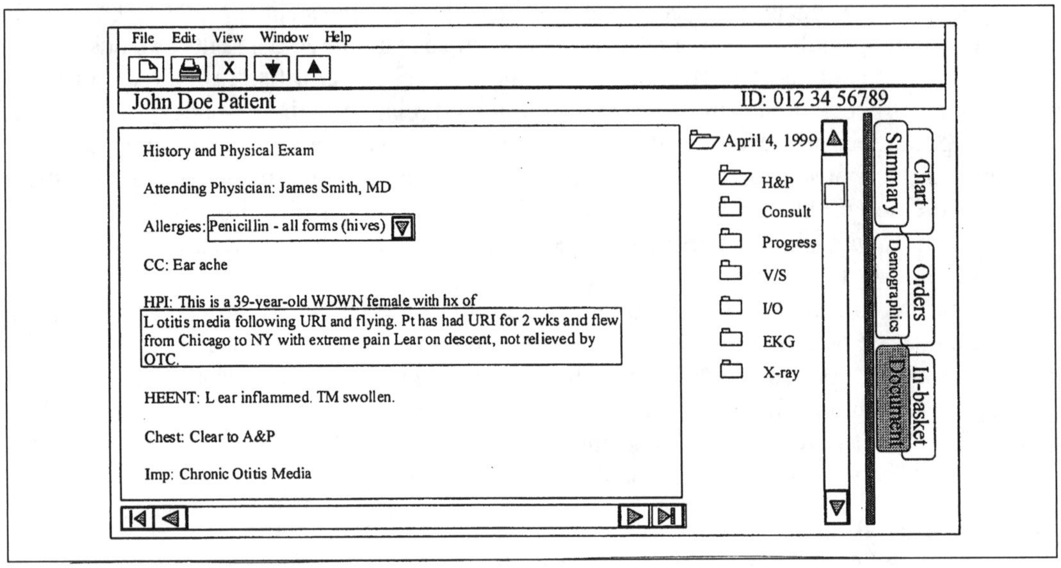

of free text and separate the words or phrases into little packets (called *parsing*). The programs then assign computer codes to the individual packets, thereby codifying the text for storage, analysis, and later retrieval. NLP is not required for adoption of an EHR, but it is an important component of EHR research for future improvements.

EHR Components for Hospitals

Today's state of the art has made it difficult for hospitals to find the best solution for their needs. However, many hospitals have structured a migration path that is starting to work. In some respects, even having a migration path where it is clear that the hospital has direction and a well-conceived plan for what EHR components will be implemented, and when, may be a factor that aids in clinician acceptance and adoption of pieces or parts of an EHR.

The value curve illustrated earlier in figure 15.1 suggests that the foundation for achieving value from an EHR is the ability to have data displayed, retrieved, and documented. Most EHR component applications, however, focus on a specific clinical function, rather than overall value function. In other words, a point-of-care (POC) charting system or online documentation for nursing provides basic data display, data retrieval, and documentation and workflow functionality and may add decision support functionality as well (but only for certain nursing functions). Alternatively, a similar application may be designed to support data display, retrieval, documentation, and decision support for physicians. Although a results review component is currently available for physician use, few documentation systems have been designed for use by physicians in the acute care area of a hospital other than those associated with the ordering function. Hence, EHR components for hospitals are still quite departmentally focused.

Figure 15.5. Example of results review screen

| Last | Next |

| MRI: 123-456 | Name: Patient Name | | DOB: 01/01/1940 | Sex: M |

Laboratory Results: 03/12 10:25:30

| 03/12/03 | 3 days ▼ | All labs ▼ | Display | Clear |

Collected: 12/14	Iron/Iron Binding Capacity			Updated: 03/11	
Iron (Iron)		23	L	33–150	UG/DL
Iron Binding Capacity (IBC)		139	L	210–400	UG/DL
Collected: 06/02	Urea Nitrogen			Updated: 03/10	
Plasma Post Dialysis					
Urea Nitrogen (UN)		18		8–20	MG/DL

Results Management

Access to data (results review) is the most fundamental function clinicians want as they approach information system adoption. Interest in better access to data crosses all departments and users, and provides the most immediate value to the clinician. Even if the data are simply diagnostic study results, transcription, and/or scanned documents that have been stored and then viewed online or even printed out for use by the clinician each time access to data is needed, there still will be a significant benefit. More than anything else, the data will be available when needed. In the hospital, this function is typically called results review. Many hospitals are attempting to make this the primary source of diagnostics studies results and are encouraging clinicians to retrieve the results directly online.

The results review function is relatively easy to implement because many diagnostic study results are already in machine-readable form. In fact, most HISs already include this functionality. Moreover, many hospitals are making this functionality available to physician offices through a Web portal, although many offices also still request faxes. Figure 15.5 provides an example of a results review screen.

It is important to be aware that results review is often fairly "flat." This means that the results may be provided only as a print file, essentially as if they were on a piece of paper. Although this makes them look familiar, the results management function, or the ability to put laboratory results and other data into a repository as discrete data and perform graphing and other manipulations to review results in different modes and combine results with other data is not feasible from a system that only displays results. The ability to combine medication and laboratory results data, for instance, is increasingly recognized as a patient safety technique. Many medications commonly used have recommendations for routine laboratory monitoring intended to reduce the risk of developing an organ toxicity or electrolyte imbalance. Studies have found, however, that such monitoring is not always performed, and this may be because not only can laboratory results not be integrated with medication data, but the reminder capability to perform such monitoring is not available through a CPOE system (Matheny et al. 2008).

At a minimum then, results review addresses the value of data display, or accessibility. Results management systems also allow manipulation of the data.

Point-of-Care (POC) Documentation

POC documentation is the step where clinicians use the EHR to document, or chart, their findings and actions. As previously noted, currently these components have primarily been designed for nursing documentation. In many cases, the nursing documentation is further categorized into separate modules, where some hospitals may start with certain assessment templates, then add additional assessment templates, and finally add alerts and prompts associated with standard assessments. There are many different types of assessments, some of which are identified in table 15.1. Each assessment includes a critical action point. Automating the alerts means the nurse does not have to remember each separate standard and its critical value. Instead, the nurse can focus on doing the assessment using clinical knowledge, with the computer tracking and monitoring for criticality. When standards change, which they often do, online systems can be updated. The assessments can be used further to generate orders for physician review and approval (Ligon and de los Reyes 2005).

Other nursing documentation that has been automated includes nursing interdisciplinary consultations, vital signs, intake and output, plan of care, problem list, POC testing and specimen labeling, shift reports, and patient education. Hospitals also have found success with providing access to clinical reference tools and incorporating nurse staffing and patient acuity to automate nurse staffing functions (King et al. 2004).

Hospitals are further investigating the ability to manage an enterprise patient safety program through automated warnings when a patient's vital signs indicate an oncoming crisis or physical deterioration. This allows across-the-hospital surveillance of spikes in temperature, hemodynamic instability, potential adverse drug reactions, or dangerous blood glucose levels (Rogoski 2005).

Outside of the physician's own office, physician documentation of items other than orders (and what is typically dictated) has been more of a challenge—not only in gaining cooperation to use but in designing suitable tools. Steps are being taken, however, to both design physician documentation tools and to analyze their impact on quality of documentation. A key issue with templates and other constructs currently is that they focus on one patient problem, where frequently the patient has multiple problems (Schnipper et al. 2008). In

Table 15.1. Examples of automated nursing assessment results and other prompts

Assessment	Action
Admission assessment	Orders for physician review and approval
Home medication order sheet	Orders for continued medications for physician review and approval
Functional status screens	Orders for physical therapy, speech therapy, or occupational therapy for physician review and approval
Body mass index calculations for obese surgical patients	Special treatment and preparation protocols
Alcohol-use screen	Alcohol withdrawal protocol
Smoking assessment	• "Stop-smoking" patient education • Nicotine withdrawal protocol
High risk for falls	Special alerts
History of congestive heart failure	Patient education
Multidisciplinary needs assessment	Automatic notification to chaplain, case management, nutrition services, enterostomy therapy, infection control
Immunization screening	Orders for pneumococcal and influenza vaccinations for physician review and approval
Lab test orders requiring fasting	"Hold tray" order
Radiology procedures requiring special patient preparation	Specific preparation information and timing information and/or alert

Source: Ligon and de los Reyes 2005.

addition, documentation tools need to be able to be easily kept up to date and current with evidence-based medical practice; they need to support the making brief, concise, and succinct notes; they need to organize and structure data; and they have to afford comprehensible and consistent support (Stetson 2008).

Patient Safety

The issue of patient safety was first raised by the Institute of Medicine (IOM) in its National Roundtable on Health Care Quality, largely as a result of the work of Bates and others who published medication error findings as early as 1997. The IOM has subsequently released a number of reports addressing patient safety, including: *To Err is Human* (2000), *Crossing the Quality Chasm* (2001), and *Patient Safety: Achieving a New Standard for Care* (2003). Subsequently, various other organizations have focused on this issue with various purposes and degrees of effectiveness. What has occurred, however, is significant attention placed on what has come to be described as the need for **closed loop medication management**. Figure 15.6 illustrates the components of current medication management, reflects the

Figure 15.6.   Medication management

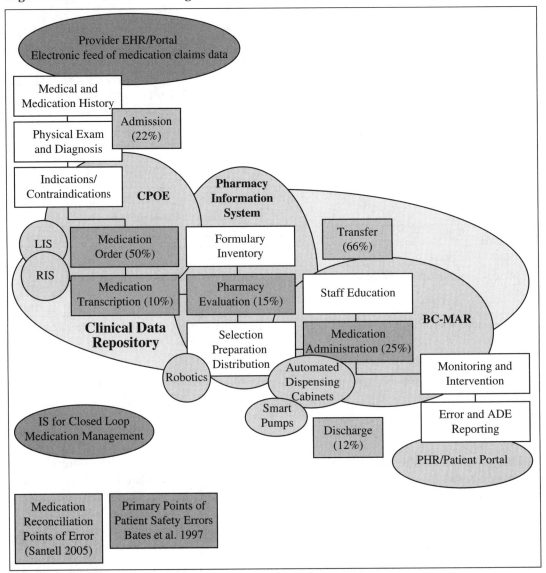

Source: Compiled from data published by Bates et al (1997) and Santell (2005).
Illustration: Copyright © 2007, Margret\A Consulting, LLC. Reprinted with permission

proportion of errors made at each point, and identifies information system applications that may reduce errors and improve patient safety.

To Err is Human asserted that 98,000 people die each year in U.S. hospitals as a result of medical mistakes that are preventable. According to the publication, such mistakes can range from receiving an incorrect procedure, prescription, or medication to being served a meal that violates dietary restrictions set by the patient's physician (Kohn 2000). For example, many drug names are mistaken because of handwriting that is difficult to read or names that sound alike. The drug codeine, which is used to treat moderate pain or to control a serious cough, is sometimes misread as cardene, a drug used to treat high blood pressure and chest pain. In citing this example, The Leapfrog Group notes that the problem is not carelessness but, instead, that highly qualified people are working under stress in a setting with many complex processes. The Leapfrog Group is an organization founded by the Business Roundtable with support from the Robert Wood Johnson Foundation. It comprises more than 150 public and private companies that provide healthcare benefits to approximately 34 million healthcare consumers. The Leapfrog Group provides contractual incentives to hospitals to adopt CPOE, evidence-based hospital referral, and intensive care unit (ICU) physician staffing (Leapfrog Group 2004).

Another common medication error is in recording dosage amounts (such as recording. 1 g instead of .01 g). The Joint Commission now requires a leading zero as a measure to help overcome this type of error. Components of the ordering process are sometimes omitted, resulting in medication errors. For example, drug name, dose, and frequency may be included, but not route, which may not always be apparent from the dose amount. CPOE systems that include required fields help overcome this type of error, although also potentially make writing an order a more time-consuming process.

Another type of medication error that occurs is at transitions of care. Recognizing this, the Joint Commission mandated that starting in January 2006, all healthcare organizations that prescribe medications "accurately and completely reconcile medications across the continuum of care" and specifically that at every transition of care accurate lists of medications pretransition and posttransition be compiled and compared to one another." This process has been called **medication reconciliation**. CCHIT has made basic medication reconciliation a criterion for its 2007 inpatient product certification, with more extensive criteria required for products certified in 2008.

Electronic/Bar Code Medication Administration Record Systems

A significant element of online documentation for nursing has been electronic medication administration records (EMAR). Some EMAR systems are essentially preprinted forms generated by the pharmacy system on which medication administration information is recorded in legible form and used by nurses to guide their actual administration. Documentation of the administration is still conducted on that paper form but is improved by making the medication legible. Another form of EMAR is sometimes referred to as bedside medication verification (BMV). In these applications, a computerized dispensing system is used at the bedside, where the drug may be visually compared with a picture on the computer, other drug knowledge information is available to the nurse, and where the device enables unit dose dispensing.

Positive patient identification via use of bar codes or radio frequency identification (RFID) has been added to many EMAR systems (then called bar code medication administration record [BC-MAR] systems). In this case, the entire medication administration record process is automated from the point of retrieving information on what medications are to be administered to documenting the actual administration or exception, as outlined in figure 15.7.

Figure 15.7.   BC-MAR process

1. On patient admission, the hospital gives the patient a bar-coded identification bracelet to link the patient to his or her EHR.

2. When ready to administer the medication, the nurse scans the patient's bar code, which causes the computer to retrieve the patient's EHR.

3. When the patient's EHR displays the medication to be administered, it is retrieved (as a unit dose prepackaged with its own bar code) and scanned.

4. The computer compares the drug that is scanned with the drug that is on the medication administration record. If it is a match, the nurse administers the medication or documents an exception. An exception may include patient refusal or patient not being present. (See step 5.) If it is not a match, the computer displays an error message (for example, wrong patient, wrong dose, wrong drug, or wrong time to administer drug). The nurse can then make the necessary adjustments.

5. Some systems also generate a computerized reminder about what medications patients are scheduled to take and when. This may be generated immediately after all medications are scheduled to be administered and alert nursing personnel that someone may have been missed. This may occur, for example, when the patient is not on the nursing unit at the time medications are normally passed because the patient is having a diagnostic study performed elsewhere in the hospital or is undergoing physical therapy. Some systems automatically advise the nurse when it is appropriate to administer the drug and in what dose so that drugs are not doubled up or skipped altogether.

Electronic/Bar Code Medication Administration Record Challenges

Hospitals should be aware that there are many challenges to acquiring such systems:

- If the hospital does not yet have a computerized provider order entry (CPOE) system, the transcription into the pharmacy information systems and resultant EMAR/BC-MAR system still must take place manually, which has been found to a source of error in itself.

- The BC-MAR system also depends on the ability to have bar-coded unit doses available. The Food and Drug Administration (FDA) has required that all human drug products and biological products have bar codes on the package that identifies the drug or biological. However, this relates only to the package, which may be the bottle of pills in the pharmacy. If the hospital does not purchase drugs in unit dose form, or does not have a unit dose packaging system and qualified staff to perform this function, the ability to use BC-MAR is not feasible. For small and rural hospitals, this can be a significant challenge. Purchasing drugs in unit dose form is generally more expensive. Not all small hospitals stock all the drugs being ordered, as their utilization may not be frequent enough and their shelf life too short to warrant retaining in inventory. Many small and rural hospitals have to supplement their drug inventories with drugs from local retail pharmacies. It is possible to purchase a unit dose drug packaging system, but this is yet another application that adds cost and time to the process. Finally, not all drugs are easily bar coded. Drugs administered through IV bags, especially in the intensive care unit when multiple bags are piggybacked onto a single IV, can be challenging to apply a unit dose bar code to.

- Another challenge, and the reason to engage a pharmacist early in the process, is that the naming conventions of the drugs used in the EMAR/BC-MAR may not be the same as the drug names in the pharmacy system. Pharmacy systems generally record drug names using the National Drug Code (NDC), which is a naming convention used in naming packages of drugs. The name of the manufacturer, brand name, serial number, and other such information all are elements embedded in this code. However, when providers enter medications into CPOE systems and when nurses record these medications on a MAR, they may use terminology that is more clinically relevant. In some cases this may be a proprietary naming convention; in other cases it may the RxNorm that has been recommended by the federal government for use in EHRs. A closed-loop medication management system with CPOE, up-to-date pharmacy system, and BC-MAR would enable mapping to occur automatically so that there is equivalency between the two naming conventions. If the systems are stand-alone or only generated from a pharmacy system without the mapping on the naming conventions, the result can be confusing.

Medication Errors

Another potential pitfall in gaining adoption of EMAR/BC-MAR systems is that they may appear to increase errors. It is important to define terms associated with errors carefully and recognize that although there may be more errors reported by the systems than currently accounted for, there are likely not more actual errors, but better reporting.

Errors should be classified by their type, including those that are not errors; adverse reactions that may have been anticipated; and near-misses. Different hospitals use different definitions for these concepts, often driven by required reporting systems. The following definitions are supplied by the Agency for Healthcare Research and Quality (AHRQ):

- *Adverse drug event*: In some reporting systems, this is a widely encompassing term referring to actual errors, near-misses, and adverse drug reactions. In other reporting systems, adverse drug event refers solely to harm caused by an actual error in medication management. The source of the error may be from one or more sources, not only medication administration. In implementing an EMAR/BC-MAR system, one of the most frequent increases in error is due to timing. Many of these systems identify a timing error as one with a narrow window. It is important to reach agreement on what an acceptable window of time is; if the window is smaller than previously due to other reporting requirements, workflow and processes should be studied to determine the impact of this change in definition. Because timing can be impacted by many factors, including that the patient was not available at the time the medication was to be administered, at least one group of researchers has proposed a "missing dose day" as the quality summary measure of medication omission (FitzHenry et al. 2005).

- *Near-miss*: An event or situation that did not produce patient injury but only because of chance. This good fortune might reflect robustness of the patient (for example, a patient with penicillin allergy receives penicillin, but has no reaction) or a fortuitous, timely intervention (for example, a nurse happens to realize that a physician wrote an order in the wrong chart). EMAR/BC-MAR systems may be able to identify some of these near-misses when an alert or reminder is invoked in the clinical decision support component of the application.

- *Adverse drug reaction*: An adverse effect produced by the use of a medication in the recommended manner. In many cases, these may be anticipated. These effects range from nuisance effects (for example, dry mouth with anticholinergic medications) to severe reactions (for example, anaphylaxis due to penicillin when the patient had never previously taken penicillin and therefore it was unknown that the patient was allergic).

Workarounds

In addition to policies that define errors, another potential pitfall to be considered is that relating to adherence to procedures. As the EMAR/BC-MAR systems become more sophisticated and especially where they more significantly change workflow, it is important to (1) engage nursing staff in all aspects of workflow and process changes prior to and during implementation, and (2) ensure that these changes are monitored either for adherence or for potential need to make adjustments. Unfortunately, many systems are installed with a specific workflow change that staff have not been engaged in understanding or having any input into. As a result, staff find workarounds to solve either real or perceived problems in workflow. The result can be significantly less patient safety improvement than anticipated and even increases in productivity issues. For example, some pharmacy dispensing systems may require the nurse to unload the medications and stock them into the COW or kiosk for administration, altering nursing workflow, increasing time, and potentially assuming a role typically played by pharmacy technicians. The ideal scenario would be that the pharmacy delivers trays for each COW or kiosk.

Phillips and Berner (2004) identified a number of ways nurses have found to "beat the system" when they find issues. Koppel et al. (2008) also found a number of the same workarounds as they documented 15 different ways nurses failed to use the BC-MAR systems as intended, with as many as 31 types of causes. Workarounds included everything from affixing copies of patient identification bar codes to the nursing unit so they could "wand" the patient there instead of at the bedside to scanning a single medication package multiple times (such as at the grocery checkout counter where the purchase is for five of the same item). Reasons for such workarounds were cited as unreadable medication bar codes, malfunctioning scanners, failing batteries on the COW, and so on.

It is important to plan thoroughly for EMAR/BC-MAR implementations. The American Hospital Association, Health Research and Educational Trust, and the Institute for Safe Medication Practices (2002) have compiled an excellent tool titled Assessing Bedside Barcoding Readiness for this purpose.

The following are items that must be considered in implementing EMAR/BC-MAR systems:

- Learning curving

- Nurse resistance to change

- Lack of portability of equipment

- Technology problems relating to hardware, software, or wireless network capability

- Definition of what results in a reportable medication error

Figure 15.8. CPOE

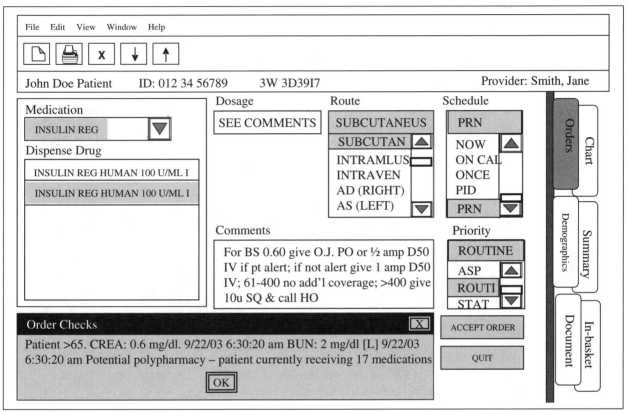

Computerized Provider Order Entry

CPOE is not to be confused with **order communication,** which is a nursing service function of transcribing orders handwritten by a physician (or other provider authorized to write orders in the hospital) into a computer system for distribution to respective ancillary department systems.

CPOE is the process whereby providers directly enter orders, making them more accurate and legible, and receiving back any alerts or reminders that they would act on in real time and that would help reduce errors, particularly medication errors. Figure 15.8 illustrates an order-entry screen that includes an order check, which is basically a reminder or an alert. A reminder or alert notification can be generated by a given order entered for a medication that might be contraindicated because of an allergy or another medication or might be inappropriate for a procedure for which the patient is being prepared. The alert also may be a notification that another medication order is about to expire. The alert might be a more global one, such as in figure 15.7, which reminds the provider about the patient's current laboratory result status and number of medications already being taken. In provider offices that have a CPOE system, reminders can be even more global for health maintenance checks, such as when it is time for an annual Pap smear or to inquire about progress being made on a smoking cessation program.

Alerts and reminders should be used judiciously. In some cases, organizations have created so many alerts and reminders that they practically appear with every order and there may be multiple alerts with just one order. Many providers find this annoying and time-consuming. The phenomenon has even been given a name: alert fatigue.

Great care also should be taken to create alerts and reminders in a manner that follows the organization's business rules. For example, it might be necessary to respond to some reminders, but permissible to dismiss others. Organizations might choose to establish audits on alerts that are dismissed or require documentation of the rationale for overriding an alert. Different organizations are approaching this documentation differently, some suggesting that alerting is still an immature science and is no different than a provider reviewing a reference that typically is not documented. Alternatively, other hospitals believe that the dialogue helps all members of the care team understand what is happening and reduces calls and questions (Rollins 2005). Many hospitals are finding limited opportunities for safely turning off frequently overridden drug–drug interaction alerts (van der Sijs et al. 2008).

Like EMAR/BC-MAR, CPOE does not require an EHR, but the level of clinical decision support that makes CPOE most effective generally is found when many of the components of an EHR exist. However, that is also the primary issue with CPOE. Many CPOE systems have limited clinical decision support. As such, many providers view performing order entry as a clerical function. In addition, some CPOE systems have been implemented with little attention to existing processes that provide adequate control points. A growing body of literature is questioning the role of CPOE in actually facilitating medication errors (Koppel et al. 2005; Han et al. 2005; Koppel et al. 2008).

Challenges to CPOE Systems

As suggested earlier, hospitals have had variable success with CPOE systems. Order entry is particularly challenging for physicians to adopt because of substantial workflow changes. Order-entry functionality may vary in inpatient and ambulatory settings, but, in general, the challenges and benefits are similar. If well designed and incorporating order sets as well as prompts, reminders, and alerts, the order-entry function can generate quality and cost improvements for the healthcare organization.

The challenge is that physicians sometimes find themselves required to enter more information at the time the order is being created than is typical for paper ordering. For example, the source of a microbiology specimen or the number of refills that may be given is an element that other professionals, such as the nurse or pharmacist, may have incorporated in their functions when communicating or receiving the order. Physicians also may have communicated some of this information at another time, such as via a follow-up phone call from a nurse or in response to a page from the pharmacist. Physicians often are unaware of the cumulative effect of such communications. Furthermore, they may be unaware that the need for subsequent checking is resulting in treatment delays.

Organizational policies on the discontinuance of certain types of orders, countersignature requirements, or adherence to a managed care formulary that may have been enforced only informally now are enforced directly through the order-entry system, contributing to the time factor for physicians.

Some physicians reluctant to adopt order entry have attempted to transfer it to house staff or nursing personnel. Although CPOE is not the only answer to medication errors (and some hospitals are finding that more errors are actually stemming from other parts of the medication preparation and administration processes), it can contribute to reducing their risk, for example, with real-time alerts to drug–drug or drug–food contraindications, inappropriate dosage or route, and reduced selection of erroneous drugs with similar names. It also can improve cost-effectiveness, for example, by offering recommendations for less costly but equally efficacious drugs and ensuring that the sequencing of medication administration and lab tests does not contribute to erroneous test results or delays. Finally, CPOE may save the physician time in the long run, for example, by not having to return phone calls about illegible refill orders or incomplete documentation.

For CPOE to be successful, physicians must be involved in the process of designing the CPOE system to ensure that it meets their needs and to understand its benefits. Organizational policies and business rules must be established to address physician requirements and whether transfer of responsibility to another provider may be permitted. There is tremendous liability in allowing a physician to give someone else his or her password so that that individual can enter orders in the physician's stead; this must be strictly prohibited.

CPOE Case Study
The flow of work varies considerably among care settings. In the inpatient setting, physicians write orders for various services or tests and procedures, which are completed by other clinical staff or ancillary personnel. In fact, it is difficult to obtain a service or conduct a test or procedure without appropriate documentation in the health record. Although the physician may visit a patient only once or twice a day, the healthcare team caring for the patient attempts to tightly coordinate all resources and services for patient care. Although this is beneficial, certain information needs may not be addressed appropriately in this scenario. For example, the needs of case managers or utilization managers may not be addressed during routine documentation, which can lead to inefficiencies in workflow.

In contrast to the location-centered focus of the inpatient record, workflow in the ambulatory environment is patient centric, but the record is not. All members of the healthcare team attempt to expedite an outpatient visit and all associated workflow so that the patient and the healthcare team can finish their work within the constraints of the visit time. To do so, the record is often "taken apart," or compiled in separate pieces, sometimes never to come together. For example, it is common for a multispecialty clinic to have multiple chart rooms and multiple charts for each patient, depending on the specialty areas in which they are being treated. Obviously, a centralized EHR would contribute greatly to coordinated care in such a situation. This may be why EHR systems have matured and grown more in the ambulatory environment despite the greater change required in workflow.

See appendix D.2 for a case study of a CPOE implementation project.

Clinical Decision Support

Clinical decision support (CDS) is incorporated into many of the EHR components but also may be acquired as a separate module to provide a body of CDS rules that are accessible to any and all other components. In addition to the CDS that may come with such software or that the hospital acquires from other commercial sources, the system may include different types of analytical tools that can help create new CDS based on the experience of the organization (and hence incorporating predictive modeling, the highest level on the EHR value curve).

The computer science industry sometimes uses the general term *artificial intelligence* (AI) to describe the process to create new rules based on existing evidence. Many clinicians are offended by this term and believe the emphasis needs to be on using clinical expertise and scientific evidence to support clinical decision making with the aid of an EHR. Hence, *clinical decision support system, expert system*, or *evidence-based medicine (EBM) systems* are more popular terms.

As previously described, CDS systems supply alerts and reminders, perform outcomes analyses, and support other knowledge management activities. From basic to complex, the technology that supports these functions of CDS systems may be categorized as rules engines, general statistical analyses, search engines, and expert systems that incorporate a variety of analytical tools to uncover new meaning.

Rules Engines

Rules engines provide a variety of reminders and alerts, clinical practice guideline advice, and benchmarking. Rules engines operate on discrete data that are generally processed as unique transactions or as aggregate data analysis.

Online Transaction Processing

When data for a single transaction are processed, the processing may be described as online transaction processing (OLTP). OLTP basically involves transactions for a single set of data, such as entering vital signs for a patient, retrieving laboratory results for a patient, being alerted to a drug–drug interaction, being advised that there is further information elsewhere, and so on. OLTP generally occurs in a clinical data repository (CDR).

Online Analytical Processing

Some EHR systems stop there, but fully comprehensive EHR systems may "learn clinician user preferences" and even generate new rules based on evidence of care patterns from many patients. The processing required on data to provide such new knowledge is often referred to as online analytical processing (OLAP), often requires a database optimized for such a purpose called a clinical data warehouse (CDW), and may be distinguished separately from a rules engine by the term *expert system* (discussed later in this chapter). Some CDWs are directly connected to the EHR and its CDR so that the clinician-specific user preferences can be continuously updated; in other cases, the warehouses are separate and require specific downloads of data, such as for outcomes analysis and processing of new CDS rules that clinicians may then review and approve before they are incorporated into the CDS system and everyday use in OLTP.

Reminders and Alerts

Reminders and alerts are provided by rules engines that perform a complex set of if–then comparisons against data to provide information specific to the data being entered. Reminders may prompt clinicians for specific information, notify them of certain conditions, or simply provide a link to additional information based on certain criteria. They frequently are displayed on the workstation in data-entry screens or in printouts of results. Alerts are distinguished from reminders only in that alerts are deemed more critical by the system developers and often are provided to the clinician in more obvious ways (for example, in a different color, by flashing on the screen, or as a pop-up box). An alert may even activate a clinician's beeper to signal that something urgent has occurred. However, alerts also can be more passive than active. An example of a passive alert may be an icon that signifies additional information about a medication condition that the provider may want to review.

Clinical Guideline Advice

Clinical guideline advice is essentially a logical pathway or set of recommendations about options clinicians can follow depending on the particular clinical situation. As previously noted, these may have been used in paper form in the past but are most effective when used at the POC in an EHR system. As each element of data is entered, a series of branching occurs to direct the clinician to capture other data, consider other information, or offer specific alternatives for consideration. The ability to modify the guideline according to the context in which data are entered is referred to as context-sensitivity.

Benchmarking

Benchmarking is a function of a database that compares specific, internal data to comparable general data, often from an external research database. It serves different purposes, some or all of which may be incorporated into a clinical decision support system. Clinical benchmarking is used to urge clinicians on to higher levels of performance, to change and standardize practice patterns, and to reduce overutilization of high-cost care, ancillaries, and tests. Other types of benchmarks include community health benchmarks, operations performance benchmarks, cost and efficiency benchmarks, and contracting benchmarks.

Benchmarks are often purchased from consultants and publishers such as Milliman & Robertson. Professional associations such as the American Medical Association, American College of Physicians, and others are sources of benchmarks.

Statistical Analysis

Statistical analysis tools include those tools available in the over-the-counter market, such as word-processing, spreadsheet, and database systems. They also include statistical analysis tools such as SPSS (Statistical Process for the Social Sciences), BMDP (Biomedical Data Package), and others.

Search Engines

Tools to search databases include structured query languages (SQLs). These tools provide the ability to obtain selected data from a database based on specific user-defined parameters. Examples of SQLs used in EHR products include Oracle, Sybase, Microsoft SQL Server, and Informix. Report writers are important tools for formatting and presenting information derived from databases.

Figure 15.9.   Model of an expert system

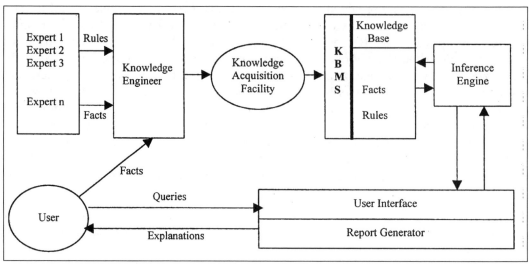

Expert Systems

Expert systems are programs that use a set of rules to construct a reasoning process. In fields outside healthcare, an expert system is referred to as artificial intelligence (Bidgoli 1997, 387). An expert system "learns" based on the continual addition of data. Its use is based on encoded concepts derived from experts in the field. As a result, expert systems provide the kind of problem analysis and advice that an expert might provide if he or she were present as a consultant (Abdelhak et al. 2001). Figure 15.9 shows a model of an expert system.

Expert systems use various types of rules-based processing schemes to provide knowledge (Siwicki 1996), including:

- *Symbolic reasoning* is a method of deduction that follows an explicit line of inferences.

- *Fuzzy logic* is a rules-based system that mimics human thought, enabling a computer to "think" in inexact terms rather than in a definitive, either–or manner.

- *Artificial neural network* (ANN) is a highly mathematical methodology that learns from many examples to properly categorize or characterize new examples.

- *Data mining* is a technique that uncovers new information from existing information by probing mammoth data sets.

- *Genetic algorithm* examines data and determines by programmed stipulations which data best match a stated goal and which data do not.

Implementing CDS

Just as with any other component of the EHR, it is important to ensure proper implementation of CDS systems. The Healthcare Information Management and Systems Society (HIMSS) has developed an Implementers' Guide (Osheroff, et al. 2005) that urges hospitals to follow a formal process for improving outcomes with clinical decision support. All stakeholders need to be involved. Goals of the program and specific clinical objectives need to be clear. The ability of supporting information systems need to be assessed to determine that they can supply the necessary data for CDS. Various approaches to CDS interventions need to be identified, assessed, developed, and tested before being put into practice. The CDS program needs to be monitored on an ongoing basis to ensure it achieves its goals to improve clinical outcomes.

Other Health Information Technology in Hospitals

Although many other applications of health information technology (HIT) are used in hospitals, and have been used for many years, some HIT applications are just now being more widely implemented or implemented as a result of EHR system capability. Following is a selection of examples.

Picture Archiving and Communication Systems (PACS)

PACS have been implemented originally as a means to better store radiology images. They have reduced reliance on radiology film and enhanced viewing capability. Initial challenges in implementing PACS were viewing devices, lighting, and workstation ergonomics in the radiology department, then integration with the radiology information system, and finally network bandwidth as the images were made accessible at the POC (*ADVANCE* 2005b). However, as EHRs become more prevalent, PACS have been playing a more critical role in clinical decision support. Being able to couple alerts and reminders with viewing of images has made a powerful difference in quality of care. The result also has had a profound impact on storage requirements for hospitals. As a result of their size, digital image archiving and storage area networks (SANs) have become key elements for hospitals (Collins 2005; Balassone and Bowers 2005). PACS have also been a boon for providing clinical expertise to remote locations. Teleradiology, which takes advantage of PACS technology, currently is one of the most cost- and clinically effective uses of technology in healthcare.

Patient-Flow Management System

The ability to determine where a patient is at all times in a facility and to link staff requirements to patient location can be a challenge. For example, knowing when the patient has been prepared for surgery can improve the time management of an anesthesiologist. Linking patient location to the EMAR can assist nursing in documentation of medications not administered. Although these systems originated in the emergency department (ED), they, and Joint Commission requirements for improved patient flow throughout the hospital, have made them key enterprisewide systems (Jensen 2004).

Emergency Department Diagnostic Aids

Another HIT application that grew out of ED needs is diagnostic decision support. Although not yet widely used in the inpatient environment, systems that help support differential diagnosis are becoming incorporated into ED systems (Britto 2005).

Supply Chain Management Systems

Supply chain refers to the ability to requisition, inventory, and track usage of supplies. New supply chain management systems linked to EHRs can help capture data for invoice matching, usage tracking, contract compliance, and rebate attainment. Such systems have helped reduce day-of-surgery delays and cancellations and enhanced safety outcomes (Pendergrass 2005). They also support device registries used to identify patients in the event of a device recall.

Patient Education

Patient education is now a fairly standard product in many EHR systems. However, unique patient education offerings are still under development. The case study in appendix D.3 presents a unique patient education example.

Conclusion

It is clear that the acute care hospital environment is in a state of change with respect to its information systems. It is an exciting opportunity as well as a challenge to make the most of legacy systems and incorporate new applications and technology. This chapter has focused on applications for hospitals, but it is clear that the presentation layer that forms the human–computer interface must utilize technology synchronized to the applications. It also is essential to ensure proper planning and attention to process improvement. As systems approach the top of the EHR value curve, they become much more sophisticated and closer to being clinical tools in addition to information tools. Effective use of such systems requires care and diligence in their design and maintenance.

References and Resources

Abdelhak, M., et al. 2001. *Health Information: Management of a Strategic Resource,* 2nd ed. Philadelphia: W.B. Saunders.

American Hospital Association, Health Research and Educational Trust, and the Institute for Safe Medication Practices. 2002. Assessing bedside bar-coding readiness. www.medpathways.info/medpathways/tools/content/3_2.pdf.

Amatayakul, M., and M. Brandt. 2003. Cut, copy, paste: EHR guidelines. *Journal of AHIMA* 74(9):72,74.

Balassone, M.T., and G.H. Bowers. 2005. Storing diagnostic images. *ADVANCE for Health Information Executives* 9(5):57–60.

Bidgoli, H. 1997. *Modern Information Systems for Managers.* San Diego, CA: Academic Press.

Britto, J. 2005. Technologies that improve the clinical process. *ADVANCE for Health Information Executives* 9(12):21–24,73.

Bufton, M. G. 1999. Electronic health records and implementation of clinical practice guidelines. In *Electronic Health Records: Changing the Vision*, edited by G.F. Murphy, M.A. Hanken, and K.A. Waters. Philadelphia: W.B. Saunders.

Certification Commission on Health Information Technology, Functionality Criteria for 2007 Certification of Inpatient EHRs, www.cchit.org.

Chan, W. 2002. Increasing the success of physician order entry through human factors engineering. *Journal of Healthcare Information Management* 16(1):71–80.

Collins, E.E. 2005. Digital image archiving. *ADVANCE for Health Information Executives* 9(11):27–30,44.

Curtis, E.H. 2004. *Studies in EHR Implementation: Computerized Physician Order Entry.* Chicago: American Health Information Management Association.

Dimick, C. 2008. Documentation bad habits, shortcuts in electronic records pose risk, *Journal of AHIMA* 79(6): 40–43.

Dullea, R.G. 2005 (Mar.). Rolling along: Update on mobile cart technology. *ADVANCE for Health Information Executives* 9(3):55–56.

Elson, R.B., J.G. Faughnan, and D.P. Connelly. 1997. An industrial process view of information delivery to support clinical decision making: Implications for system design and process measures. *Journal of the American Medical Informatics Association* 4(4):266–278.

FitzHenry, F., et al. 2005. Measuring the Quality of Medication Administration. *AMIA Annual Symposium Proceedings.*

Food and Drug Administration. 2004 (Feb.). FDA issues bar code regulation. www.fda.gov/oc/initiatives/barcode-sadr/fs-barcode.html.

Franklin, B.D., et al. 2007. The impact of a closed-loop electronic prescribing and administration system on prescribing errors, administration errors, and staff time: a before-and-after study, *Quality and Safety in Health Care*; 16:279–284.

Han, Y.Y., et al. 2005. Unexpected increased mortality after implementation of a commercially sold computerized physician order entry system. *Pediatrics* 116(6):1506–1512.

Hardin, J.M. 2002. Expert systems and decision support. In *Health Information Management: Concepts, Principles, and Practices,* edited by K.M. LaTour and S. Eichenwald-Maki. Chicago: American Health Information Management Association.

Hayes, B.M. 2004. *Studies in EHR Implementation: Patient Education and References, St. Vincent, Indianapolis.* Chicago: American Health Information Management Association.

Institute of Medicine. 2003 (July 31). Letter Report: *Key Capabilities of an Electronic Health Record System.* Washington, DC: National Academies Press. www.nap.edu/books.

Jensen, J. 2004. United hospital increases capacity usage, efficiency with patient-flow management system. *Journal of Healthcare Information Management* 18(3):26–31.

Joint Commission. 2006 (Jan. 25). Sentinel Event Alert Issue 35. Oakbrook Terrace, IL, Joint Commission.

King, L.A., A. Wasdovich, and C. Young. 2004. Transforming nursing practice: Clinical systems and the nursing unit of the future. *Journal of Healthcare Information Management* 18(3):32–36.

Kohn, L.T., et al., ed. 2000. *To Err is Human: Building a Safer Health System.* Washington, DC: National Academies of Medicine, Institute of Medicine.

Koppel, R., et al. 2005. Role of computerized provider order entry systems in facilitating medication errors. *Journal of the American Medical Association* 293:1197–1203.

Ligon, K.J., and A.E. de los Reyes. 2005. Nursing goes high-tech. *ADVANCE for Health Information Executives* 9(4):33–38.

Koppel R. et al. 2008. Workarounds to barcode medication administration systems: their occurrences, causes, and threats to patient safety, *Journal of the American Medical Informatics Association* 15(4).

Leapfrog Group. 2004. Patient safety practices. www.leapfroggroup.org.

Matching monitors and displays to applications. 2005a. *ADVANCE for Health Information Executives* 9(3):50–52.

Matheney, et al. 2008. A randomized trial of electronic clinical reminders to improve medication laboratory monitoring, *Journal of the American Medical Informatics Association* 15(4).

McDonald, C.J., and W.M. Tierney. 1998. Computer-stored medical records: Their future role in medical practice. *Journal of the American Medical Association* 259:3433–3440.

Nelson, N.C., et al. 2005. Detection and prevention of medication errors using real-time bedside nurse charting. *Journal of American Medical Informatics Association* 12(4):390–396.

Osheroff, J.A., et al. 2005. *Improving Outcomes with Clinical Decision Support: An Implementers' Guide.* Chicago. HIMSS.

Pendergrass, A. 2005. Supply chain generates newfound savings. *ADVANCE for Health Information Executives* 9(8):47–49.

Phillips, M.T., and E.S. Berner. 2004. Beating the system: Pitfalls of bar code medication administration. *Journal of Healthcare Information Management* 18(4):16–18.

Planning for PACS. 2005b. *ADVANCE for Health Information Executives* 9(1):52–56.

Quinsey, C.A. 2007. Managing forms in the legal health record. *Journal of AHIMA* 78(7): 58–59.

Rogoski, R.R. 2005. The enterprise take on patient safety. *Health Management Technology* 9(8):12–22.

Rollins G. 2005. The prompt, the alert, and the legal record: Documenting clinical decision support systems. *Journal of AHIMA* 76(2):25–28.

Siwicki, B. 1996 (Apr.). Although only a handful of health care organizations are applying the technology, artificial intelligence holds great promise for revolutionizing information systems. *Health Data Management,* 47–52.

Schnipper J.L., et al. 2008. "Smart forms" in an electronic medical record: documentation-based clinical decision support to improve disease management. *Journal of the American Medical Informatics Association* 15(4).

Stetson, P.D. 2008. Preliminary development of the physician documentation quality instrument, *Journal of the American Medical Informatics Association* 15(4).

Turchin, A., et al. 2008. Evaluation of an inpatient computerized medication reconciliation system. *Journal of the American Medical Informatics Association* 15(4).

Van der Sijs, H., et al. 2008. Turning off frequently overridden drug alerts: limited opportunities for doing it safely. *Journal of the American Medical Informatics Association* 15(4).

Chapter 16
Ambulatory Care EHR Applications

When a physician office, clinic, or other ambulatory care organization sets about acquiring an electronic health record (EHR), there are certainly many vendor offerings and choices of product types, but the EHR is generally a more self-contained system than those for acute care settings. In some respects, this makes the selection and implementation simpler, although the system itself may actually be more comprehensive and clinically robust than that for the acute care environment. This chapter:

- Recognizes differences and similarities between elements of EHRs for acute vs. ambulatory settings

- Describes the EHR for use in the ambulatory setting

- Offers suggestions for a migration path suitable for an ambulatory setting

- Distinguishes electronic prescribing (e-prescribing) from computerized provider order entry (CPOE)

Ambulatory vs. Acute Care EHR Systems

Although every EHR is intended to capture data from multiple sources and to be used at the point of care for clinical decision making and there is the desire for seamless exchange of data across the continuum of care via health information technology (HIT), there are significant differences between acute care and ambulatory care settings in their IT infrastructure, workflows, and processes that necessarily make their EHRs different in several respects and also a challenge with which to achieve interoperability.

Existing IT Infrastructure

One difference between implementing an EHR in an ambulatory setting vs. an acute care setting actually has nothing to do with the EHR itself, but with the existing infrastructure, although as time goes on even this difference is diminishing. Clinics and hospitals generally have some information systems already; however, clinics typically have fewer systems. Even where a hospital has deployed a best-of-fit acquisition strategy, the components comprising the system are highly pervasive. As previously noted, few hospitals are willing to replace all the elements of their existing IT infrastructure. Alternatively, many clinics approaching an EHR have only a practice management system (PMS) or billing system. If the PMS is fairly new, the vendor may have an EHR module that will fit well. If it is fairly old, its useful life is virtually nothing and most clinics, at least after they determine the incremental cost of acquiring a new PMS integrated with the EHR, will acquire the fully comprehensive PMS/EHR system.

Interoperability and Workflows

The result of the infrastructure differences makes it easier for a clinic to achieve interoperability within its own setting. Having observed this, however, it must be recognized that such a scenario still may leave the clinic with interoperability issues between its PMS/EHR and lab and other systems it may have internally, and certainly with external source systems, such as a reference lab, commercial lab, imaging center, and the hospital where its physicians admit patients.

Interfaces with Source Systems

Most EHR vendors, however, are well aware of the need to interface with labs and have created such interfaces with many of the major lab systems. The major commercial labs are also well aware of the need to interface their systems and provide a significant level of support for this. As previously discussed, of course, an interface does not necessarily achieve full interoperability. The interface may only transfer a print image of the lab result into the EHR. Ideally, a lab interface should enable the transmission of an order for a lab test to be transmitted to the lab and for the lab results to be returned in discrete format. The same would be true for the results of diagnostic imaging, although, of course, the diagnostic image itself would come across as a digital image.

Interfaces with Hospital

Creating an interface between the hospital and clinic is more challenging. Not only are the workflows and processes different, but the predominant strategy has been to provide a physician portal where data from the hospital can be viewed or downloaded as an image of a document. Some hospital system vendors have created templates where physician offices can enter data for scheduling an admission or surgery via the portal. However, in such cases, the office's PMS or EHR does not supply demographic data directly through an interface; it must be keyed in separately. Of course, hospitals may also provide remote access to members of their medical staff so they may gain access to the entire patient's EHR and its functionality. Again, however, this requires a separate process apart from the office's EHR. From the hospital back to the office, some hospitals are providing kiosks for physicians to connect to their PMS to enter professional charges, although these have not been very popular. Instead, physicians are using PDAs or smart phones to capture this information and then connect the devices to their office systems or arrange for wireless transmission once they are back in the office.

As a result of the less-than-satisfactory means to achieve interoperability between physician office and hospital, or even between an outpatient system and inpatient system where different vendor products are used, some integrated delivery networks (IDNs) of hospitals and physician practices are considering a rip and replace strategy to acquire an EHR from the same vendor. Still, and especially for practices that are not a part of an IDN, the decision typically is made to acquire a separate product for the office, as there are not a lot of products on the market that afford both true integration and comprehensive functionality. All too often, a hospital information system (HIS) vendor acquires an ambulatory care vendor or establishes an exclusive relationship with an ambulatory care vendor, writes a custom interface between the two products, and calls it integrated. This rarely meets the expectations anymore of physicians who have studied the marketplace and understand the level of sophistication available in other products.

Ambulatory Interoperability Strategies

Given the issues with interoperability between the ambulatory and acute care environments, the inevitable question is: Should we wait? (This question is being asked by both the acute and ambulatory "sides" of the fence.) There is certainly growing momentum for achieving interoperability, although the degree to which the vendors in a free-market environment will actually achieve interoperability is uncertain. Most industry observers suggest that each organization needs to assess its goals for an EHR. If the primary goal is to exchange data across the continuum of care, waiting or giving up some functionality to acquire a product from the same vendor may be appropriate. On the other hand, many others believe functionality is key and there are sufficient workarounds, including interfaces and Web-based portals or clinical messaging, to exchange the information that is truly needed. One physician put it this way: "I spend 80 percent of time seeing patients in the office and rarely need more than 20 percent of data from the hospital, so I don't want a system that only gives me 20 percent of the functionality I want in return for exchanging only 20 percent of data."

What data truly need to be exchanged must be considered in making the selection decision. This may vary by the nature of the physician's specialty. Neither a hospital nor a physician office needs or wants all the information held by the other for a given patient. Most want key data, such as data from a problem list, medication list, allergies, and immunizations, as well as the ability to view recent lab results. Physician offices do not need all of a patient's vital signs to repose in its EHR, and hospitals do not need endless records of visits for flu shots. In addition, it must be recognized that the physician office–hospital connection is not the only point of desirable connectivity. Even in a small town where there is only one hospital and a small number of physicians, virtually all of whom are members of the hospital's medical staff, patients may well obtain tertiary care from another hospital or receive emergency care in other parts of the country. There is also nursing home or home healthcare to be considered. In areas with more healthcare organizations, it is unlikely that only one vendor will be represented, so achieving true interoperability with all vendors in the mix of all sites of care will be a long time in coming.

In summary, then, although there are advantages to the simpler infrastructure of the physician office environment for acquiring an EHR, interoperability is becoming an important issue and must be evaluated in light of all other elements in the selection of an ambulatory care EHR. However, there are means to exchange data that do not depend on use of only one vendor product.

Data Presentation and Use Processes

Where the nature of data and processes surrounding its use vary between acute and ambulatory care environments, equally important in both environments is how data are presented to the user and how data are used in clinical decision making. Chapter 15 provides a thorough discussion of the presentation layer for data retrieval and documentation, as well as a comprehensive description of how computers achieve clinical decision support (CDS).

What reviewers of both acute and ambulatory care EHRs may actually find when they review systems is that the ambulatory care EHR integrates functions much more closely. Where a hospital EHR may be composed of point-of-care (POC) charting, electronic or bar code medication administration record (EMAR/BC-MAR), CPOE, picture archiving and communication systems (PACS), and so on, these may be separate applications that require separate log-ons. If there is **single sign-on** (SSO) that permits one log-on for access to every application the user is authorized to access, there still may be a different look and feel to each application. Some hospitals are using middleware designed to make applications look more similar, but this still does not serve to totally integrate data. In an ambulatory EHR, the various functions are truly integrated and much less likely to have different presentation styles.

EHR Functionality

What functions an EHR supports clearly will be different between the ambulatory and acute care environments. Data collected, processes, and workflows are different by the nature of patients served. A hospital will have a dense and large volume of information about a patient for a relatively short period of time, where clinics will have many small and often unrelated sets of information about a patient spread over potentially a very long period of time. This impacts everything from whether clinics assign an account number to each visit (which they generally do not) to the need for chart conversion (which is generally more likely in a clinic than a hospital).

Data entered into a hospital EHR must be available for all members of the care team to view, and must be date and time stamped to identify the time an entry was made and by whom. Any error that is made must be annotated properly. Because things happen quickly in a hospital, it is conceivable that an erroneous entry could be relied on by another caregiver for subsequent action, even when the error is caught as quickly as the very next time the author of the erroneous entry documents.

Although diligence in authenticating the author of an entry in an ambulatory EHR is required by HIPAA, state licensing laws, and other requirements, the fact of the matter is that in many small practices, it is primarily the physician who enters data into a chart. In some offices, even the medical assistant or nurse who rooms a patient, takes vital signs, and inquires of the reason for the visit does not record information other than perhaps vital signs into the chart. He or she may write all other information on scratch paper for the physician. As a result, some clinic EHRs do not have robust means to switch from one user to another, annotate errors, or even permit more than one user to access the EHR at a time. These are important functions to evaluate when a physician office or clinic is reviewing vendor offerings.

Alternatively, many ambulatory EHRs include all functionality in a tightly integrated manner and can provide multiple data points simultaneously in a single view or set of windows, where this is frequently not the case for a hospital EHR. This significantly impacts the type of human–computer interface devices chosen for the respective environments. Another element of data integration relates to patient identification. Clinics are likely to take a digital picture of the patient and refer to it as well as engage in verbal communication for positive identification. On the other hand, hospitals are beginning to use bar code technology to support positive identification because the patient may not always be able to communicate verbally and his or her face may not be clearly visible at all times.

Finally, the ability for the clinic to quickly achieve a "paperless" state is much more likely than for a hospital, where the hospital frequently must exist in a hybrid state for potentially several years. For a clinic, this means that a chart conversion strategy is essential. Some clinics scan all previous records or at least records of its active patients. Other clinics abstract key data from active patients' records to have available in clinical decision support. Still other clinics use a combination of chart conversion strategies and some even decide not to undertake conversion of old charts, but to pull old charts for a period of time. Physicians themselves may abstract pertinent information from the old charts during or immediately before/after a visit to eliminate their subsequent pulling. There are advantages and disadvantages to each strategy.

Most hospitals, however, face a situation where not all data are available electronically because certain applications have not yet been implemented, acquired, or may not even be available in the suite of products offered by the vendor. As a result, some data must be recorded on paper and other data may be entered electronically (or are generated electronically from a source system). Various strategies to address the legal health record and overcome the hybrid condition are described in chapter 14.

Ambulatory EHR Functions

There are several ways ambulatory functions might be categorized with respect to information sources and uses. Figure 16.1 displays key clinical processes in a sequence as they might logically occur in a visit or separate from a visit.

Figure 16.1. Key clinical processes

Visit-Specific Functions
1. Appointment scheduling, diagnostic studies scheduling, insurance verification, chart preparation
2. Patient check-in
3. Patient intake and documentation of vital signs, reason for visit, history, and so on.
4. Review results (including images), other encounter data, other provider and patient-supplied data
5. Clinical documentation of history and physical exam, encounter notes
6. Develop care plan for patient consistent with clinical guidelines
7. Medication management, including new prescriptions (to retail, community, and mail-order pharmacies), changes and cancellations, managing samples, approving refills/renewals, fill status notification
8. Order entry, including tests, surgery, procedures, referrals, admissions
9. E/M and other coding support
10. Charge capture
11. Supply patient instructions, summary of visit, personal health record
12. Checkout
Non-Visit-Specific Functions
a. Medical messaging, including triage, results, refills, release of information, referrals
b. Chronic disease management
c. Support for health maintenance, including immunizations
d. Retrieve data for drug/device recall, HEDIS and other reporting, quality measures
e. Quality assurance, including clinical, financial, and administrative
f. Quality improvement

Copyright © 2008, Margret\A Consulting, LLC. Reprinted with permission.

Another way to categorize EHR functions might be by the functions performed on the data. Figure 16.2 illustrates this approach.

Either or both of the categories of EHR functionality should be considered in acquiring an ambulatory EHR. These have been derived from the works of the Institute of Medicine (IOM) EHR System Capabilities by Time Frame and Site of Care (IOM 2003), Health Level Seven (HL7) EHR-System Functional Descriptors (2007), and the Certification Commission on Health Information Technology (CCHIT) Certification Criteria for Ambulatory EHR Products (2007). Such works also should be reviewed in making EHR vendor selections.

Of course, the EHR does not provide each of these functions separately, but as integrated functionality throughout a sequence of screens and displays designed to address the workflow and processes of the respective users. As such, there frequently will be a scheduling or in-basket function from which any given patient's record can be retrieved; a patient

Figure 16.2. EHR functions for ambulatory care environments

1. **Patient data capture functions**
   a. Capture and record patient medical history
   b. Capture and record patient medication history
   c. Receive diagnostic studies results
   d. Record clinical documentation
   e. Record temporary notes to self or others
   f. Capture key health data for minimum data sets
   g. Capture external clinical documents
   h. Capture images from PACS and other medical devices
   i. Capture patient-originated data
   j. Capture and display advance directives

2. **Patient data management functions**
   a. Manage problem list
   b. Manage medication list
   c. Manage allergy and adverse reaction list
   d. Manage patient-specific care plans, guidelines, and protocols
   e. Capture variances from standard care plans, guidelines, and protocols
   f. Trend data from multiple sources (e.g., labs, meds impact on labs)

3. **Prescription/ordering functions**
   a. Manage medication formularies
   b. Write prescriptions
   c. Approval refills/renewals
   d. Receive refill notifications
   e. Drug, food, allergy, lab interaction checking
   f. Drug-condition/indications checking
   g. Patient-specific dosing and warnings
   h. Order diagnostic tests
   i. Order referrals

4. **Clinical decision support functions**
   a. Receive results notification
   b. Receive support from standard assessments
   c. Receive support from patient context-enabled assessments
   d. Receive information on most cost-effective services, referrals, devices, and so on to recommend to patient
   e. Support clinical trial recruitment
   f. Support for health maintenance, preventive care, and wellness
   g. Support automated surveillance for ADE, disease outbreaks, bioterrorism
   h. Support chronic disease management
   i. Support drug/device recall
   j. Manage rules presentation: passive, context-sensitive, mandatory, reference

(continued)

Figure 16.2.   (Continued)

5. **Patient support functions**

   a. Provide patient-specific instructions

   b. Generate patient reminders

   c. Provide patient-friendly summary

   d. Provide access to patient education materials

   e. Support home monitoring/tracking capability

6. **Clinical workflow functions**

   a. Schedule and manage clinical tasks (work queues, personnel, rooms, equipment)

   b. Provide personalized in-basket/dashboard support

   c. Automatically generate administrative data from clinical record

   d. Enable printout of documents when necessary

   e. Enable deidentification of protected health information when necessary

   f. Enable specialized views of data

   g. Support multimedia: images, waveforms, scanned documents, pictures, sounds

7. **Administrative and reimbursement functions**

   a. Automatically generate administrative and financial data from clinical record

   b. Provide rules-driven financial and administrative coding assistance

   c. Manage external accountability reporting/outcomes measures

   d. Contract management

8. **Electronic communication and connectivity functions**

   a. Enable transfer of data to notifiable registries (reportable diseases, immunizations)

   b. Provide a current directory of provider information

   c. Manage provider identifiers

   d. Manage (external) trading partners: retail pharmacy, insurer, lab, radiology

   e. Provide secure Web messaging

   f. Support remote access

   g. Provide secure authentication

   h. Provide access management and audit trail services

   i. Enforce patient privacy and confidentiality

   j. Ensure integrity, data retention, and availability

   k. Manage system versioning (change control)

   l. Support interoperability through compliance with data interchange standards and agreements

   m. Support data comparability through use of controlled vocabularies

summary screen that typically launches various functions within the patient's record; documentation templates for recording notes and entering orders; windows or pop-up boxes that supply alerts and reminders and support various actions, such as the transmission of an order to an ancillary system, a prescription to a retail pharmacy, or a claim to a payer; and some form of report writer, including predesigned reports and the ability to create new reports.

Scheduling, Registration/Check-In, In-Basket, and Checkout

Scheduling, registration/patient check-in, in-basket, and checkout are related functions. Although scheduling always occurs first and checkout always occurs last, whether a patient visit is scheduled in advance or the patient is a walk-in, the registration/check-in and in-basket functions along with potentially additional other functions vary by EHR capability and preferred workflow of the clinic.

Scheduling

The scheduling function is used to locate and record the time the patient is to be seen. Some ambulatory EHR systems provide a patient portal that permits patients to request an appointment; some even permit patients to schedule an appointment.

Some scheduling systems prompt staff to initiate a benefits eligibility inquiry. Clinics may do this for all or only a selection of patients. Many clinics use a direct data-entry (DDE) function made available by some of the benefits carriers. Some PMS/EHR products support eligibility inquiry and response using the HIPAA transaction standards (ASC X12 270/271 Eligibility Inquiry and Response).

Currently, most clinics find the DDE form of inquiry to be cumbersome and not available for all benefits plans, yet yielding more complete information for a given patient. This is anticipated to change as the Council for Affordable Quality Healthcare (CAQH) is working to make it easier for physicians (and hospitals) to access eligibility and benefits information for their patients at the point of care. CAQH is a not-for-profit alliance of health plans and networks that promotes collaborative initiatives to help make healthcare more affordable, share knowledge to improve the quality of care, and make administration easier for physicians and their patients. Its Committee on Operating Rules for Information Exchange (CORE) is working on a program where providers will be able to submit a request, using the electronic system of their choice, to obtain a variety of coverage information for any patient and from any participating health plan. Providers will receive more consistent and predictable data, regardless of health plan (CAQH 2006).

After a patient is scheduled, some clinics are promoting use of an online patient self-administered history assessment (Wenner 1994). If the patient has access to the Internet, this may be made available through a secure portal in advance of the visit. If the patient does not have access to the Internet, the patient may be asked to arrive earlier than the scheduled appointment so the assessment can be performed at a kiosk in the waiting room. Some clinics are even setting up special carrels where patients can enter their information in private and receive assistance from staff, if necessary. Although such a process is quite new and not yet broadly adopted, many clinics are starting to realize that it is a useful way for a fairly comprehensive—and consistent—set of data about the patient to be entered into the EHR. The assessment is context-sensitive, so only questions related to the encounter are asked (for example, males would not be asked for pregnancy information, a person with a recurring appointment for a chronic condition would not be asked for a complete history at every visit). The result is that patients can take their time to answer all pertinent questions, and the data are entered in discrete form ready for use in the EHR. When the provider is ready to see the patient, the information gleaned from the assessment can be validated and any additional documentation added as necessary. This also reduces the amount of data entry the physician must perform, freeing time for discussion with the patient.

Registration

The registration function generally occurs immediately prior to or at the time of check-in. At the time of check-in, all pertinent registration functions, if not previously performed, can be conducted or information updated as necessary. The patient's check-in updates the in-basket function with the patient's arrival information.

Many clinics take digital pictures of their patients to incorporate into the EHR as a means of positive patient identification. They also may have a card or document scanner in the check-in area to scan the patient's insurance card and potentially other documents the patient may need to sign or bring with them for incorporation into the EHR. Automated processes, however, also may be used for signing a notice of privacy practices or authorization for release of information. Niche vendors sell informed consent and patient education systems, where a standardized, automated informed consent is prepopulated with demographic information and walks the patient through the key elements of the consent process, then captures an electronic signature through an ID and password given the patient in advance (Burke 2005).

Patient-Provided Documentation

The incorporation of patient-provided documentation into the EHR, such as from a personal health record (PHR), should be a matter addressed in the clinic's policies.

Some clinics accept virtually any and every document the patient may bring from other providers. Other clinics, however, are more discriminating, accepting only documents they have specifically requested and sometimes accepting them only directly from another provider. In other cases, the physician may review documentation brought to the visit by a patient and select what will be scanned into the EHR or will summarize key factors as a note, returning the documentation to the patient.

In addition to what may be incorporated into the EHR, it is a good idea to have a policy describing the communication with the patient that is appropriate to accompany incorporation or rejection of such documents. Some patients may view provision of such documents as a HIPAA amendment function, when often the content is not directly related to existing documentation and not appropriately considered an amendment. Providers are concerned about liability for accepting a voluminous set of documents that they must spend time reading and which may contain information they do not address in a particular visit. Many legal experts believe it is best to return these documents to patients, suggesting the documents are their personal records and should be kept for their own reference and used as a way to jog their memory about what they might want to discuss with their providers. As the PHR gains greater popularity, is more often supported directly by a provider organization, and as PHR may even serve as the consent management function of a health information exchange

(HIE), providers needs to keep abreast of changes in both the legal/regulatory environment and consumer empowerment movement.

In-Basket Function

The in-basket is a function that provides workflow information to various system users based on their needs. It works as a highly structured paper in-basket on the desk or a personal scheduling and reminder system. In the physician office setting, the in-basket alerts the medical assistant or nurse to the patient's arrival for an appointment, the physician when the patient has been roomed and ready to be seen, the office manager (and potentially all users) regarding how long the patient has been waiting, and so on. It also lists results to review, prescription refills to be approved, transcribed reports to be authenticated, and so on. Some in-baskets have telephone auto-dial features to facilitate calls to patients, and most also incorporate e-mail. Some in-basket functionality permits physicians to record their professional services conducted in the hospital. Figure 16.3 displays an example of an in-basket screen.

Figure 16.3.   Example of an in-basket screen

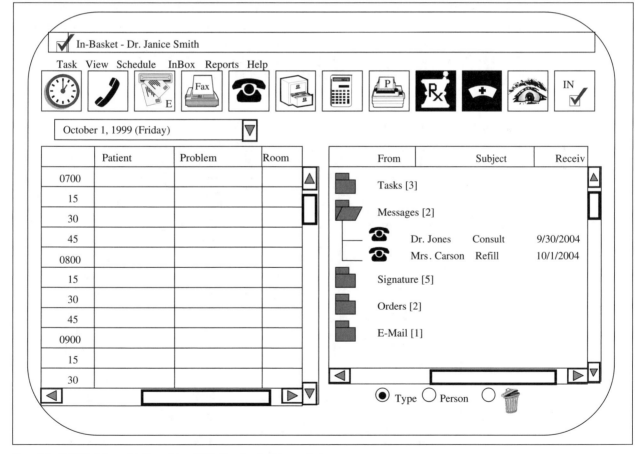

Checkout

Many physician offices do not have a checkout process. Some think they are too small and do not need this function. Very large clinics believe too many patients wander away from the examining rooms without understanding where to go to be checked out. With an EHR, however, checkout can be managed better and in multiple locations, if necessary. Functions performed at checkout include having the patient schedule the next appointment, obtain instructions, and pay the bill (or co-pay portion of the bill). Just as with scheduling, all these activities can be automated and performed from any location. They generally contribute to enhanced patient satisfaction as well as improved cash flow and potentially increased revenue for the clinic.

Patient Summary

Physicians are likely to view the **patient clinical summary** as one of the most desired functions in an EHR. A patient summary usually displays basic demographic information, a problem list, a current medication list, and a listing of recent visits and results available for review. Figure 16.4 shows an example of a patient summary screen. Although a patient summary may be easily generated by an EHR and retrievable online, some physician offices are using a patient summary worksheet generated by the patient's health plan, such as the Blue Care Connection Initiative, as an intermediary step between paper records and full adoption of an EHR (MEDecision 2007). When the worksheet includes up-to-date reminders for chronic disease management, this can improve physician performance in adhering to accepted standards of care (Wilcox et al. 2005).

Figure 16.4.   Sample patient summary screen

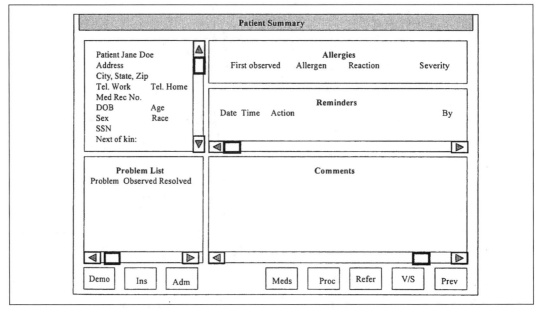

The current medication list may be compiled in a number of ways. For example, physicians may enter medications directly through a prescribing function or history-taking function, or nurses taking intake information may contribute to it and add to it from prescriptions written by the physician during the visit and from visit notes. In such cases, the medication list will contain all the medications the clinician believes the patient is taking, including over-the-counter (OTC) drugs.

A medication list also may be compiled through a subscription service to a pharmacy benefits management consolidator, such as SureScripts/RxHub. This company supplies an e-prescribing gateway that is a standardized communication framework that links prescribers, pharmacies, pharmacy benefits managers (PBMs), and health plans for the purpose of sharing prescription benefit information and exchanging prescriptions electronically (SureScripts/RxHub 2008). A subscription to this or other similar service may provide a consolidated list of all medications for which the patient has filed a claim. (Thus, if the patient paid by cash or credit card in full for filling a prescription, there would be no claim and the transaction would not be included in this list. Also, OTC medications would not be included, although one large retail pharmacy chain is attempting to capture such information through its point-of-sale merchant function.)

Documentation Templates

Although documentation for the EHR can occur through writing on paper that is later scanned or dictating a note that is later transcribed and electronically fed into the EHR, most clinics want their EHRs to support as much structured data entry as possible. Such structured data is essential for the CDS function. To aid in entering structured data, templates are used to guide data collection. Templates are generally built around care plans, clinical guidelines, protocols, or pathways that have been created by the EHR vendor, using either publicly or commercially available sources, or through their own clinical design team or user community.

Care plans, clinical guidelines, protocols, or pathways are important clinical workflow devices. Although they have been used on paper for some time, their use is cumbersome and essentially a reference device. Their use in an EHR can bring them alive and support not only information and workflow, but also documentation. Some experts draw distinctions among these terms, as follows:

- Care plans tend to refer specifically to treatment plans created for individual patients.

- Guidelines are generally considered recommendations based on systematic statements or clinical algorithms of proven care options. They are often developed by professional organizations, payers, and government agencies (such as the Agency for Healthcare Research and Quality [AHRQ]).

- Protocols tend to be more detailed care plans based on investigations done by professional societies, drug companies, or individual researchers.

- Pathways, or care maps, delineate standardized, day-to-day course of care for a group of patients with the same diagnosis or procedure to achieve consistent outcomes. Pathways are often developed by the local facility or health plan (Bufton 1999).

Physicians have routinely developed care plans, although the plans may not be documented explicitly as such in the health record. In hospital records, evidence of the physician's care plan is generally found at the conclusion of the history and physical examination report as the "plan," and in the orders for care. In the inpatient setting, nurses also routinely develop care plans. In the paper environment, these may have been recorded on temporary forms and were not incorporated into the permanent health record. As nursing documentation systems have come about, the care plan is being incorporated into nurses' notes. Nurses also have begun to adopt more formalized clinical guidelines, protocols, or pathways of their own. In the ambulatory environment, physicians develop care plans that they often evidence in their encounter notes.

Physicians are just beginning to recognize the enormous variation in how they treat patients and are adopting clinical guidelines, protocols, or pathways that have been developed through research or other formal analysis of what makes best practices. This is often referred to as **evidence-based medicine**. Of course, some variability is inherent in treating the human condition. Some cases of variation even in similar patients lead to important medical discoveries. However, much of the variation in physician practice is due to differences in physician training, not keeping current with diagnostic and therapeutic modalities, or the pressure of seeing so many patients in a day. This is especially true for primary care physicians who face a huge variety of diagnostic challenges and cannot possibly be expected to keep up with all the latest drugs and treatment protocols. Where the average physician may see 20 or so patients a day, some primary care physicians may see two, three, or even four times that number of patients in a day—especially during flu season or at back-to-school times.

Although much of the documentation in the ambulatory EHR is performed by the physician or midlevel provider (such as physician assistant, nurse practitioner, or nurse midwife) during a patient encounter, it should be pointed out that documentation occurs at other times and by other clinicians. Telephone encounters, e-mail encounters (called **e-visits** [Colwell 2004], for which some payers are starting to provide some reimbursement), refill and renewal documentation, recall management, and other purposes of documentation are needed. Each different type of clinician also performs other functions, works differently, and has different needs from the EHR. Certainly, physical therapists, laboratory technicians, nutritionists, and many other clinicians who may work in ambulatory settings (and, of course, in hospitals) have their own unique data retrieval and documentation requirements.

A prime example of the variability of EHR needs is in highly structured note documentation. This may not suit some physicians but may suit other physicians, as well as nurses, quite well. Moreover, it may suit some situations better than others, such as for documenting a physical examination vs. a consultation. Drawing tools and anatomical diagrams also are documentation options. Figure 16.5 provides an example of a drawing tool incorporated into a template for an eye examination for use by ophthalmologists.

Some specialties tend to use diagrams more than other specialties (for example, ophthalmologists use them frequently). Incorporating images also must be considered. Images would include those from radiology, potential macroscopic and microscopic laboratory specimen images, waveforms from electrocardiograms and other medical devices, and pictures of a patient's skin rash, disfigurement, or other condition for before-and-after comparisons. All these functions and forms of data must be evaluated against the costs

Figure 16.5.   Example of structured data-entry screen with drawing tools

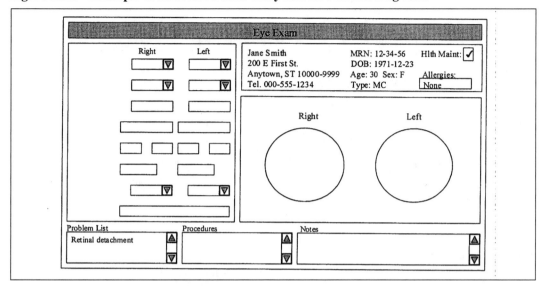

associated with the storage of data, retrieval time, and physician time spent working with data. Following is a case study:

> In reviewing one EHR system, it was noted that no drawings were included. A dermatologist was asked whether the ability to draw diagrams showing the locations of skin conditions or their appearance was missed. The dermatologist responded that in the paper environment such diagrams were made and everyone was aware that such tools were available through the EHR system, but people were not inclined to learn to use them and the results were not missed. The expressed fear was not so much the learning curve that would be required but, rather, that more time would be spent making "pretty pictures" than was warranted. Alternatively, the ophthalmologists in this practice were still drawing on paper that was scanned into the EHR. They, too, expressed concern about spending time drawing. As a result, the software was going to be modified to simplify the drawing tools and incorporate some drawing macros.

An EHR should be capable of presenting various views of the same data. Again, because clinicians work in different ways and sometimes it is desirable for a given clinician to view data in multiple ways, the ability to view data in narrative, table, flowchart, or graphic form should be considered. It also may be desirable to be able to cut and paste (or more accurately copy and paste) data from one place to another. For example, in sending laboratory results to a referring physician, one may want to copy a graph into an e-mail message.

The ability to graph and flowchart is especially important as patients are introduced to EHR system use. Customized views, reports, and instructions may be developed for them and used during the patient encounter as well as to supply the patient with information for a personal health record (PHR) or instructions for care.

Table 16.1.   Functions of CDS systems

Function	Example
Alerting	Highlighting a critical blood potassium level
Reminding	Annual flu vaccine
Critiquing	Rejecting duplicate diagnostic test orders
Interpreting	Diagnosing atrial fibrillation on ECG
Predicting	Predicting mortality risk from a severity-of-illness score
Diagnosing	Listing a differential diagnosis for patient with chest pain
Assisting	Modifying antibiotic choice for patient with renal failure
Suggesting	Generating suggestions for mechanical ventilator weaning

Source: Carter 2001, 182.

Clinical Decision Support

Carter (2001) suggests that "if the [EHR] is the clinician's black bag for the 21st century, the most powerful instrument contained within is clinical decision support (CDS)." Carter also summarizes the functions of CDS systems, as illustrated in table 16.1.

CDS is not without its controversies or concerns. These include everything from annoyance to accuracy. To overcome issues associated with CDS, the clinician should routinely use the EHR at the point of care, becoming accustomed to the various active and passive forms of CDS. Active CDS is that which requires action. It may be a pop-up box or field that must be completed before advancing to the next field, screen, or chart completion. These are typically the forms of CDS that are considered most annoying. They be studied thoroughly to determine their necessity. In the most customizable EHR systems, active CDS can be tailored to specific user preferences so that primary care physicians may have more than specialists, or new physicians to the practice may have more than established physicians. Passive CDS is the form of CDS that aids or guides a user. It is the structure of a template, an icon that appears on a screen that leads to further information, or a pop-up box concerning differential diagnosis. None of these forms of passive CDS require action; they are simply informational.

Sufficient structured data also must be available to ensure that the CDS has all the necessary data to operate properly. CDS software must be kept up to date and reviewed regularly for accurate and current information. An assessment of the impact of CDS also is helpful. When clinicians can see it helping to improve patient safety and quality of care, they are more inclined to use it.

Data Analysis and Report Generation

The functions described above are typically associated with a patient visit or the conclusion/follow-up to a visit. There also are many nonvisit functions that EHR systems can support. An important element of such nonvisit functions is the ability to work with the data being collected, analyze them, and develop reports from them. This is the essence of many of the new external reporting programs (for example, report cards, benchmarking), disease management functions promoted by health plans, and pay-for-performance incentive programs, also increasingly supported by health plans. Additionally, there are functions relevant only for internal use, such as managing workload, evaluating coding quality, recredentialing staff, or customizing patient education material. Data analysis functions also may be as simple as generating letters to remind patients about upcoming appointments or the need for appointments/screenings, send drug recall notices, request patient satisfaction surveys, or mail newsletters or announcements.

Although most EHR systems acquired by physician offices have some ability to generate some reports, not all EHR systems have the ability to easily conduct sophisticated analysis. As previously noted, it may be necessary to move data into a clinical data warehouse, which is a database optimized for analytical processing in order to process a large sampling of data or even the universe of data for a given patient population. Very few clinics have the staff or financial resources to support a clinical data warehouse, although many contribute data to external warehouses, in the form of the Medicare claims data file, disease registries, etc. However, there is growing interest in being able to do more with the data captured during patient care visits and to validate the accuracy of data submitted to health plans and other services. As such, report writing tools, analytical or data mining software, and statistical analysis systems are being acquired and used either against the EHR's repository or by dumping data into a separate database.

As a prelude to any data analysis, the data itself must undergo an assessment to ensure they are appropriate for analysis. A controlled, and ideally standardized, vocabulary should be used to make valid comparisons. The system's metadata may need to be reviewed to determine what changes may have been made to such a vocabulary and when so as to be able to limit the scope of data included to those that will be consistent. The accuracy of the data entry should be validated. If a field is optional, what is the frequency with which data are entered? If narrative documentation is permitted, how frequently are narrative notes made instead of using the discrete data field? If narrative notes can be converted to discrete data, is the conversion accurate?

The result of data analysis can be insightful and powerful. At one provider location, data analysis was used to create new alerts, analyze physician ordering patterns to reduce cost, and reengineer laboratory specimen turnaround times (Ebidia et al. 1999).

Analysis of data from an EHR, of course, also can be used to support clinical research. Some EHR products include the ability to manage data for clinical trials and even to prompt physicians to recruit patients for clinical trials.

Ambulatory EHR Migration Path

Although the ambulatory EHR is generally more comprehensive and self-contained than the modular acute care EHR, there still may be a need to plot a migration path for a clinic or physician office.

In some cases, an ambulatory setting may not be able to afford a fully robust EHR but wants to achieve some of the benefits of automation. Physician resistance may be particularly strong so that a clinic may decide to move at a slower pace and introduce a less intrusive component first. There may be evidence that the hospital's EHR vendor is working on developing an EHR for the ambulatory environment, and it may make sense to acquire a stand-alone module to address only e-prescribing or clinical messaging temporarily. There may be organizational reasons why an EHR should not be acquired until a merger or acquisition has taken place. There may be significant disagreement over what product to acquire, or a large shareholder may be promoting a less-than-desirable product. Whatever the reason, it may be appropriate to be selective about the path a clinic takes to the EHR. Even if the ultimate goal is the comprehensive EHR, it may take a while to develop the technical infrastructure and operational elements that need to be in place. Alternatively, it may be that the ambulatory environment is very large, with its own lab, pharmacy, and radiology departments and will need multiple applications to comprise its EHR, similar to a hospital environment.

As with any EHR migration path, clinics need to address applications, technology, and operations. Dependencies among each application, technology, and operation as well as among applications, technologies, and operations need to be understood. Some of the areas physician offices trip over include:

- *Buying hardware before selecting an EHR:* It cannot be emphasized enough that different vendor applications work better with certain types of server configurations, human–computer interfaces, and so on. The amount of bandwidth and storage depends on the volume and type of images. Some examples of questions to consider in plotting the migration path include: How much paper will be scanned for backfilling and going forward? How soon will a PACS be acquired or images from an imaging center be incorporated? Are additional clinic sites anticipated that would require a larger network?

- *Buying a stand-alone system that is not standards compliant or CCHIT certified:* There are actually many interesting, niche systems that can get an office started on e-prescribing, patient history assessment, clinical messaging, EHR-light products, and so on, but they are not HL7 or NCPDP compliant for later incorporation into an EHR. These may be Web based and can complement an EHR going forward but will not be integrated with the EHR. However, when a practice looks at an EHR to achieve the full benefits of quality, patient safety, productivity, etc., and expects to reap benefits for doing so, such as in pay-for-performance program, it is virtually essential to buy a CCHIT-certified product, as many of these programs require such use of certified products.

- *Starting down the EHR path without engaging all stakeholders, including the board and staff:* This is a common misstep because, frequently, the office may not even recognize it is starting down the EHR path until too many disparate applications have been acquired. Attending to operational elements of identifying a project manager, compensating a medical director of information systems, establishing standard practices across sites or even physicians, engaging nurses and administrative staff, and addressing documentation policy are early steps in a migration path to EHR.

- *Engaging in self-development or beta testing with a vendor, thinking this will save money and be a way to acquire a "real" system on the cheap:* Although a small number of these endeavors have been successful, with several hundreds of vendors having entered and left the marketplace, this is not for the faint of heart.

Appreciating the impact on the clinic and the potential for a homegrown EHR to "fit" with any commercial products later need to be part of migration path planning in this environment. Many practices also do not appreciate the time and effort it takes to implement a fully functional EHR, let alone one that is only in beta version and that will, by definition, have many bugs to be worked out.

EHR Components

EHR components ambulatory care environments may consider, or at least should understand, include: e-prescribing (vs. CPOE), clinical messaging (vs. portals), and EHRs acquired through ASP (vs. community) offerings.

E-Prescribing vs. CPOE

It is important to point out that CPOE is also a function of an EHR in an ambulatory environment. Although it is not a separate module in such a system, the function of ordering a lab test, making a referral, or issuing any other, nonmedication order is as much CPOE as its acute care counterpart. In many cases, however, such ordering entails not only the documentation of what was ordered for a patient, but also clinical messaging to an external party rather than to an internal, ancillary system. Such clinical messaging is described here.

E-prescribing is a special case of CPOE in the ambulatory environment. It refers to the writing of a prescription to be filled by a retail, community, or mail-order pharmacy, instead of the ordering of a drug from a clinical pharmacy that is a department of a hospital. There are several important distinctions between CPOE relating to medication ordering in a hospital and e-prescribing in the ambulatory world:

- A prescription is written for a drug that may or may not be included in the patient's drug benefits. If it could be known that a drug is on- or off-formulary for a patient and what the patient's copayment would be for the drug, the physician writing the prescription could make the necessary change in the drug of choice with the patient and prior to the patient's going to the pharmacy. Such knowledge will reduce phone calls from pharmacies back to the physician and will decrease wait time for patients. Alternatively, most benefit plans pay for almost any drugs ordered in the hospital and the few that are not covered are well known. Access to a benefits formulary, then, is often not a function of CPOE, but it is an important function of e-prescribing.

- Many e-prescribing systems currently produce either a legible prescription, having been generated by the entry of discrete data into the application, or an electronic fax (e-fax) of the legible prescription. The paper copy can be handed to the patient. The e-fax goes directly to the pharmacy of the patient's choice. Of course, an order for a drug in a hospital is not given to the patient. (If the order is faxed internally to the clinical pharmacy in the hospital as a means of communication, it is done so because there is no order communication system or the pharmacy needs a facsimile of the wet signature. It is not faxed outside the hospital.)

- New standards have been adopted for the transmission of prescriptions to retail, community, and mail-order pharmacies. Promulgated by the National Council for Prescription Drug Programs (NCPDP) and called SCRIPT, these standards will be required under the Medicare Modernization Act of 1003 by 2009, for any electronic prescription written for Medicare Part D beneficiaries. Because this represents a sizeable proportion of all prescriptions, more than 95 percent of all retail chain, community, and mail-order pharmacies have adopted this standard and most e-prescribing vendors are planning to adopt them for all e-prescribing systems (SureScripts/RxHub 2008). The NCPCP SCRIPT standard being adopted for e-prescribing, however, is only used in the retail, community, and mail-order environment. Hospital pharmacy information systems use the message format standard from HL7 to receive and send communications between the CPOE and the pharmacy system. Although there is an effort to "harmonize" HL7 and NCPDP SCRIPT, until that has occurred and been adopted by the vendors in their products, the two standards essentially are incompatible. This means that a physician cannot use the e-prescribing system from the office for writing hospital medication orders, or vice versa.

- Another issue relating to e-prescribing is that of authentication. Although all states have laws permitting electronic signature on prescriptions for all but controlled substances, following Drug Enforcement Administration (DEA) requirements, states require a wet signature for controlled substances. The DEA has proposed a ruling that would enable e-prescribing for controlled substances with special considerations for heightened security. See chapter 10 for additional information.

E-prescribing systems are applications that support a variety of prescribing functions. Some are as simple as supplying a drug reference database that actually does not generate a prescription. Others generate a prescription but do not do any CDS, such as drug–drug checking. Still others can be synchronized with a PMS to obtain patient demographics and possibly drug allergy information that can be checked against the drug prescribed. Some can be synchronized with an external system, such as SureScripts/RxHub, that provides formulary benefit information. Finally, the most robust e-prescribing systems conduct the NCPDP transactions and provide comprehensive drug–allergy, drug–drug, and drug–lab checking based on a patient's EHR data.

For an e-prescribing application to transmit the new prescription or refill approval transactions to a retail, community, or mail-order pharmacy of the patient's choice, it must support the NCPDP standards and link to an e-prescribing gateway (EPG), or network. SureScripts/RxHub currently is the primary network that operates in 40 states, with most of the major pharmacies and many of the e-prescribing and EHR vendor applications. Other states and locations may have local or regional networks covering a much smaller segment of the market. Figure 16.6 illustrates the variety of transactions that can occur within the realm of e-prescribing.

Clinical Messaging vs. Portals

Clinical messaging is the secure transmission of clinical information from one entity to another, including providers to providers, patients to providers, payers to providers, and

Figure 16.6.   E-prescribing transactions

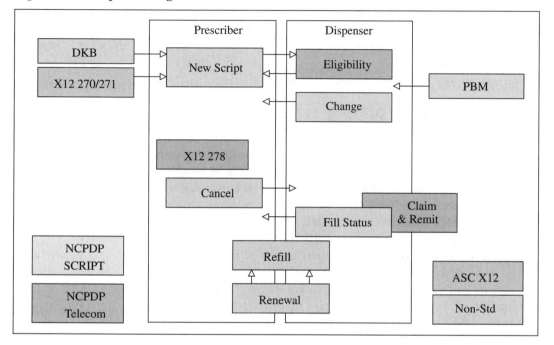

among members of a healthcare community, such as within a regional health information organization (RHIO) or other HIE organization. The company, Axolotl, claims to have invented and registered the term, although many other vendors are using it to describe the same functionality.

A key element of clinical messaging is the security afforded by the process. Although e-mail could be used to conduct clinical messaging, sending e-mail containing clinical information in the clear through the Internet is generally not advisable. Instead, the concept of clinical messaging is to support easy communication of messages in a safe manner.

Several companies serve as communications channels for clinical messaging. Medem is one of the largest of such companies and was created by the American Medical Association and several other medical societies. Its site is free and provides personal health records (PHRs) for patients, disease management and medication adherence programs, and online consultation. Other companies charge for more sophisticated services than provided by Medem. If an organization already has a Web site, it can either set up a private portal for just its physicians and patients or insert a link to clinical messaging service from Medem or other companies.

Each company providing clinical messaging does so in a slightly different manner. Some are clearly Web portals, which are sites on the Web that provide personalized capabilities to their visitors. Others are only a means to encrypt e-mail, and still others are virtual private networks or other point-to-point network connections that transmit content directly into a system configured to accept it.

Where clinical messaging is essentially the secure exchange of e-mail messages, which may be facilitated through a portal, portal technology may also provide more functionality. A portal is literally an entranceway. It may provide entrance to an e-mail server; or it may provide entrance directly into an application. So, physicians from their offices may connect to a provider portal offered by their hospital and actually enter orders or retrieve lab results. Portal technology is more sophisticated than simple secure messaging.

ASP vs. Community Offering for EHR

Yet another consideration for ambulatory care providers to acquire an EHR is an ASP or a community offering. Most healthcare organizations (acute or ambulatory) acquire an EHR through direct licensing with a vendor or **value-added reseller (VAR)**. However, some vendors and VARs also offer an **application service provider (ASP)** model of EHR. This is typically a version of their EHR that may be as customizable as their primary version and is provided via a subscription fee service, so it is both a type of EHR and an EHR financing mechanism. Various features of the ASP model have been described previously.

However, some providers, in conjunction with their vendors, are offering a somewhat different version of an ASP. Commonly called a community model, it is a means to acquire licenses through another provider. It offers many of the same benefits of an ASP, such as elimination of the hassles of data center maintenance and staff support. However, because it is offered by a provider via additional licenses instead of a vendor or VAR as a true ASP, there is one **Active Directory** (component of the Windows operating system that manages identification of data and their relationships within a system) and one repository of data, although the providers obtaining such licenses have their data physically partitioned within the repository and are the only individuals afforded access. Such an arrangement logically separates the data, but may not physically separate the data. In general, customization is limited to the customization performed by the primary provider or to that which can normally be provided individual users.

The advantages to the community offering are the ability for physicians to use the same product as their hospital, to have the ability to share data seamlessly with their hospital, and to acquire an EHR with little overhead. However, there are some concerns surrounding the community offering. These include the fact that it is only access control technology separating the clinic's data from the hospital's data, the level of service a hospital typically not in the business of providing IT services can actually support, and questions relating to Stark Law and the Anti-Kickback Statute (although exceptions and safe harbors have been permitted—refer to chapter 1).

Conclusion

Clearly, the vast array of EHRs, niche products, components, and forms of offerings are promoting adoption of EHRs in the ambulatory arena. It is not surprising, then, that a RAND Corporation study in 2005 found the acceleration of EHR adoption among ambulatory providers significantly higher than that among hospitals. In fact, with the level of EHR available to ambulatory settings, it may be the physicians driving hospital adoption rather than the other way around in the near future. Although adoption still remains fairly low, at about 17 percent nationwide (DesRoches, et al. 2008), in some locations it is considerably higher. For example, according to a 2007 statewide EHR survey by Stratis Health, Minnesota's Medicare Quality Improvement Organization, 64 percent of adult primary care practices have either fully implemented or are in the process of implementing EHRs.

References and Resources

Allscripts Healthcare Solutions. 2005. *The Electronic Physician: Guidelines for Implementing a Paperless Practice*. Chicago: Allscripts.

Amatayakul, M., and S.S. Lazarus. 2005. *Electronic Health Records: Transforming Your Medical Practice*. Denver: Medical Group Management Association.

Amatayakul, M., C. Woolley (RxHub), and K. Whittemore (SureScripts). 2005 (Sept. 8). Medicare HIT Policies: Medicare and Part D ePrescribing Issues: Toward a Seamless System for Better Outcomes. Presentation at HIT Summit, Washington, DC.

American Health Information Management Association. 1998 (May 6). Application and Interface Strategies in the EHR. Audio Seminar. Chicago: AHIMA.

Axolotl, Corp. 2005 (Aug. 24). Clinical Messaging. www.axolotl.com/solutions/physicians/cm.

Bachman, J.W. 2003. The patient–computer interview: A neglected tool that can aid the clinician. *Mayo Clinic Proceedings* 78:67–78.

Bufton, M.G. 1999. Electronic health records and implementation of clinical practice guidelines. In *Electronic Health Records: Changing the Vision*, eds by G.F. Murphy, M.A. Hanken, and K.A. Waters. Philadelphia: W. B. Saunders. pp.249–268.

Burke, M. 2005. Rethinking informed consent. *ADVANCE for Health Information Executives* 9(8):10.

Carter, J.H. 2001. *Electronic Medical Records: A Guide for Clinicians and Administrators*. Philadelphia: American College of Physicians–American Society of Internal Medicine.

Certification Commission for Health Information Technology. 2008, CCHIT Certification Criteria for Ambulatory EHR Products Chicago: CCHIT.

Colwell, J. 2004 (Dec.). How two practices are taking patient visits online—and getting paid for them. *ACP Observer.* www.acponline.org/journals/news/dec04/evisit.htm.

Council on Affordable Quality Healthcare (CAQH), Committee on Operating Rules for Information Exchange (CORE). 2006. Promoting Interoperability: Online Eligibility and Benefits Inquiry. www.caqh.org.

Daigrepont, J.P. 2004. *Automating the Medical Record,* 2nd ed. Chicago: American Medical Association.

DesRoches CM, et al. 2008 (June 18). Electronic health records in ambulatory care—a national survey of physicians. *N Engl J Med* 359: 50–60.

Ebidia, A., C., Mulder, B., Tripp, M.W., Morgan. 1999. Getting data out of the electronic patient record: Critical steps in building a data warehouse for decision support. Toronto, Ontario, Canada: University of Toronto Department of Medicine Shared Information Management Services (SIMS) University Health Network.

Health and Human Services, Office of the Secretary. 2005 (Oct. 11). Centers for Medicare and Medicaid Services. Proposed rule: Medicare program; Physicians' referrals to health care entities with which they have financial relationships; exceptions for certain electronic prescribing and electronic health records arrangements. *Federal Register,* 45 CFR Part 411.

Health and Human Services, Office of the Secretary. 2005 (Oct. 11). Office of Inspector General. Proposed Rule: Medicare and state health care programs: Fraud and abuse; safe harbor for certain electronic prescribing arrangements under the Anti-Kickback Statute. *Federal Register,* 42 CFR Part 1001.

Health Level Seven. 2007. EHR System Functional Model. www.hl7.org/ehr.

Institute of Medicine. 2003 (July 31). *Letter Report: Key capabilities of an Electronic Health Record System.* Washington, DC: National Academies Press. www.nap.edu/books.

Keet, R. 2003 (June 12). Clinical Messaging Systems and E-Health Automation. Mountain View, CA: Axolotl Corp.

Lapp, T. 2003 (Sept.). Paperless system: The cure for the harried physician. *Family Practice Report* 9(9). www.aafp.org.

Lowes, R. 2004 (Mar.). Phones driving you crazy? *Medical Economics* 81:65.

MEDecision, 2007 (Sept 24). MEDecision Patient Clinical Summary Delivered to Health Care Service Corporation Member Portal.

Medem. 2006. The Medem Network: Connecting Physicians and Patients Online. www.medem.com.

Medicare Prescription Drug, Improvement, and Modernization Act of 2003 (Dec. 8). Public Law 108–173. www.cms.hhs.gov/medicarereform/MMAactFullText.pdf.

Middleton, B., K. Renner, and M. Leavitt. 1997. Ambulatory practice clinical information management: Problems and prospects. *Healthcare Information Management* 11(4):97–112.

National Committee on Vital and Health Statistics. 2004 (Dec. 8–10). Testimony to Senate Subcommittee on Standards and Security, Washington, DC.

Osheroff, J.A., et al. 2005. *Improving Outcomes with Clinical Decision Support: An Implementer's Guide.* Chicago: Healthcare Information and Management Systems Society.

RxHub LLC. 2002 (Aug.). The Challenges of Today's Prescribing Process. www.rxhub.net.

Schwartz, D. 1998. Creating a benchmark database. *Health Management Technology* 19(1):65–66.

Stratis Health 2007 (Oct. 3). Press Release: Significant Increase in Electronic Health Record Use in Minnesota Clinics.

SureScripts. 2008 (July 1). Retail Pharmacies and Largest Pharmacy Benefit Managers Announce Merger of E-prescribing Networks—Improving Safety, Accuracy, Efficiency of Prescription Medicines for Patients Nationwide.

Wenner A.R., M. Ferrante, D. Belser. 1994. Instance medical history. *Proceedings of the Annual Symposium on Computer Applications in Medical Care*: 1036.

Wilcox A, et al. 2005. Use and Impact of a Computer-Generated Patient Summary Worksheet for Primary Care, *AMIA Annual Symposium Proceedings*: 824–828.

Chapter 17
Growing Momentum for Health Information Exchange

A number of events in the past few years have highlighted the need to be able to better share health information across the continuum of care. The Institute of Medicine (IOM) report, *To Err is Human,* published in 1999, probably did more to raise the nation's collective consciousness concerning patient safety and the need for health information exchange (HIE) than any other single event. When confronted with the fact that "every day, tens if not hundreds of thousands of errors occur in the U.S. healthcare system," despite that many are "near-misses" or do not result in harm, the nation reacted to the wake-up call.

Subsequent events, such as the hurricane disasters of 2005, where individuals were left unable to get at prescription information, let alone their actual medications, reemphasized the need for the transportability and ubiquity of health information.

The federal government has responded to these issues by taking on a number of initiatives and providing increased federal funding for private-sector initiatives to explore health information exchange opportunities. This chapter:

- Discusses the impetus for HIE in the U.S. and the elements required to promote such exchange

- Describes the basic forms of HIE organizational structures, architectures, and services

- Reinforces the need for data stewardship in HIE services

- Identifies state, regional, and local activities in achieving benefits and overcoming challenges for HIE organizations

- Describes the federal government's concept of a nationwide health information network

Key Words

Data stewardship	HIE organization	Nationwide health information network
Health data stewardship	HIE participation agreement	Person identification
Health information exchange	Identity management	Personal health information
Health information service provider	National health information infrastructure	Record custodian
HIE data sharing agreement		Record locator service
		Stewardship

Health Information Exchange in the U.S.

The Department of Health and Human Services (HHS) Web site on Value-Driven Health Care (2008) states:

> "The health care 'system' in America is not a system. It's a disconnected collection of large and small medical businesses, health care professionals, treatment centers, hospitals, and all who provide support for them. Each player may have its own internal structure for gathering and sharing information, but nothing ties those isolated structures into an interoperable national system capable of making information easily shared and compared."

Need for Value-Driven Healthcare

As embarrassing as the preceding statement may appear to be, the fact remains that many indicators suggest the need for significant improvements in the U.S. healthcare system. According to World Health Organization (WHO) Core Health Indicators (2005), the U.S. spends more on healthcare, both as a proportion of gross domestic product (GDP) and on a per-capita basis, than any other nation in the world. Current estimates from the Centers for Medicare and Medicaid Services (CMS) National Health Expenditure Data (2008) put U.S. healthcare spending at approximately 16 percent of GDP, with the U.S. spending a projected $2.26 trillion on healthcare, or $7,439 per person in 2007, up from $5,635 in 2003 (Anderson et al. 2005). In comparison, Canada spent $3,003 per person and the Netherlands $1,886 in 2003.

However, although there is some controversy over exact numbers and their meaning, the quality of outcomes for the level of spending (that is, value) is generally poor. WHO in 2000 ranked the U.S. healthcare system first in both responsiveness and expenditure, but 37th in overall performance and 72nd by overall level of health (among 191 member nations included in the study). The Central Intelligence Agency (CIA) World Factbook (2008) ranked the U.S. 43rd in the world for lowest infant mortality rate and 47th for highest total life expectancy. A study conducted by Nolte and McKee for *Health Affairs* in 2008 found that between 1997 and 2003, preventable deaths declined more slowly in the United

States than in 18 other industrialized nations. Despite these outcomes, the National Health Interview Survey, released annually by the Centers for Disease Control and Prevention's (CDC) National Center for Health Statistics (NCHS) reported that approximately 66 percent of survey respondents said they were in "excellent" or "very good" health in 2006.

Identifying causality for healthcare outcomes and then instituting corrective action is certainly very difficult. However, several factors have been identified as potentially contributory to reduced value in the U.S. For example, the IOM (2004) has observed that the U.S. is the only wealthy, industrialized nation that does not have a universal healthcare system, with the U.S. Census Bureau (2007) identifying 16 percent of the U.S. population without health insurance coverage.

Technology for Value-Driven Healthcare

Of interest with respect to use of information technology (IT), Anderson et al for *Health Affairs* (2006) suggests that there are a number of areas in which the U.S. is lagging behind that may be contributory to less than stellar healthcare value. Table 17.1 summarizes cost/outcomes (value) and technology use findings for a sample of countries.

Information Silos

As has been discussed throughout this book, there are many factors that have related to slow adoption of IT. One relating in particular to more widespread adoption of technology to support use of evidence-based guidelines across the continuum of care is that the U.S. healthcare systems remains a cottage industry despite its level of spending. Many providers, whether they are solo practitioners, practice in a group, or are employed by a healthcare organization, view themselves as independent of other providers in how they work and what they do. *Health Affairs* (Sirovich et al. 2008) has also studied discretionary decision making by primary care physicians and the cost of U.S. healthcare, finding that efforts to improve the value of U.S. healthcare have focused largely on fostering physician adherence to evidence-based guidelines. They found that use of evidence-based guidelines, fostered through the use of IT, were important with respect to outcomes, but not necessarily important to cost. Physicians often used their discretionary bent to order tests or perform

Table 17.1. Technology and value-driven healthcare

Indicator	U.S.	Canada	Netherlands
Medical spending per person[a]	$5,635	$3,003	$1,886
Infant mortality rate (# deaths/ 1,000 live births)[b]	6	5	4
Life expectancy at birth (# years)[b]	78	81	79
Use of EHR by primary care physicians[c]	28%	23%	98%
Computerized system to alert physicians to potential drug dose or interaction problems[c]	23%	10%	93%

Sources of data:
a. Anderson, G.F., et al. for Health Affairs 2005 (2003 data)
b. CIA The World Factbook (2008 estimated data)
c. Anderson, G.F., et al. for Health Affairs 2006 (2003 data)

other interventions irrespective of cost. In fact, a Massachusetts Medical Society survey in 2005 found widespread distrust and lack of knowledge in use of evidence-based guidelines to manage quality and cost.

Such a cottage industry mentality or discretionary posture has carried over to various departments in hospitals, each also operating highly independently, whether they are the lab and radiology, or internal medicine and oncology. In some cases, departments in hospitals are actually found to run better when they are independent and outsource work to separate companies. For example, it is not uncommon now to find laboratory, pharmacy, radiology, and emergency departments outsourced.

Needless to say, information systems also have focused on individual functions and the operations of only their respective departments or users. Reference has been made to information silos, or stovepipes. Indeed, the definition of EHR includes recognition of the need to collect data from multiple sources for use in clinical decision making at the point of care. Although providers recognize the need for, and may often be frustrated by the lack of, data from across disparate sources, the fact remains that, until recently, little has been done to support more seamless exchange of health information. In fact, it is almost as if a provider's view is "I need your data to treat our patient, but you can't have my data."

Further complicating the picture is the notion that the information is the provider's property. Patients had little say in how their information was managed until the HIPAA legislation provided privacy rights regarding protected health information. Although patients have always been required to authorize release of information to another provider, they are frequently required to pay for their own copies. Incorporating patient-generated or even other provider-generated information supplied by the patient has been discouraged. Absent laws until HIPAA requiring providers to permit access to their health information, patients frequently were turned down when they requested access to records held by their physicians. In fact, one of the top complaints filed with the Office of Civil Rights (OCR) under the HIPAA privacy rule has been "denied access to records" (*Health Information Compliance Insider* 2005).

Office of the National Coordinator for Health Information Technology

In April 2004, President Bush called for widespread adoption of interoperable EHRs within 10 years and established the Office of the National Coordinator (ONC) for Health Information Technology. An important element of ONC is to effectively communicate with the public concerning the federal HIT initiatives. Figure 17.1 is the vision for HIT, as described by President Bush, which was published on ONC's Web site. ONC also created a message about the value of HIT directed to consumers, provided in figure 17.2.

Strategic Framework
In the President's Executive Order 13335, the national coordinator was required to report within 90 days of operation on the development and implementation of a strategic plan to guide the nationwide implementation of HIT in both the public and private sectors. In July 2004, *The Decade of Health Information Technology: Delivering Consumer-centric and Information-rich Health Care: Framework for Strategic Action* was delivered. The framework includes four major goals, each with a corresponding set of strategies. The strategies also describe specific actions that will advance and focus future efforts. These goals and strategies as summarized in the strategic framework's executive summary are provided in figure 17.3.

Figure 17.1.   Consumer message on president's vision for HIT

In April 2004, President George W. Bush revealed his vision for the future of healthcare in the United States. The President's plan involves a healthcare system that puts the needs of the patient first, is more efficient, and is cost-effective. The President's plan is based on the following tenets:

- Medical information will follow consumers so that they are at the center of their own care.
- Consumers will be able to choose physicians and hospitals based on clinical performance results made available to them.
- Clinicians will have a patient's complete medical history, computerized ordering systems, and electronic reminders.
- Quality initiatives will measure performance and drive quality-based competition in the industry.
- Public health and bioterrorism surveillance will be seamlessly integrated into care.
- Clinical research will be accelerated and postmarketing surveillance will be expanded.

Together, these tenets will revolutionize healthcare, making it more consumercentric, and will improve both the quality and the efficiency of healthcare in the United States.

Source: ONC 2005b.

Figure 17.2.   ONC's consumer message on value of HIT

We Need to Bring Every Doctor, Outpatient Office, Hospital, and Nursing Home into Information Age

- Our medical research is the world's best. We have state-of-the–art diagnostic and procedural technology. But we lack the ability to get critical clinical information to the doctor at the point of care.
- Vital data sit in paper records that are hard to access or combine. We rely on paper files and handwritten notes to the pharmacist.
- Information gets lost. Problems with drug interactions are not systematically checked. Preventable medical errors are made—and patients get hurt.
- IT is changing American industries. But healthcare hasn't kept up. At the end of the 1990s, most industries were spending about $8,000 per worker for IT. But the healthcare industry was investing only about $1,000 per worker.

The Benefits Health IT Can Bring to Our Nation—Fewer Mistakes, Lower Costs, Less Hassle, Better Care

- It is estimated that HIT can reduce healthcare costs up to 20% per year by saving time and reducing duplication and waste.
- It is also estimated that HIT can reduce medical errors by providing complete patient histories, computerized ordering, and electronic reminders.
- HIT enables true partnerships and collaborations with doctors. Consumers make more informed choices about treatment options and doctors become more involved in their care.
- Electronic health records not only save lives:
  - They reduce errors such as when a pharmacist can't read a physician's handwriting, or when the wrong drug is prescribed by the physician.
  - They save time in that patients don't have to give their address, insurance information, and other basic information again and again.
  - They reduce duplication and waste by showing physicians when tests or treatments may not be necessary.
  - They make it easier for consumers to get care from different physicians by making sure that their information follows them throughout their care.
  - They give us better information to track public health problems and advance clinical research.
  - They protect privacy by making sure that only authorized people see the medical record.

Source: ONC 2005d.

Figure 17.3.   Goals and strategies of the ONC framework for strategic action

Goal 1: Inform Clinical Practice.   Informing clinical practice is fundamental to improving care and making healthcare delivery more efficient. This goal centers largely around efforts to bring EHRs directly into clinical practice. This will reduce medical errors and duplicative work, and enable clinicians to focus their efforts more directly on improved patient care. Three strategies for realizing this goal are:

- *Strategy 1. Incentivize EHR adoption.*   The transition to safe, more consumer-friendly and regionally integrated care delivery will require shared investments in information tools and changes to current clinical practice.

- *Strategy 2. Reduce risk of EHR investment.*   Clinicians who purchase EHRs and who attempt to change their clinical practices and office operations face a variety of risks that make this decision unduly challenging. Low-cost support systems that reduce risk, failure, and partial use of EHRs are needed.

- *Strategy 3. Promote EHR diffusion in rural and underserved areas.*   Practices and hospitals in rural and other underserved areas lag in EHR adoption. Technology transfer and other support efforts are needed to ensure widespread adoption.

Goal 2: Interconnect Clinicians.   Interconnecting clinicians will allow information to be portable and to move with consumers from one point of care to another. This will require an interoperable infrastructure to help clinicians get access to critical healthcare information when their clinical and/or treatment decisions are being made. The three strategies for realizing this goal are:

- *Strategy 1. Foster regional collaborations.*   Local oversight of health information exchange that reflects the needs and goals of a population should be developed.

- *Strategy 2. Develop a national health information network.*   A set of common intercommunication tools such as mobile authentication, Web services architecture, and security technologies are needed to support data movement that is inexpensive and secure. A national health information network that can provide low-cost and secure data movement is needed, along with a public-private oversight or management function to ensure adherence to public policy objectives.

- *Strategy 3. Coordinate federal health information systems.*   There is a need for federal health information systems to be interoperable and to exchange data so that federal care delivery, reimbursement, and oversight are more efficient and cost effective. Federal health information systems will be interoperable and consistent with the national health information network.

Goal 3: Personalize Care.   Consumer-centric information helps individuals manage their own wellness and assists with their personal healthcare decisions. The ability to personalize care is a critical component of using healthcare information in a meaningful manner. The three strategies for realizing this goal are:

- *Strategy 1. Encourage use of Personal Health Records.*   Consumers are increasingly seeking information about their care as a means of getting better control over their healthcare experience, and PHRs that provide customized facts and guidance to them are needed.

- *Strategy 2. Enhance informed consumer choice.*   Consumers should have the ability to select clinicians and institutions based on what they value and the information to guide their choice, including but not limited to, the quality of care providers deliver.

- *Strategy 3. Promote use of telehealth systems.*   The use of telehealth—remote communication technologies—can provide access to health services for consumers and clinicians in rural and underserved areas. Telehealth systems that can support the delivery of health care services when the participants are in different locations are needed.

(continued)

Figure 17.3.   (Continued)

Goal 4: Improve Population Health.   Population health improvement requires the collection of timely, accurate, and detailed clinical information to allow for the evaluation of healthcare delivery and the reporting of critical findings to public health officials, clinical trials and other research, and feedback to clinicians. Three strategies for realizing this goal are:

- *Strategy 1. Unify public health surveillance architectures.*   An interoperable public health surveillance system is needed that will allow exchange of information, consistent with current law, between provider organizations, organizations they contract with, and state and federal agencies.

- *Strategy 2. Streamline quality and health status monitoring.*   Many different state and local organizations collect subsets of data for specific purposes and use it in different ways. A streamlined quality-monitoring infrastructure that will allow for a complete look at quality and other issues in real-time and at the point of care is needed.

- *Strategy 3. Accelerate research and dissemination of evidence.*   Information tools are needed that can accelerate scientific discoveries and their translation into clinically useful products, applications, and knowledge.

Source: Thompson and Brailer 2004

Key actions to implement the Framework for Strategic Action were further identified:

- Establishing a health information technology (HIT) leadership panel to evaluate the urgency of investments and recommend immediate actions

- Ensuring private-sector certification of HIT products

- Funding community health information exchange (HIE) demonstrations

- Planning the formation of a private interoperability consortium

- Requiring standards to facilitate electronic prescribing

- Establishing a Medicare beneficiary portal

- Sharing clinical research data through a secure infrastructure

- Committing to standards

Interoperability

Clearly, a major theme of the Framework for Strategic Action and subsequent activity has been interoperability. As previously described, basic interoperability is the capability of software and hardware on different machines from different vendors to share data. Organizations focusing on HIT interoperability have gone beyond this basic definition to describe not only more technical capability but also the human factor elements of interoperability. Figure 17.4 includes four different organizations' additional refinements to the definition of interoperability within healthcare.

As the first National Coordinator for Health Information Technology, David J. Brailer, MD, PhD stressed the importance of interoperability as "an essential factor in using HIT to

Figure 17.4.   Definitions of interoperability for healthcare

- The ability to exchange patient health information among disparate clinicians and other authorized entities in real time and under stringent security, privacy and other protections (ONC 2005b).

- The ability of different information technology systems and software applications to communicate, to exchange data accurately, effectively, and consistently, and to use the information that has been exchanged (NAHIT 2005).

- The ability of health information systems to work together within and across organizational boundaries in order to advance the effective delivery of healthcare for individuals and communities (HIMSS 2005).

- At the application level, interoperability means the capacity of a connected, authenticated user to access, transmit and/or receive/exchange usable information with other users (Connecting for Health 2005).

improve the quality and efficiency of care in the U.S." He observed that "interoperability and health information exchange are techno-speak jargon for health care information that is treated as a required element of diagnosis and therapy, albeit one that jealously guards patients' privacy and confidentiality." It could be observed that Dr. Brailer, who is both a physician and an economist, may be suggesting that market demand has not done enough to overcome the lack of interoperability:

> Without interoperability and health information exchange, health information will remain in proprietary silos, in which the health care enterprise hopes to gain competitive advantage by imposing high costs on consumer switchover and by exercising market leverage over small niche players such as solo physicians and community hospitals.

Finally, Dr. Brailer concluded that "interoperability and HIE are best understood as business concepts rather than technical concepts," with a need for:

- Uniform business processes

- Uniform privacy laws

- Uniform patient identification

- Controlled medical terminology

- Commonly accepted business transaction definitions (HHS 2005a)

Strategic Plan

ONC has undertaken many initiatives to advance use of health information technology in general and EHR specifically, to promote health information exchange, and to create the concept of a nationwide health information network. Further consistent with Executive Order 13335, on June 3, 2008, ONC released the ONC-Coordinated Federal Health IT Strategic Plan: 2008–2012. Although the Strategic Framework was quite broad, encompassing both public and private sector initiatives, the Strategic Plan is more narrowly focused on specifically what federal government activities are necessary to achieve the technology infrastructure envision in the Executive Order. Certainly consistent with the Strategic Framework, the Strategic Plan has two primary goals. The goals and related objectives of the Strategic Plan are described in figure 17.5.

Figure 17.5. Goals and Objectives in the ONC-Coordinated Federal Health IT Strategic Plan: 2008–2012

Goal 1: *Patient-focused healthcare:* Enable the transformation to higher quality, more cost-efficient, patient-focused healthcare through electronic health information access and use by care providers, and by patients and their designees.

> *Objective 1.1—Privacy and Security:* Facilitate electronic exchange, access, and use of electronic health information while protecting the privacy and security of patients' health information
>
> *Objective 1.2—Interoperability:* Enable the movement of electronic health information to where and when it is needed to support individual health and care needs
>
> *Objective 1.3 – Adoption:* Promote nationwide deployment of EHRs and PHRs that put information to use in support of health and care
>
> *Objective 1.4—Collaborative Governance:* Establish mechanisms for multistakeholder priority-setting and decision-making to guide development of the nation's health IT infrastructure

Goal 2: *Population health:* Enable the appropriate, authorized, and timely access and use of electronic health information to benefit public health, biomedical research, quality improvement, and emergency preparedness.

> *Objective 2.1—Privacy and Security:* Advance privacy and security policies, principles, procedures, and protections for information access and use in population health
>
> *Objective 2.2—Interoperability:* Enable the mobility of health information to support population-oriented uses
>
> *Objective 2.3—Adoption:* Promote nationwide adoption of technologies and technical functions that will improve population and individual health
>
> *Objective 2.4—Collaborative Governance:* Establish coordinated organizational processes supporting information use for population health

Data Source: Marc Overhage, MD, PhD, Indiana Health Information Exchange, MAeHC-20Mar05.
Illustration: Copyright © 2008, Margret\A Consulting, LLC. Reprinted with permission of author.

Health Information Exchange Organizations

A major tenet of the Framework for Strategic Action and the Strategic Plan is the need for formal efforts for HIE through the creation of organizations that would enable such activity.

HIE Terminology

As with EHR and EMR, terms associated with HIE have different meanings to different people. The National Alliance for Health Information Technology (Alliance) was tasked by ONC to develop consensus definitions for terms associated with HIE and their definitions for network terms are illustrated in figure 17.6.

It is observed that these terms are somewhat inconsistent with terms used by ONC. ONC (2007) describes a HIE as "an entity that enables the movement of health related data among entities within a state, a region, or a non-jurisdictional participant group." In order to ensure proper understanding and in an effort to be both as generic as possible as well as to be consistent with consensus process, this chapter uses the term **health information exchange** (HIE) to refer to the generic exchange of data as defined by the Alliance, and uses the term **HIE organization** to refer to any entity that has been organized for the purpose of overseeing and governing the exchange of health-related information among

Figure 17.6.   Network Terminology from The National Alliance for Health Information Technology

> **Health Information Exchange (HIE)**: The electronic movement of health-related information among organizations according to nationally recognized standards
>
> **Health Information Organization**: An organization that oversees and governs the exchange of health-related information among organizations according to nationally recognized standards
>
> **Regional Health Information Organization (RHIO)**: A health information organization that brings together healthcare stakeholders within a defined geographic area and governs HIE among them for the purpose of improving health and care in that community

organizations according to nationally recognized standards, including organizations called local health information organizations (LHIO), regional health information organizations (RHIO), connected communities, or any other such term.

Another concept ONC identifies is a **health information service provider** (HSP). This is a company or other organization that supports one or more HIE organizations by providing them with operational and technical health exchange services.

HIE Organization Goals and Governance

HIE organizations are forming all over the country. The eHealth Initiative, a non-profit organization with a mission to drive improvement in the quality, safety, and efficiency of healthcare through information and information technology, tracks funding of HIE organizations and has identified 130 active and five "dropped" organizations that closely align with the definitions identified earlier. The Healthcare Information Management and Systems Society (HIMSS) also tracks HIE organizational activity, but considers HIE organizations from a much broader perspective, including, for example, statewide immunization registries as a form of HIE organization. In 2008, the HIMSS State Dashboard identified 390 active HIE organizations, 120 that had "expired," and 94 that were being proposed.

Irrespective of the actual numbers, the fact there is such a wide discrepancy in numbers and that several HIE organizations have already stopped functioning is telling: this is as yet an immature activity. The federal government, as well as private sector, provider organizations (especially provider organizations), has put a lot of money into nurturing HIE organizations. They differ widely in their goals, governance, and financial structures.

Some of the earliest and most financially viable HIE organizations focused their goals on aiding the exchange of the HIPAA financial and administrative transactions (for example, claims processing, eligibility verification). The New England Healthcare EDI Network (NEHEN) and Utah Health Information Network (UHIN) are examples. Others that are also well established are more a spin-off of the integrated delivery network, but without common ownership. For example, the Indiana Health Information Exchange (IHIE) has been in existence for many years, exchanging data within the Indianapolis community of providers. The Massachusetts Simplifying Healthcare Among Regional Entities Initiative (MA-Share) is another example of a long-standing organization operated by the Massachusetts Health Data Consortium and focused their goals on supporting specific HIE projects, such as sharing data among emergency departments and forming an e-prescribing gateway.

Many of the newer HIE organizations are heavily funded by grants from the federal government. Those that are most successful appear to be focused on meeting specific HIE

Figure 17.7.   HIE architectural models

HIE MODEL	ILLUSTRATION
• **Consolidated:** multiple independent enterprises agree to share resources using a central repository	
• **Federated:** – **Consistent datases**: multiple independent enterprises agree to connect and share specific information **managed centrally** but with **independent repositories**	
– **Inconsistent datases**: multiple independent enterprises agree to connect and share specific information in a **point-to-point** manner	
• **Switch:** a service that enables the exchange of information across multiple independent enterprises that have unilateral agreements to exchange data and in which there is no access to personal health information	
• **Patient managed:** patients "carry" their own electronic records or subscribe to a service that enables the patient to direct exchange of data	
• **Hybrid:** (not illustrated) combination of any of these models	

Data Source: Marc Overhage, MD, PhD, Indiana Health Information Exchange, MAeHC-20Mar05.

Illustration: Copyright (c) 2008, Margret\A Consulting, LLC. Reprinted with permission of author.

needs between hospitals and physician offices—enabling access to patient demographic data, laboratory results, etc. In fact, the more successful HIE organizations seem to be homogeneous (that is, composed primarily of providers, rather than a mix of providers, health plans, employers, etc.) and highly focused on a narrow band of functionality administered through a fairly simple technological infrastructure (for example, provider portal). Those HIE organizations that have attempted to be broader in scope and provide "all things to all people" are struggling more to identify a sustainable business model.

HIE Architectures

In addition to defining their goals and governance models, HIE organizations also need to find the technical architecture that will best serve them. Overhage (2005) has proposed that there are five possible architectural models, one of which has two "flavors." These models and an illustration of how they work are provided in figure 17.7.

Consolidated Model

The earlier HIE organizations have tended to be of the consolidated architectural type. In this model, data are contributed to a central data repository and managed centrally. In most cases, however, the data repository was more like a data warehouse, with independent data vaults. Much like a bank managing its safe deposit boxes, access to the data was highly controlled. Because of the centralized management, strong security controls were applied—and accepted by the users.

Federated Models

Today, largely due to the perception and concerns by the general public that a centrally managed structure is less private and secure for their data, the consolidated model has fallen out of favor and the federated model is becoming more prevalent. Interestingly, however, two forms of federated model have come into existence, with the "consistent database" model being essentially the same as the consolidated model of data being stored in separate data vaults, yet still centrally managed. Still, many HIE organizations are attempting to utilize the inconsistent database approach—both for privacy and because they believe it will reduce the start-up costs of centralizing on a common database structure. The result is essentially a centrally managed point-to-point network.

Hybrid Model

In many HIE organizations there is a hybrid of both consolidated and federated approaches, simply because some existing infrastructure of one type or another already exists and additional HIE services are added to that structure.

Switch Model

The switch form of HIE organization is one in which there is no access by the switch to the information exchanged. As a form of HIE organization, the switch would be the most private and secure; however, as most HIE organizations are finding, it is virtually impossible today to exchange data without having some access to the information exchanged in some cases. The e-prescribing state of affairs is a good example of this.

E-prescribing could almost be considered a special type of nationwide health information network. There is one primary vendor (SureScripts/RxHub) that is capable of supplying network connectivity (it calls an e-prescribing gateway) across almost all physicians and retail pharmacies. Each physician who wants to exchange prescription transactions is certified for use of the gateway. Part of the certification process is to prove identity, supply DEA information, and agree to abide by the requirements for privacy and security. Ideally, the physician would have an e-prescribing application (which may be a part of an EHR or a standalone system) that would generate a prescription transaction that has been standardized by the National Council for Prescription Drug Programs (NCPDP). This then would be transmitted, through the secure gateway, to the retail pharmacy, which would have a pharmacy information system that can accept NCPDP standard transactions. The prescription transaction would then flow directly into the retail pharmacy's pharmacy information system and enable dispensing of the drug to the consumer. E-prescribing also enables electronic refill and renewal processing and other useful prescribing-related transactions. However, the NCPDP standard has undergone various revisions over the years and any given physician or pharmacy may use a system that has a version that is different than someone else's. In addition, not every physician and retail pharmacy has the capability to accept such a transaction yet. One of the functions, then, of the e-prescribing gateway is to convert the transaction to a version compatible with the sender's or receiver's system or even to convert it to a fax, as applicable. Although the conversion process is automated, it is conceivable that a human would have to intervene in some cases to ensure that the conversion is correct or a fax might be returned for some reason. Hence, the need to access the information in the transaction negates the fact that the e-prescribing gateway could be considered a switch, which is intended to not ever have access to any information it exchanges.

Although this may seem like a long-winded description about something that largely does not exist, the details are important to understand—both from the perspective of understanding how e-prescribing works as well as to appreciate the level of concern there is surrounding the privacy and security of HIE.

Patient-Managed Model

The patient-managed architecture is a special case of either one of the federated models or the hybrid model. This is discussed further in chapter 18.

HIE Services

Although there are potentially many services that an HIE organization can provide, those which are basic, or fundamental, to enabling data sharing among disparate organizations generally relate to the ability to identify the individual about whom information is sought, find where that information may be located, ensure that only authorized entities or systems have access to the data sought in accordance with the individual's consent, and send the data in a secure manner that is logged and auditable.

Registry and Directory Services

For whatever architecture an HIE organization may have, there needs to be a way to identify participants, which may include individual providers, representatives of payer organizations, and patients/consumers, as well as organizational entities and their information systems. It is highly likely that some of the data to be exchanged across an HIE will not be triggered only by a person but by the availability of data. For example, lab results may not only be specifically requested by a provider, but returned directly to a provider's information system when they become available after an order has been placed. A registry service would register all users, systems, etc. and keep an index, or directory, of who they are. This is more than a master person index, as it must serve an entire HIE organization, and may, itself, be a system of registries or federated directories.

Person Identification

Because the U.S. Congress has prohibited the development or funding by the federal government of a unique patient identifier (at least until such time as federal privacy legislation is passed), ensuring that the HIE organization can identify the right patient as it seeks to exchange information is a process of identity matching. This process can be anything from a basic comparison of data elements using an exact match of demographic information (for a very small, stable environment) to the use of sophisticated mathematical or statistical algorithms (as in most HIE environments).

Figure 17.8.   Record Locator Service (RLS) process

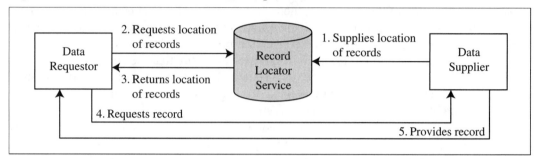

Record Locator Service

Once an individual's identity is confirmed, the HIE organization must next locate where there may be information. A **record locator service** (RLS) is used for this purpose. It is essentially a series of pointers. In a consolidated HIE architecture, all individuals (users and patients) as well as all inbound data could be assigned an internal identifier that would then operate much as a master person index. However, in the federated model, there must be the ability to identify the individual (user and patient) but where information may be located. Figure 17.8 illustrates how a RLS would operate in a federated HIE.

Identity Management

Identity management is a process that operates to ensure individuals who have been identified are who they say they are, that they have authority to do what they want to do, and that their actions are tracked. This process is essentially the typical security functions of authorization, authentication, access control, and audit control.

In distinguishing between **person identification** and **identity management**, it should be noted that there is a difference between identify and identity. *Identify* is an action, in which you determine who people are and perhaps assign them an identifier for future reference. *Identity* is a status. It is proof of who a person is, and in the case of HIE, what they may do.

Consent Management

As part of ensuring you have the right person, right location, and right record, identity management provides the assurance of right authority to access the HIE network and its functions. However, a special case of authority is being adopted by most HIE organizations. This is consent management, where not only is a user authorized to have specific access, but the individual patient/consumer has the authority to provide specific consent directives. Hence, Dr. Smith may be authorized to use an HIE network, has authenticated himself or herself to the network, and is granted access to clinical data where there is an identified treatment relationship with the individual. However, Mary Jones the patient may provide specific consent directives that indicate that Dr. Smith may access all of her medical but not genetic information, and only if Mary is in the emergency department of a hospital.

The basic forms of consent directives include opt-in and opt-out:

- *Opt-in*: Data may not be exchanged by default unless the individual consents

- *Opt-out*: Data may be exchanged by default unless restricted by the individual

Although these basic forms of consent directive appear simple to deploy, they actually are not, and in many cases, individuals appear to have a preference for a "quilted" form of consent, where a subset of data can be exchanged with individual consent based on institution, data user, data producer, and situation, such as in the example of Dr. Smith and Mary Jones. However, having made this observation, most HIE organizations still are able only to manage an all or nothing (all opt-in or all opt-out) consent management process; many are deciding on an opt-out structure exclusively.

Secure Data Transport

Obviously, a basic service provided by an HIE organization must be the actual transmission of the data. This is the technical networking service that provides appropriate bandwidth, latency, availability, ubiquity, and security.

Advanced Services

More advanced services are those that enhance utility of the HIE organization and provide greater benefits for participants. Depending on its business model, an HIE may decide to provide basic services to all participants and generate its revenue to sustain provision of those basic services through more advanced, special services. One service some HIE organizations is providing is more sophisticated data exchange, where they may provide vocabulary mapping, data extraction, and data quality management. Deidentification and data aggregation services of various types are fairly common. Data warehousing and analytics may be offered. Add-on lines of business might include billing and clearinghouse services, transcription, coding/revenue cycle management, EHR hosting, public health surveillance, and many others.

HIE Organizational Agreements

Finally, all of the above services would be described in a formal **HIE data sharing agreement** and/or **HIE participation agreement**. This would spell out in detail who the participants are, what services the organization will provide, how the organization will be architected, how the organization will be funded, and address other legal matters of ownership, liability, risk mitigation, and so on.

Data Stewardship

As suggested by the description of basic services, HIE has its own "five rights," much like for medication management or EHR. For HIE, the five rights might include right user (person, entity, system, or patient/consumer), right location, right record, right authority, and right consent. Such "rights" might well be considered under the rubric of health data stewardship. **Stewardship**, in general, is personal responsibility for taking care of something one does not own. For example, a bank takes care of funds individuals put into savings accounts. **Data stewardship** has become an important function in corporate America—where management of the corporation's data assets is critical for competitive advantage. In healthcare, the American Medical Informatics Association (AMIA) (2007) has defined **health data stewardship** as encompassing "the responsibilities and accountabilities associated with managing, collecting, viewing, storing, sharing, disclosing, or otherwise making use of personal health information."

It should be observed that this definition extends beyond HIPAA's protected health information to **personal health information**, which includes health information that may be held by individuals themselves or in commercial PHR systems that are not subject to HIPAA.

However, even AMIA's definition may not encompass all the data stewardship responsibilities and accountabilities that are necessary to support value-driven healthcare. For example, as data for the National Hospital Quality Measures ("Core Measures") are collected and used to evaluate quality of care, provide pay-for-performance incentives, etc., there is a need not only to protect the privacy and security of those data, but to ensure the quality of the data and how well analytics are performed to draw conclusions about cost/quality. The general public has focused on privacy and security concerns. As the new data breach notification laws are being invoked, there is much more publicity surrounding loss, theft, or other breaches. However, there is nothing equivalent for ensuring that data are documented, collected, and used properly. The quality of the data and how well they are analyzed directly contributes to the knowledge that builds evidence-based guidelines. Data that do not adhere to a common data dictionary, are incomplete, or not interpreted correctly can have a deleterious effect on an individual's health. So, health data stewardship should do all the things AMIA defines, but there also needs to be respect for the data as "assets" that contribute to the well-being of individuals treated in the healthcare delivery system as well as the financial viability of the organizations established to provide such treatment.

In 2007, the ONC was interested in identifying steps to enhance protections for what it called "secondary uses" of health data as it increasingly worked with large pools of data, such as the Core Measures. In December 2007, the National Committee on Vital and Health Statistics (NCVHS) returned a set of recommendations, including that the term "secondary use" should not be used to describe the full range of uses of health data, as such terminology was believed to promote the idea that such uses were less important and potentially less in need of protection. NCVHS also called, again, for federal privacy legislation that would extend and enhance the requirements of HIPAA to all uses and users of personal health information. Specific recommendations also were made relating to the attributes in table 17.2.

Benefits and Challenges of HIE

Data stewardship is different than being a **record custodian**, who has responsibility for ensuring proper record management and being able to attest to the fact that compilation of the records occurred in the normal course of business. Data stewardship is not limited to one person, group of people, or department in an organization, but is the responsibility of all users for all uses. Without good data stewardship, the benefits of any health data collection will not accrue beyond merely documentary evidence of care delivered. Certainly there are many more benefits for patient safety, quality, productivity, cost, research, and education. These can be enhanced further as HIE ensures data are available across the continuum of care; can be easily and accurately compiled for quality measurement, reporting, and improvement; and clinical and population research and disease prevention and control are aided by access to more timely and complete information.

HIE Benefits

Benefits of HIE are cited for patients, providers, consumer, and payers, and include:

- Savings, with research projecting savings to the U.S. economy of $78 billion (Walker 2003)

Table 17.2.   NCVHS Health Data Stewardship

Data Stewardship Attributes	Summary of Recommendations
Accountability/Chain of Trust	Heighten attention on how business associates and their agents use health information, either in identifiable or deidentified form
Transparency	Achieve greater clarity in notices of privacy practices and other documents required for use in exchange of data
Individual Participation	Utilize HIPAA requirements for authorizations and consent appropriately, and ensure that the Federal Trade Commission exercises its authority over non-HIPAA covered entities in their use of privacy notices
HIPAA Deidentification	Utilize the safe harbor or statistical process required by HIPAA to ensure proper deidentification of health information
Security Safeguards and Controls	Apply fully the HIPAA Security Rule requirements, especially with respect to auditing access logs, recognizing increased risk in an HIE and NHIN environment
Data Quality and Integrity	Apply principles of data quality and integrity to ensure precision, accuracy, reliability, completeness, and meaning to data collected
Oversight of Data Uses	Consider applying a joint oversight to uses of data for quality and research, as these uses blend into one another, yet have significantly different data protection requirements

Source: NCVHS, Enhanced Protections for Uses of health Data: A Stewardship Framework for "Secondary Uses" of Electronically Collected and Transmitted Health Data, December 2007.

- Cost containment by an estimated 8 percent to 20 percent of current spending (Middleton 2006)

- Better outcomes, through shared access to patient records letting providers spot warning signs faster to provide appropriate treatments earlier

- Improved patient–caregiver relations, through systems consistency, time savings, and bolstered credibility in caregiver services

- Streamlined workflow, with less time spent on administrative tasks

- Positive perception, where hospitals and providers are perceived by consumers to be actively working to improve the health and well-being of the community (Scalise 2005)

From the individual provider perspective, physicians involved in several of the HIE initiatives identify the ability to:

- Save time by alerting the provider to tests and procedures that other physicians have already ordered or performed on patients

- Make physicians aware of other physicians who are treating their patients, helping catch patients who may be "shopping" for controlled substances

- Have a complete drug list available for each patient to find out what medications new patients are taking and how frequently current patients are refilling their prescriptions so coaching can be provided to enhance compliance

- Access results from anywhere and view them online as needed

- Communicate more quickly and easily between physicians and hospitals (Terry 2005)

HIE Challenges

HIE organizations, however, are not without their skeptics. Some in the healthcare industry remember the failed attempts of community health information networks (CHINs), which were popular in the mid-1990s. CHINs attempted to link and exchange health information at a local level. Many believed they did not succeed because of funding and business issues. However, HIE organizations are seen as having some major advantages over their CHIN predecessors. HIEs are being promoted by the federal government both through planning and implementation grants as well as a solid national agenda focusing on value—combining both cost and quality. In addition, HIPAA, state attention to data protections, and better tools for using Internet technology contribute to a more solid infrastructure.

Molly J. Coye, MD and CEO and founder of the Health Technology Center, a nonprofit research and education organization, in discussing RHIOs is quoted as noting that "nationally, the principal barrier to RHIOs isn't technology; it's the absence of trust and a shared sense that the effort is worth the cost" (Terry 2006). Most agree that creating an HIE organization is a massive undertaking, partly because it requires competitors to cooperate. If done well, there can be great success. The Indiana Health Information Exchange worked for many years, long before CHINs, RHIOs, or other forms of HIE organizations were identified, to work together for the betterment of their community. Terry (2005) reports that it took Cincinnati health systems 7 years to form HealthBridge and then another 6 years for a significant number of area physicians to start using the network's Web portal. However, one can also point to the Santa Barbara County Care Data Exchange failure as an example of how it is essential to get the business rules for working together ironed out. Despite that, Dr. Brailer hailed from the Santa Barbara project, this HIE organization ultimately ran out of money, many saying because providers were unwilling to subscribe to an HIE service that had set up such barriers to exchanging data that providers literally could only view but not download data needed for patient care.

Hallmarks of HIE Success

The eHealth Initiative has identified the following characteristics they believe afford the greatest degree of success for state, regional, or community HIE organizations:

- Governed by a diverse and broad set of stakeholders within the region or community

- Develop and ensure adherence to a common set of principles and standards for the technical and policy aspects of information sharing, addressing the needs of every stakeholder

- Develop and implement a technical infrastructure based on national standards to facility interoperability

- Develop and maintain a model for sustainability that aligns the costs with the benefits related to HIE

- Use metrics to measure performance from the perspective of patient care, public health, provider value, and economic value (eHealth Initiative 2005)

Nationwide Health Information Network

In furtherance of interoperability, ONC's Framework for Strategic Action and Strategic Plan also described a nationwide "utility" or public infrastructure that would link disparate healthcare information systems together to allow patients, physicians, hospitals, public health agencies, and other authorized users across the nation to share clinical information in real time under stringent security, privacy, and other protections.

National Health Information Infrastructure

The NCVHS, as the nation's statutory advisory committee to HHS, first envisioned a **national health information infrastructure** (NHII) that would bring timely health information to, and aid communication among, those making health decisions for themselves, their families, their patients, and their communities. Figures 17.9 through 17.14 are scenarios described in the NCVHS report (NCVHS 2001), and continue to be valid scenarios for use of what the federal government currently is referring to as a **nationwide health information network** (NHIN). The scenarios illustrate the various stakeholders and arrays of information and knowledge that should be available, when needed, to make the best possible health decisions.

Figure 17.9.   Avoiding unnecessary care, cost, and anxiety through NHII

Scenario: Mr. S. flies across the country to start a new job. He has already chosen a medical practice in his new town because it has the same online health support service as his previous doctor, even though it is a different medical plan. He can set up appointments, get prescription refills and lab results, e-mail the doctor or nurses, and manage his personal health history. A week after he arrives, he develops fever and muscle aches. Fearing that he may have anthrax or smallpox, he e-mails his doctor a list of his symptoms, along with his itinerary over the previous 14 days. The doctor's automatic system immediately matches his itinerary against the public health database of anthrax and smallpox occurrences and runs his symptoms against his own personal health record, including his medications. It sends an urgent alert to the doctor, who sees no likely source of exposure for Mr. S., but spots a potential drug–drug interaction. She calls him and tells him that the new drug he just started could have caused an adverse reaction. She feels confident that he does not need to come in for tests or take unnecessary antibiotics. Instead, she changes his medication and asks him to e-mail her in 24 hours. The next day, his e-mail message confirms that his fever and aches are gone. Unnecessary lab tests, investigation by public health authorities, anxiety for Mr. S. and his family, and an unneeded antibiotic are all avoided. This "nonevent" is the happiest of all endings for Mr. S., his doctor, and the health of the public.

Figure 17.10.   Enhancing continuity of care and public health outreach through NHII

Scenario: Everyone benefits from automated vaccination records that are part of electronic personal health histories and medical records. Parents can track their children's immunizations over time, even if they see different physicians. Parents and doctors can receive automatic reminders when the next vaccination is due. Local vaccine reporting systems can aggregate anonymous patient data to show immunization rates by individual physician, practice group, and neighborhood. Public health officials can then compare local, state, and national rates, compare rates against CDC guidelines, and target areas for outreach and improvement.

Figure 17.11.   Avoiding adverse events through NHII

Scenario: Concerned about his persistent cough, Mr. A. visits his doctor, Dr. Z. At the end of the visit, Dr. Z. advises Mr. A. that she will transmit an electronic prescription to the pharmacy. Dr. Z. enters the medication choice in Mr. A.'s electronic medical record, which is integrated with a prescription alert system, and receives a warning that, after taking this same medication, some patients with similar health conditions have experienced adverse effects, such as a rash and muscle cramps. Dr. Z. substitutes a different medication that is equally effective, which Mr. A. can take without incident. Dr. Z's clinical practice management system also has received a general alert from the drug manufacturer to avoid prescribing Dr. Z.'s first medication choice to patients with certain health conditions. The system automatically reviews all patients' records, finds no others currently taking the medications, and updates its internal drug review program.

Figure 17.12.   Upgrading public health resources for the identification of bioterrorist threats through the NHII

Scenario: The Illinois Department of Public Health (IDPH) is notified of a credible threat that plague bacteria may be used in an act of bioterrorism. The IDPH sends out an alert through the Health Alert Network (HAN) to all local health departments. In addition, a similar alert is sent to all hospitals and emergency departments. The signs and symptoms of all forms of plague are incorporated into a software object that is then downloaded to the clinical information systems of clinicians throughout the state. Dr. T.'s system identifies two patients with a matching clinical profile in his practice. After approval by Dr. T., the system notifies the two patients by phone and their home health information system. They agree to come in later that day. That morning Dr. T. sees a patient who appears to have pneumonia and is coughing up blood. He prepares to send the patient to the hospital for x-rays and cultures when his office information systems warn him that this patient's symptoms fit the recently updated public health surveillance profile. He forwards a notice to the public health department and sends the patient to the hospital for further evaluation. The public health laboratory assists in making the diagnosis of a common pneumonia. Patterns of reports by Dr. T. and other physicians are monitored by IDPH as they continue to be alert to a potential terrorist attack.

Figure 17.13.   Improving individuals' ability to self-manage chronic conditions through NHII

Scenario: With the help of a multimedia home information center, a 50-year-old mother, Mrs. M., manages her family's health. She receives automatic alerts and e-mails from her own doctors and her daughter's, and she also receives health information tailored to her specifications. For example, the last time her daughter had an asthma attack, Mrs. M. was able to e-mail information about her daughter's condition to the physician, receive advice within 2 hours, and avoid a trip to the emergency room. Because Mrs. M. is an authorized user for her dad's personal health information manager, she and her father, who lives far away and has emphysema, are alerted simultaneously when the air quality index in his community shows high levels of pollution. Her father also has a voice-activated medication reminder service that he accesses from the information appliance in his kitchen. The reminder service tells him which pills to take when, and he confirms that he has taken the pills as directed. His daughter also can see whether he is taking his medications correctly. The medication reminder service also tracks the need for refills and automatically sends a refill request, as needed, to the mail-order prescription service.

Figure 17.14.   Responding rapidly to individual emergencies and local public health threats through NHII

Scenario: Sixty-six-year-old Mrs. F. and her sister are camping in a national park. While hiking, she experiences severe stomach and chest pains. She activates her wireless automated medical alert system, which includes a global positioning system. It alerts the closest emergency medical team, which arrives quickly. Simultaneously, Mrs. F.'s own cardiologist, Dr. Y., in another state receives the same alert. The emergency team, which has standing position to access relevant medical history in patients' online records, rushes Mrs. F. to the closest emergency room. All the necessary patient information is available to Dr. X., the physician on duty in the emergency room, when Mrs. F. arrives. After a thorough examination and tests and online consultation with Dr. Y., Dr. X determines that Mrs. F. probably has gastroenteritis, advises her to drink lots of fluids, and clears her to return to her camping trip. Mrs. F.'s electronic personal health history and medical record are simultaneously updated with the information from the emergency room visit. Dr. Y., the cardiologist, is notified that Mrs. F.'s emergency room visit is added to its database on incidents in local parks. That afternoon, health department staff identify a broken sewer line that contaminated park drinking water and caused the outbreak of bacterial gastroenteritis.

NCVHS envisioned three dimensions to the NHII. As illustrated in figure 17.15, these include the healthcare provider dimension, population health dimension, and personal health dimension. The healthcare provider dimension is, in essence, the EHR. The population health dimension refers to the health statistics reported to states and the Centers for Disease Control and Prevention (CDC). This could also include various registries for which participation is often required by state law or in which many healthcare organizations participate voluntarily. The personal health dimension of the NHII describes use of the Internet for information searching, social support, e-mail, health assessments, and other elements of personal health management, including PHRs.

Figure 17.15.   Dimensions of the NHII

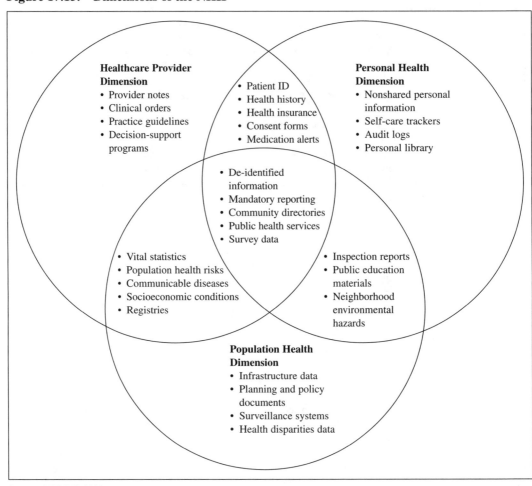

Source: NCVHS 2001.

Nationwide Health Information Network

The NHII serves as a conceptual model for achieving a nationwide health information net-work (NHIN). As such, the ONC released a request for information (RFI) in November 2004, that sought public comment regarding how widespread interoperability of health information technologies and health information exchange can be achieved through a NHIN. Five hundred and twelve organizations representing a cross-section of the industry as well as individuals submitted responses that yielded one of the richest and most descriptive collection of thoughts on interoperability and HIE that has likely ever been assembled in the U.S. Among the many opinions expressed, the following concepts emerged from most of the RFI respondents:

- A NHIN should be a decentralized architecture built using the Internet linked by uni-form communications and a software framework of open standards and policies.

- A NHIN should reflect the interests of all stakeholders and be a joint public–private effort.

- A governance entity composed of public and private stakeholders should oversee the determination of standards and policies.

- A NHIN should be patient-centric with sufficient safeguards to protect the privacy of personal health information.

- Incentives will be needed to accelerate deployment and adoption of a NHIN.

- Existing technologies, federal leadership, prototype regional exchange efforts, and certification of EHRs will be the critical enablers of a NHIN.

- Key challenges will be the need for additional and better-refined standards; addressing privacy concerns; paying for the development and operation of, and access to, the NHIN; accurately matching patients; and addressing discordant interstate and intrastate laws regarding HIE.

Subsequent NHIN Activities

As a result of the findings from the NHIN RFI, the HHS provided supplementary funding to advance nationwide interoperable HIT standards harmonization, compliance certification, and privacy and security solutions (HHS 2005b); created the American Health Information Community (AHIC); and awarded contracts for NHIN prototype development and trial implementations.

Healthcare Information Technology Standards Panel (HITSP)

The American National Standards Institute (ANSI), the nonprofit organization that administers and coordinates the U.S. voluntary standardization activities, was awarded a contract to convene the Healthcare Information Technology Standards Panel (HITSP), which would bring U.S. standards developers and other stakeholders together to develop, prototype, and evaluate a harmonization process for achieving a widely accepted and useful set of HIT standards that will support interoperability among healthcare software applications, particularly EHRs, and to advance the ability to achieve the NHIN. HITSP has subsequently developed interoperability specifications for NHIN use cases identified by the AHIC. The federal government has begun formally recognizing these standards for adoption by federal agencies now and ultimately for use in the NHIN (Executive Order 13410, 2006).

Certification Commission for Health Information Technology (CCHIT)

The Certification Commission for Health Information Technology (CCHIT), created by the American Health Information Management Association (AHIMA), Healthcare Information and Management Systems Society (HIMSS), and The Alliance (NAHIT), was awarded a contract to develop criteria and evaluation processes for certifying EHRs and the infrastructure or network components through which they interoperate. CCHIT currently continues to expand its EHR certification to specialty domains, applying greater sophistication in inspection and testing of products, and enhancing its outreach and communication services.

Health Information Security and Privacy Collaboration (HISPC)

The Health Information Security and Privacy Collaboration (HISPC) was a partnership consisting of a multidisciplinary team of experts and the National Governor's Association (NGA). It worked with approximately 40 states and territorial governments to assess and develop plans to address variations in organization-level business policies and state laws that affect privacy and security practices that could pose challenges to interoperable health information exchange. RTI International, a private, nonprofit corporation, was awarded the contract to provide oversight for this activity. The result has been a significant rise in state legislative initiatives relating to HIT and HIE.

American Health Information Community (AHIC)

The AHIC was chartered as a federal advisory body in 2005, to make recommendations to the Secretary of the U.S. Department of Health and Human Services (HHS) on how to accelerate the development and adoption of health information technology.

Since its formation, the AHIC identified four initial areas with potential for early breakthroughs in the advancement of standards that will lead to interoperability. These breakthrough areas included:

- *Consumer Empowerment*: Make available a consumer-directed and secure electronic record of healthcare registration information and a medication history for patients.

- *Chronic Care*: Allow the widespread use of secure messaging, as appropriate, as a means of communication between doctors and patients about care delivery.

- *Biosurveillance*: Enable the transfer of standardized and anonymized health data from the point of healthcare delivery to authorized public health agencies within 24 hours of its collection.

- *EHRs*: Create an EHR that includes laboratory results and interpretations that is standardized, widely available, and secure

Plans are now underway to establish a successor to the AHIC as a public-private partnership based in the private sector.

NHIN Prototypes

In addition to the efforts to advance nationwide interoperable HIT and advise on areas that could be impacted in the near term, contracts were also awarded in 2005, by HHS to four groups of healthcare and HIT organizations to develop prototypes for a NHIN architecture.

Each of the four consortia designed and implemented a standards-based network prototype to test identification and information locator services, user authentication, access control, and other security protections and specialized network functions, and the feasibility of large-scale deployment. A summary of the NHIN prototype architecture contracts was released in May 2007 by HHS. Results of the prototype projects validated that the underlying principles of the current approach to the development of a NHIN were feasible. Specifically that:

- The NHIN can be operated as a network of networks, without a central database or services

- Common standards for developing the NHIN, particularly in the way that component exchanges would interact with one another, were critical

- Synergies and important capabilities can be achieved by supporting consumers and healthcare providers on the same infrastructure

- Consumer controls can be implemented to manage how a consumer's information is shared on the network

- There can be benefits from an evolutionary approach that does not dictate wholesale replacement or modification of existing healthcare information systems.

NHIN Trial Implementations

To further the development of the NHIN, contracts were also awarded to nine broad-based state and regional HIE organizations to expand participation in testing and demonstration of NHIN core services (refer to figure 17.16). Subsequently cooperative agreements for additional participants were added in 2008.

Figure 17.16.   NHIN core service and capabilities

- **Data Services**
  - Secure data delivery
  - Data look-up, retrieval, and location registries
  - Notification of new or updated data
  - Subject-data matching
  - Summary patient record exchange
  - Data integrity and nonrepudiation checking
  - Audit logging and error handling
  - Support for secondary use of clinical data
  - Data anonymization and reidentification, as well as HIPAA deidentification

- **Consumer Services**
  - Management of consumer-identified locations for PHRs
  - Location requests and data routing
  - Consumer-controlled providers of care and access permissions
  - Consumer choice not to participate
  - Consumer access to audit logging and disclosure information for PHR and HIE data
  - Routing of consumer requests for data corrections

- **User and Subject Identity Management Services**
  - User identity proofing and/or attestation of third-party identity proofing
  - User authentication and/or attestation of third-party authentication for those connected through that HIE
  - Subject and user identity arbitration with like identities from other HIEs
  - User credentialing
  - Support of an HIE-level, nonredundant methodology for managed identities

- **Management Services**
  - Management of available capabilities and services information for connected users and other HIEs
  - HIE system security including perimeter protection, system management, and timely cross-HIE issue resolution
  - Temporary and permanent deauthorization of direct and third-party users when necessary
  - Emergency access capabilities to support appropriate individual and population emergency access needs

Source: U.S. Department of Health and Human Services, Summary of the NHIN Prototype Architecture Contracts, May 31, 2007

Sustaining the Momentum

Although much-needed emphasis and funding are currently being applied to EHR and HIE, there is always a concern about whether these initiatives will be sustained for a long enough period of time and with sufficient resources to truly make an impact. Of course, only time will tell for sure.

The ONC is responsible for coordinating all federal activities relating to HIT, including those outside HHS. Figure 17.17 lists the agencies and organizations and provides examples of some of their initiatives.

Conclusion

Clearly, much is planned and much is being accomplished at the federal government level. Community efforts also are starting to take hold. Hospital by hospital and physician by physician, EHRs and HIE are being adopted. As John Halamka (2005), chief information officer at Care-Group Healthcare System in Boston and chair of HITSP recently noted, "The challenges are not technical. They never are." The challenges, whether discussing matching and connecting patient records across unaffiliated organizations and disparate information systems or the broadest of broad NHIN, are organizational and people related. Building trust—across organizations and with patients that complete and accurate information will be available to provide the best possible healthcare with the strictest of privacy controls—is the essential element in EHR and HIE.

Figure 17.17.   Federal HIT Initiatives

- Department of Health and Human Services (HHS) guides the development of standards for health IT systems that will improve patient care and increase efficiency across the healthcare system. HHS, through several of its agencies, also provides funding to organizations engaged in building and testing health IT systems, standards, and projects.

- American Health Information Community (AHIC) is a federal advisory body, chartered to make recommendations to the Secretary of HHS on how to accelerate the development and adoption of Health IT. The AHIC pursues breakthroughs that will produce tangible value to the healthcare consumer in the near term, while building toward long-term goals for a broad and robust system.

- Office of the National Coordinator for Health Information Technology (ONC) provides leadership for the development and implementation of a nationwide health IT infrastructure allowing secure and seamless exchange of data and records. The ONC advises the Secretary of HHS on health IT policies and initiatives, and coordinates the Department's efforts to meet the President's goal of making an electronic medical record available for most Americans by 2014.

- Federal Health Architecture (FHA) was established as an eGov Line of Business in response to The President's Management Agenda calling for increased efficiency and effectiveness in government operations. The FHA is responsible for leveraging federal expertise in creating a federal framework that would be derived from a national health IT infrastructure, supporting federal activities in the development and adoption of health IT standards, and ensuring that federal agencies can seamlessly exchange health data between and among themselves, with state, local, and tribal governments, and with private sector healthcare organizations.

(continued)

Figure 17.17.   (Continued)

- Agency for Healthcare Research and Quality (AHRQ) funds HIT research and development with $166 million in grants and contracts. This money is awarded to programs across the country to support and stimulate investment in health IT, especially in rural and underserved areas. AHRQ also created the National Resource Center for Health Information Technology, which provides technical assistance and shares knowledge and findings that have the potential to transform everyday clinical practice.

- Health Resources and Services Administration (HRSA) promotes the widespread availability and use of health IT and telehealth to meet the needs of people who are uninsured, underserved, or have special needs. HRSA provides technical assistance to health centers and other HRSA grantees in adopting model practices and technologies; promotes grantee health IT advances and innovations as models; and ensures that HRSA health IT policy and programs are coordinated with those of other HHS components.

- Indian Health Services (IHS) provides care for nearly two million American Indians and Alaska natives across the United States. For three decades, the IHS has been at the forefront of health IT utilization. The IHS captures clinical and public health data using the Resource and Patient Management System (RPMS). The RPMS EHR allows providers to manage all aspects of patient care electronically, starting before the patient is ever seen and continuing through follow-up care. The IHS continues to develop its electronic systems to provide greater service and convenience to all those in the system.

- National Institutes of Health (NIH), through the National Library of Medicine (NLM), hosts an online medical database that provides up-to-date information to consumers and healthcare professionals. Called MedlinePlus, the database is free to use, provides extensive information about drugs, an illustrated medical encyclopedia, interactive patient tutorials, and the latest health news.

- Centers for Medicaid and Medicare Services (CMS)—CMS's new EHR demonstration is designed to show that widespread adoption and use of interoperable EHRs will reduce medical errors and improve the quality of care for an estimated 3.6 million consumers. Over a 5-year period, the project will provide financial incentives to as many as 1,200 physician practices that use certified EHRs to improve quality as measured by their performance on specific clinical quality measures. Additional bonus payments will be available, based on a standardized survey measuring the number of EHR functionalities a physician practice has incorporated. To further amplify the effect of this demonstration project, CMS is encouraging private and public payers to offer similar financial incentives consistent with applicable law.

- Department of Defense (DoD)—Currently, thousands of military medical providers use the DoD's EHR system, AHLTA, and nearly 300,000 outpatient visits are captured digitally every week. DoD's vision is to provide each patient with a continuously updated digital medical record from the point of injury or care on the battlefield to discharge from military clinics and hospitals in the United States. These records would be completely transferable electronically to the Veterans Health Administration as part of the Joint Patient Electronic Health Record (JPEHR).

- Veterans Health Administration (VHA) is a division of the U.S. Department of Veterans Affairs, and provides care for more than five million veterans of the United States Armed Services. The VHA's EHR system, My HealtheVet, allows patients to refill prescriptions online, and provides access to health information, links to Federal and VA benefits and resources, and the patient's Personal Health Journal. The VHA continues to add capabilities to My HealtheVet, to empower consumers to take a more active role in managing their health and healthcare.

Source: www.hhs.gov/healthit/initiatives, 2008.

References and Resources

Anderson, G.F., et al. 2006. Health care spending and use of information technology in OECD countries. *Health Affairs* 25(3): 819–831.

Anderson, G.F., et al. 2005. Health spending in the United States and the rest of the industrialized world. *Health Affairs* 24(4): 903–914.

Benner, E.S., and J. Moss. 2005. Informatics challenges for the impending patient information explosion. *Journal of the American Medical Informatics Association* 12(6):614–617.

Blair, R. 2005 (July). Strategy-driven growth. *Health Management Technology*, 20–22.

Centers for Medicare and Medicaid Services, National Health Expenditure Data, 2008.

Centers for Medicare and Medicaid Services, Specifications Manual for National Hospital Quality Measures, Version 2.3, 2008. https://www.qualitynet.org/dcs/ContentServer?cid=1141662756099&pagename=Qnet Public%2FPage%2FQnetTier2&c=Page.

Central Intelligence Agency. *The World Factbook.* 2008. https://www.cia.gov/library/publications/the-world-factbook.

Connecting for Health. 2005. The collaborative response, appendix A: Glossary of key terms. New York: Markle Foundation. www.connectingforhealth.org/resources/collaborative_response/appendices/glossary.php.

eHealth Initiative. 2005. Connecting Communities Toolkit. www.toolkit.ehealthinitiative.org.

eHealth Initiative. 2005. Key findings from the eHI 2005 annual survey of state, regional and community-based health information exchange initiatives and organizations. Washington, DC: Foundation for eHealth Initiative. www.ehealthinitiative.org/keyhighlights.mspx.

e-HIM Work Group on Patient Identification in RHIOs. 2006. Surveying the RHIO Landscape: A Description of Current RHIO Models, with a Focus on Patient Identification. *Journal of AHIMA* 77,(1): 64A–D.

Executive Order 13410: Promoting quality and efficient health care in federal government administered or sponsored health care programs. George W. Bush. August 22, 2006.

Fuler, K.H. 2005. Paying for performance. *ADVANCE for Health Information Executives* 9(3):42–46.

Halamka, J., et al. 2005. Health care IT collaboration in Massachusetts: The experience in creating regional connectivity. *Journal of the American Medical Informatics Association* 12(6):596–601.

Health and Human Services Press Office. 2005a (Oct. 6). HHS awards contracts to advance nationwide interoperable health information technology.

Health and Human Services, Press Office. 2005b (Nov. 10). HHS awards contracts to develop nationwide health information network.

Health Information Technology Adoption Initiative. 2006. www.hitadoption.org.

Health on the Net Foundation. 2004. HON Code of Conduct. www.hon.ch/HONcode/Conduct/html.

Health Information Compliance Insider. 2005 (Oct.). Expect OCR to remain focused on voluntary compliance. Marblehead, MA: HCPro.

Health Information Management and Systems Society. 2005 (Feb. 13–17). Integrating the Healthcare Enterprise (IHE). Interoperability Showcases: Delivering Interoperability in the Real World. Presentation at HIMSS conference, Dallas, TX.

Institute of Medicine. 1991. *The Computer-based Patient Record: An Essential Technology for Health Care,* edited by R.S. Dick and E.B. Steen. Washington, DC: National Academies Press, 149–150.

Institute of Medicine Committee on the Consequences of Uninsurance, 2004. Insuring America's Health: Principles and Recommendations, Washington, DC: National Academy Press.

Kappel, M., and S. Bence. 2005. Creating CommunITy. *ADVANCE for Health Information Executives* 9(6):29–32.

Krohn, R. 2004. JHIM quick study: Healthcare business intelligence and real-time decision support systems. *Journal of Healthcare Information Management* 18(3):14–16.

Loonsk, J.W. 2007 (June 21). Nationwide health Information Network Health Information Exchange (NHIE) Services. Presentation of Office of National Coordinator for Health Information Technology to National Committee on Vital and Health Statistics.

Loonsk, J.W., et al. 2006. The public health information network (PHIN) preparedness initiative. *Journal of the American Medical Informatics Association* 13(1):1–4.

Massachusetts Medical Society, 2005 (Oct.). Transparency in Health Care Cost and Quality. http://www.massmed.org/AM/Template.cfm?Section=Home&CONTENTID=14449&TEMPLATE=/CM/ContentDisplay.cfm#265,10,Q.8. Would your referrals to physicians be influenced by the current quality or cost measurement programs? (n=408).

Middleton, B. 2006. Evaluating the value of healthcare information technology: finding the diamond in the rough and tumble. AMIA Annual Symposium Proceedings. 1172–1173.

National Alliance for Health Information Technology. 2008 (May). Defining Key Health Information Technology Terms. www.nahit.org.

National Alliance for Health Information Technology. 2005 (July 5). More than 35 major organizations endorse the healthcare interoperability definition crafted by the National Alliance for Health Information Technology. www.nahit.org/cms/index.php?option=com_content&task=view&id=69&Itemid=30.

National Committee on Vital and Health Statistics. 2007 (Dec.) Enhanced protections for uses of health data: A stewardship framework for "secondary uses" of electronically collected and transmitted health data. www.ncvhs.hhs.gov.

National Committee on Vital and Health Statistics. 2001. Information for health: A strategy for building the national health information infrastructure. www.ncvhs.hhs.gov.

Nolte E. and C.M. McKee, 2008. Measuring the health of nations: Updating an earlier analysis. *Health Affairs* 27(1).

Office of the National Coordinator. 2006. Directory of federal HIT programs. www.dhhs.gov/healthit/federalprojectlist.html.

Office of the National Coordinator. 2005a (Oct. 7). American health information community potential breakthroughs. www.hhs.gov/healthit/breakthroughs.pdf.

Office of the National Coordinator. 2005b (Feb. 18). President's vision for health IT. www.dhhs.gov/healthit/presvision.html.

Office of the National Coordinator. 2005c (June). Summary of nationwide health information network (NHIN) Request for information (RFI) responses. www.hhs.gov/healthit/rfisummaryreport.pdf.

Office of the National Coordinator. 2005d (May 23). Value of HIT. www.hhs.gov/healthit/valueHIT.html.

O'Kane, M.E. 2006 (Jan./Feb.). Emerging IT enablers: Physician practice connections. *Patient Safety & Quality Healthcare,* 22–23.

Overhage, J.M. 2005 (March 20). Indiana Health Information Exchange, MAeHC.

Overhage, J.M., L. Evans, and J. Marchibroda. 2005. Communities' readiness for health information exchange: The national landscape in 2004. *Journal of the American Medical Informatics Association* 12(2):107–112.

Rollins G. 2005. Matchmaking: An interview with John Halamka on linking patient records regionally. *Journal of American Health Information Management Association* 76(4):42–43.

Roman, M. 2006 (Jan./Feb.). Ensuring successful care management. *Physician Practice Connections: Patient Safety & Quality Healthcare,* 36–38.

Scalise, D. 2005 (July). A primer for building RHIOs. *H&HN,* special suppl.

Sirovich, B. et al. 2008. Discretionary Decision Making by Primary Care Physicians and the Cost of U.S. Health Care. *Health Affairs* 27(3): 813–823.

Terry, K. 2006 (Feb. 7). The rocky road to RHIOs. *The Connected Physician.* Special Technology Section, pp. TCP8–TCP12.

Terry, K. 2005. (Nov.). Why these doctors love their RHIO. *The Connected Physician* pp. 8–12.

Thomspon, T.G., and D.J. Brailer. 2004 (July 21). *The Decade of Health Information Technology: Delivering Consumer-centric and Information-rich Health Care—Framework for Strategic Action.* Washington, DC: HHS ONC.

U.S. Census Bureau. 2007 (August). Income, Poverty, and Health Insurance Coverage in the United States: 2006.

U.S. Department of Health and Human Services, Office of the National Coordinator for Health Information Technology, The ONC-Coordinated Federal health IT Strategic Plan: 2008–2012.

U.S. Department of Health and Human Services 2007 (May 31). Summary of the NHIN Prototype Architecture Contracts: A Report for the Office of the National Coordinator for Health Information Technology.

Walker, S. 2006. Evolution of evidence-based medicine. *Physician Practice Connections: Patient Safety & Quality Healthcare* 3(1):30–34.

Wolter, J., and B. Friedman. 2005. Health records for the people: Touring the benefits of the consumer-based personal health record. *Journal of AHIMA* 76(10):28–32.

World Health Organization, Core Health Indicators, 2005. www.who.int/whosis/database/core.

Wright, C., and J. Hunt. 2006. Beyond the electronic health record: Providence Medical Group's journey to cross the quality chasm. *Group Practice Journal* 55(1):13–19.

Chapter 18
Personal Health Records

The concept of the personal health record (PHR) is not new. One of the oldest and best-known forms of PHR is probably the Medic-Alert bracelet worn to alert good Samaritans and others that the wearer is diabetic and may be experiencing an event related to this illness. Many individuals have found it useful to keep track of health information for themselves or others, especially related to immunizations, medications, and response to treatment regimens in those with chronic illness. More recently, PHRs are starting to be integrated with electronic health records (EHRs) as well as sold as stand-alone products. The federal government has taken a keen interest in personal health records as a means to support consumer empowerment for its value-driven healthcare initiatives. Likewise, health insurers and employers also are interested in supporting PHRs for this reason. This chapter:

- Describes the impact of consumer empowerment on PHRs and their role in value-driven healthcare

- Discusses the current state of PHR utilization

- Identifies the attributes and functionality of PHRs and supporting standards requirements

- Identifies policies and practices that may aid in overcoming barriers and enable adoption of PHRs

Consumer Empowerment

Consumer empowerment is the investment of power or authority in those who purchase goods and services (Rollyson 2007). With the advent of social networking made possible by Web 2.0 technologies such as blogs, wikis, and podcasts and intermediaries such as Technorati, Wikipedia, You Tube, e-Bay, and LinkedIn, to help people connect and collaborating in by far greater numbers, worldwide. It is being recognized that such technology is

---

Key Terms

Consumer empowerment	Pharmacy benefits manager	Transparency
Cyberseal	Stand-alone	Value-driven healthcare
Health record bank	Tethered	

---

moving us from the Information Age to the Connected Age (Zelenka 2007) and creating an entire new Generation V. Members of the Generation Virtual are not defined by age, gender, social demographics or geography, but by a preference for conversation (rather than communication) using digital media channels for collaboration ("we" is more powerful than "me") in global communities (Prentice and Sarner 2008). As a result, a new market force is being created, which digitizes what has always been the most powerful determinant of customer relationships—word of mouth.

A movement as far reaching as consumer empowerment enhanced through Web technologies will ultimately reach healthcare, and, indeed, it has done so! Healthcare consumerism is a natural progression from consumerism in general.

Federal Government Initiatives

The federal government, especially, is seeking to take advantage of this movement. In its **Value-Driven Healthcare** initiative, the federal government (www.hhs.gov/valuedriven) observes that:

> "Consumers deserve to know the quality and cost of their healthcare. Healthcare **transparency** provides consumers with the information necessary, and the incentive, to choose healthcare providers based on value. Providing reliable cost and quality information empowers consumer choice. Consumer choice creates incentives at all levels, and motivates the entire system to provide better care for less money. Improvements will come as providers can see how their practice compares to others."

The federal government views the steps to transparency as including that:

- The federal government, individual private employers, and health plans commit to sharing information on price and quality in healthcare. Together, the government and major employers provide healthcare coverage for some 70 percent of Americans.

- The federal government and individual private employers commit to quality and price standards developed with the medical community. This will help guarantee a fair and accurate view of the quality of care delivered by individual providers, as well as providing consistent measures for quality.

- The federal government and individual private employers commit to standards for health information technology (IT). Health IT will be important for gathering and using the best information for consumers. These standards are also crucial to the goal of achieving EHRs for all Americans.

- The federal government and individual private employers commit to offering plans that reward consumers who exercise choice based on high quality of care and competitive price for healthcare services.

The federal government has followed through with the Centers for Medicare and Medicaid Services (CMS), offering a PHR to patients with Medicare Advantage or Medicare Part D coverage, through its www.mymedicare.gov site. CMS is also partnering with a group of health plans for a program designed to encourage Medicare beneficiaries to use PHRs. This program, whose participants include HIP USA, Humana, Kaiser Permanente, and the University of Pittsburgh Medical Center, will run as a pilot, for 18 months, in which CMS will collect data to get a sense of how consumers use PHRs. With the data in hand, CMS will then pick out which features it likes best. CMS also will use study data to design outreach and education efforts intended to boost PHR use.

The Department of Veterans Affairs (VA) offers the PHR, My Health_e_Vet, to veterans and their families in an opt-in arrangement. This is essentially a gateway to veteran health benefits and services, providing links to federal and VA benefits and resources, the Personal Health Journal, and online VA prescription refill. In the future, registrants are expected to be able to view appointments, copayment balances, and key portions of their VA medical records online.

Health Plan Initiatives

Health plans are also getting on the consumer empowerment bandwagon with PHRs (both commercial and self-developed) being offered by several BlueCross BlueShield plans. Aetna has also launched a PHR developed by a subsidiary of the insurer (O'Donnell 2006). America's Health Insurance Plans (AHIP) and BlueCross BlueShield Association (BCBSA) have also engaged in a collaborative process to identify standard data elements and a consumer-facing, Web-based portability model for PHRs expected to be unveiled by December 2008 (Conz 2007).

Whether health plans promote PHRs or also create payer-based health records, payers and payer-affiliated disease management organizations can bring vast amounts of patient data, clinical analysis tools, best practice and best process protocols based on specialty society norms, and their own experience with huge numbers of similar patients to be able to cost-effectively communicate routinely with patients and their caregivers to encourage compliance and behavior modifications when necessary (St. Clair 2005).

Although not precisely a PHR but certainly a form of consumer empowerment is the recent movement by payers to reimburse providers for e-visits. An e-visit is an exchange of secure e-mail with a provider; e-visits may be reimbursable through insurance coverage (using CPT code 0074T). Several of the BlueCross BlueShield plans and some other health plans are reimbursing between $20 and $30 for an e-visit (Terry 2006). Physicians are finding that where they thought this would result in a deluge of e-mails and one more uncompensated drain on their time, patients are actually articulate in e-mail, and the provider gets much better information than when the patient plays "telephone tag" with nurses as intermediaries. Many patients are even willing to pay for the visit themselves if it means they do not have to take time off from work or pay a babysitter. Several medical societies (for example, American Medical Association, American College of Physicians), malpractice carriers (for example, The SCPIE Companies), and PHR vendors who also support e-visit functionality (for example, Medem) have developed guidelines for appropriate parameters for e-visits (Colwell 2004).

Employer Initiatives

Employers have become engaged in promoting healthcare consumerism. At the end of 2006, a group of companies announced a "plan to create a massive data warehouse that could eventually give all their employees online access to their personal health records" (Hoover 2006). They called this "Dossia." The sound bite for this announcement read "Fed up with rising health care costs, Intel, Wal-Mart, and others think giving employees digital records will help." The goal was to let employees compare costs, availability of services, and to some extent performance across care providers, putting more power into their hands. This same article observed that separately, a few other major companies, such as Microsoft, have their own initiatives underway. Two years later, Dossia is still under development, with toned-down language indicating that employers are creating Dossia to provide consumers with an important new health benefit: a lifelong PHR they own and control; suggesting that "Soon complete information about your medical history information that you alone control will be available whenever you need it: for routine doctor visits, when you get sick away from home, in an emergency or even after a fire or natural disaster that could destroy paper records" (www.dossia.org). There have also been cautions expressed about legal and policy issues that employers should check into when promoting PHRs (Goldman 2007).

Vendor Initiatives

Microsoft (Health Vault), Google (Google Health), and AOL founder Steve Case (Revolution Health) also are all undertaking PHR development that promises direct-to-consumer functionality. As well, there have been many other PHR products on the market, and PHR systems are being developed by EHR vendors for providers to support.

Health Record Banking Initiative

One other initiative that is worth noting is something of a hybrid between an EHR, a patient-managed HIE architecture, and a PHR. Although all of the preceding PHR initiatives have the goal of integrating consumer empowerment with PHRs and HIE organizations, the health record banking initiative is designed to maintain EHRs within a health record bank that would be managed solely by the consumer.

The concept of a **health record bank** has strong analogies to a financial bank where the patient/consumer has control over deposits and withdrawals (Wolter 2007), but should not be misconstrued to be related to health savings accounts or other forms of healthcare banks that enable consumers to administer health reimbursement. The health record banking model is based on the principles that every consumer has a right to control a permanent, tamper-proof copy of his or her aggregated medical record, that only the consumer may decide who can see his or her health data, and that any monetary value derived from using the consumer's medical data should belong to the consumer, rather than to a third party who acts without the consumer's authorization (McCallie 2007).

The Health Record Banking Alliance has been formed by William A. Yasnoff, MD, PhD and serves to promote community repositories as an effective and sustainable solution for electronic health information, provide assistance to communities building health record banks, and promote necessary legislation and regulation consistent with community health record banks. Several states have investigated the use of the health record banking model for their HIE organizational structure. The concept is not new and has also been described by several other HIT vendors.

Current Status of PHR Utilization

Although some may suggest that the ability for consumers to drive healthcare in its present state is an oversimplification of the potential impact (Shreeve 2007) and one industry observer has suggested that consumer-directed healthcare is more a move to shift costs to consumers (as well as creating personal accountability for healthcare purchases) (Krohn 2007), the combination of consumer empowerment and transparency has certainly impacted individuals' interest in PHRs.

In attempting to take the pulse of just how widespread interest and use of PHRs is in the general public, there are many surveys that offer insights, although often with different perspectives and significantly different findings. In general, however, it appears that consumers say they are interested (from 65 percent [Connecting for Health 2006] to 84 percent [HarrisInteractive 2004] of those surveyed think a PHR is a good idea), do seek health information from the Web (from 43 percent [CHCF 2008] to 60 percent [Health Industry Insights 2006] say they have a paper-based PHR), and do maintain personal or family records of care (42 percent of those surveyed [HarrisInteractive 2004]), but have increasing concerns about privacy that appear to keep them from adopting electronic PHRs in general and Web-based PHRs in particular (80 percent of those surveyed are concerned about identity theft and 77 percent fear their information may get into the hands of marketers [Connecting for Health 2006]). As many as 77 percent of adults would like reminders via email from their doctors when they are due for a visit or some type of medical care and 74 percent would like to use email to communicate directly with their doctor (HarrisInteractive 2006).

There is also a significant need for education and for providers to be supportive of the concept of PHR. A study conducted for the California Health Care Foundation (CHCF 2008) found that there was strong interest in online PHRs (40 percent of those surveyed) and that use of technology by their doctor would influence their choice of doctor (70 percent of those surveyed), yet 31 percent believed their doctor did not offer technology, 17 percent were concerned about security/confidentiality, 15 percent do not know how to use the functionality, 14 percent do not have the necessary technology to use the functionality, and 11 percent never heard of the functionality. Despite strong interest, however, individuals are also not using—the albeit limited—technology available to them. The HarrisInteractive survey from 2006 found that only 4 percent of adults were using their doctor's email reminder system whereas 3 percent had it available to them but were not using it.

PHR Definition, Attributes, and Functionality

AHIMA defines the PHR as "an electronic, universally available, lifelong resource of health information needed by individuals to make health decisions. Individuals own and manage the information in the PHR, which comes from healthcare providers and the individual. The PHR is maintained in a secure and private environment, with the individual determining rights of access. The PHR is separate from and does not replace the legal record of any provider" (AHIMA 2005).

Connecting for Health (2006) observes that "PHRs encompass a wide variety of applications that enable people to collect, view, manage, or share copies of their health information or transactions electronically. Although there are many variants, PHRs are based on the fundamental concept of facilitating an individual's access to and creation of personal health information in a usable computer application that the individual (or a designee) controls." Connecting for Health offers a version of PHR dimensions that suggests there are at least five dimensions that characterize PHRs. The following dimensions and their discussion were adapted from Connecting for Health:

- *Sponsor*: Who is supplying the PHR for the individual—provider, payer, employer, HIE, affinity group (for example, a professional organization or disease-related group), or commercial vendor? There may be different functions supplied by different sponsors and possibly different privacy and security concerns raised.

- *Integration*: Is the PHR **tethered** (that is, connected largely to a provider, but possibly to a payer or other sponsor) or **standalone** (that is, independent of any sponsor, also considered "commercial")? If tethered to a HIPAA covered entity, the consumer may feel more confident of the privacy and security protections; although standalone commercial products may actually afford more security for fear of going out of business due to a breach. A corollary to this question may better be—how will the data in the PHR be used? There are at least two vendors offering Web-based EHRs in which they clearly state that the product is provided free of charge to the provider in return for the ability to mine the data collected for marketing and other purposes.

- *Platform*: How is the PHR supplied from a technical standpoint? This may be Web-based, provided in a download, CD, or other format for use on a desktop, via a portable method, (for example, flash drive), or on paper. Each platform has its own set of advantages and disadvantages for privacy, security, convenience, price, and so on.

- *Data Source*: Often the source of the data (that is, provider, payer, consumer, other) is related to the sponsor, although it can also be mixed. Closely related to the data source should be the ability for the consumer to exercise control over who is provided access.

- *Business Model*: How is the PHR funded? Options include licensed, as any other software, fee for use, also called subscription—frequently used to acquire a Web-based product, advertisements (refer to "Integration" section earlier in this chapter), and value. The value proposition is one many sponsors are considering, as value may improve process efficiency, brand loyalty, messaging, and behavioral change and outcomes improvement.

CMS also defines "a PHR [as] a confidential and easy-to-use tool for managing information about your health. It is usually an electronic file or record of your health information and recent services…You control how the information is used and who can access it. They are usually used on the Internet so you can look up your information wherever you are." Interestingly, the California HealthCare Foundation, in issuing "Personal Health Records: Employers Proceed with Caution," notes: "A PHR can exist in many different forms, both electronic and paper. It can be as simple as a form created by an individual to record important medical information or as complex as a Web-based system accessed and populated by patients, healthcare providers, insurers, pharmacies, employers, and companies providing health-related content.

Despite these well-crafted, yet somewhat different definitions, however, others in the industry are hesitant to offer a definition. The National Committee on Vital and Health Statistics (NCVHS 2006) notes that "PHRs are broadly considered as a means by which an individual's personal health information can be collected, stored, and used for diverse health management purposes. There is no uniform definition, and the concept continues to evolve. Lack of consensus makes collaboration, coordination, and policymaking difficult." NCVHS concluded that "it is not possible, or even desirable, to attempt a unitary definition at this time." NCVHS, however, did identify a set of attributes it thought important for PHRs.

Likewise, the standards development organization, Health Level Seven (HL7) notes that its PHR-System Functional Model does not attempt to define the PHR, but rather identifies the features and functions in a system necessary to create and manage an effective PHR. HL7 also makes a clear distinction between a PHR and a PHR system, where PHR is the underlying record that the software functionality of a PHR system maintains. This distinction is consistent with its EHR System Functional Model in which it defines the attributes of an EHR system, but does not explicitly define EHR.

PHR Attributes

Without a consensus-based, let alone standards-based, definition of PHR, it may be most appropriate to consider attributes for a PHR as any individual or organization attempts to use or support such an initiative. There does appear to be more of a consensus in the industry on attributes for PHRs than definitions.

AHIMA organizes PHR attributes into six categories:

- Ownership of the PHR, which is by the individual or designee

- Functions, including supporting individual health education and decision making, selected retrieval by providers, and many others

- Format may be paper, electronic (personally held or Web-based), or a hybrid; and appropriate content is recommended to include all medical and clinical information from all providers, personal identification, genetic information, and more

- Privacy, access, and control are strictly controlled by the individual

- Maintenance and security provide for an audit trail and recommended backup and regular refreshment

- Interoperability helps achieve easy, accurate, and consistent exchange with others (as authorized by the individual)

A complete description of these attributes is available in AHIMA's e-HIM Personal Health Record Work Group report on the role of the PHR in the EHR. (See appendix C.5.)

Connecting for Health and NCVHS have also offered attributes of a PHR that are highly consistent with those from AHIMA.

PHR Standards

Health Level Seven (HL7)

The HL7 PHR-System Functional Model, released in November 2007, is currently in Draft Standard for Trial Use format. The functional model identifies what a PHR should be able to do. It is illustrated in figure 18.1.

Healthcare Information Technology Standards Panel (HITSP)

Although not a standards development organization, the Healthcare Information Technology Standards Panel (HITSP) is the organization that identifies interoperability specifications based on the American Health Information Community (AHIC) use cases designed to promote development of a nationwide health information network (NHIN). AHIC has

Figure 18.1.   HL7 PHR system functional model, DSTU

Personal Health	PH.1.0	Account Holder Profile	
	PH.2.0	Manage Historical Clinical Data and Current State Data	
	PH.3.0	Wellness, Preventive Medicine, and Self Care	
	PH.4.0	Manage Health Education	
	PH.5.0	Account Holder Decision Support	
	PH.6.0	Manage Encounters with Providers	
Supportive	S.1.0	Provider Management	
	S.2.0	Financial Management	
	S.3.0	Administrative Management	
	S.4.0	Other Resource Management	
Information Infrastructure	IN.1.0	Health Record Information and Management	
	IN.2.0	Standards-Based Interoperability	
	IN.3.0	Security	
	IN.4.0	Auditable Records	

Source: Health Level Seven 2007. Copyright © 2007 by Health Level Seven, Inc.

developed a use case for consumer empowerment published by HHS Office of the National Coordinator for Health Information Technology (ONC 2007). How consumers would receive and access clinical information is one of the scenarios developed by AHIC in this use case and is illustrated in figure 18.2.

Figure 18.2.   AHIC use case for consumers to receive and access clinical information

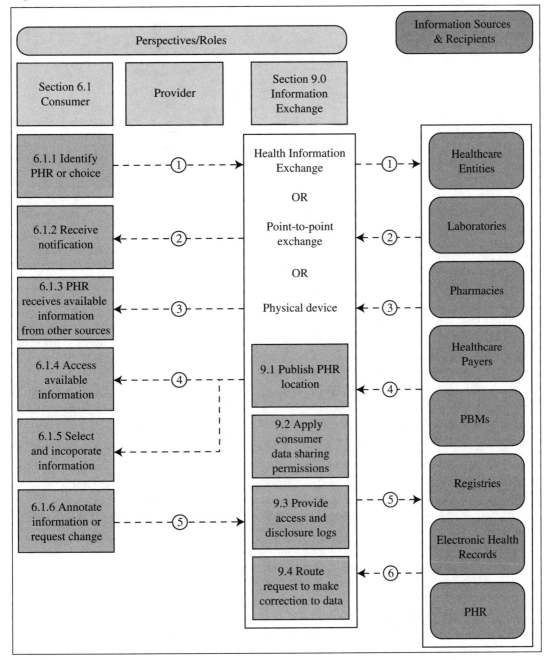

Source: U.S. Department of Health and Human Services Office of the National Coordinator for Health Information Technology, June 18, 2007.

Figure 18.3.   HITSP consumer empowerment interoperability specification roadmap, V2.1, recognized for implementation

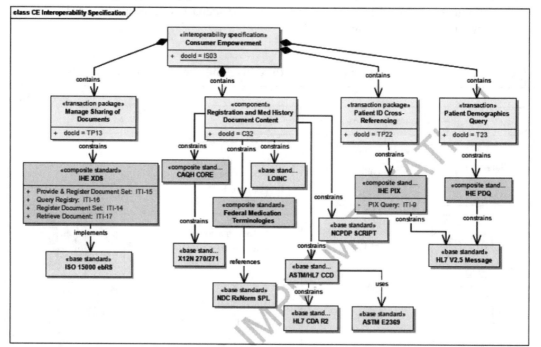

HITSP then has taken this use case and identified standards that should be used to carry out the use case scenario. The standards are identified in the HITSP Consumer Empowerment Interoperability Specification (I.S.) V2.1 Roadmap illustrated in figure 18.3. (A complete list and description of all standards included is provided at www.hitsp.org.)

It should be noted that this I.S. is the version that has been recognized for use in federal procurements by the federal government (by Executive Order 13410, 2006; Recognized by HHS Secretary Mike Leavitt, January 23, 2008). A V3.0 was released on December 13, 2007, that expands the scope of the use to Consumer Empowerment and Access to Clinical Information via Networks.

ASTM International Continuity of Care Record and HL7 Clinical Document Architecture Combine to Form the Continuity of Care Document

One other set of standards that is important to recognize for their contribution to PHRs is the combination of ASTM International's Continuity of Care Record (CCR) and HL7's Clinical Document Architecture (CDA) that form the Continuity of Care Document (CCD).

ASTM International is an international standards development organization, based in the United States. It produces standards for many different industries and has been active in health informatics standards since the early 1970s. Teaming up with ASTM's E31 Committee on Health Informatics, the Massachusetts Medical Society, American Academy of Family Physicians, and HIMSS recognized the need to organize and make transportable a set of basic information about a patient's healthcare that can be provided to referring physicians.

The CCR is a specification of content for an organized, transportable set of basic patient information consisting of most relevant and timely facts about a patient's condition, especially for use in referrals and transfers of patients across the continuum of care. It is a defined set of core data in specified XML code that can be prepared, transmitted, and viewed in a browser, an HL7 CDA (Clinical Document Architecture)-compliant document, secure e-mail, any XML-enabled word-processing document, and other multiple formats. It also can be printed as a paper document and stored on a portable storage device for use as a PHR.

Developers of the CCR content specification hasten to emphasize that it is not an EHR. It is not a record of a patient's lifelong health status and healthcare, it does not provide interactive clinical decision support, it is not universally accessible, and it does not have a universal patient identifier or record locator service.

HL7 is an American National Standards Institute (ANSI)-accredited standards development organization created in 1987, which primarily produces standard protocols for processing clinical and administrative data.

The HL7 CDA is a document markup standard that specifies the structure and semantics of "clinical documents" for the purpose of exchange. A CDA document is a defined and complete information object that can include text, images, sounds, and other multimedia content.

The result of the harmonized ASTM CCR and HL7 CDA is the CCD. Although it may be rendered in XML, it may also be rendered as a PDF file. A key element of the CCD that makes it a desirable structure for PHRs is not only the standard data content but that all data may be sourced to their original author. When data are sourced, access controls on the data enable viewing but not alteration. The potential lack of data integrity in a PHR has been a major concern of providers—and frequently the solution is not well known or understood. It is also the reason that many PHRs are constructed so that the consumer can supply information, side-by-side, with other sourced data. For example, if the source of a prescription is a specific provider or a **pharmacy benefits manager** (PBM) reporting a drug claim, a consumer may want to annotate they are taking only half the dose, or stopped taking it halfway through the prescribed treatment regimen, or experiencing an adverse reaction. This provides valuable information associated with the drug, but does not alter the fact that the drug was prescribed by a certain provider and filled by a pharmacy.

PHR Policies and Practices

Although the value of PHRs may be of strong interest to various sponsors for many different purposes, and there are many physicians who view them as extremely valuable to both their patients and themselves when their patients are able to provide them with information from disparate sources in a structured and legible manner, there are also concerns that worry some physicians.

David Lansky, executive director of the Personal Health Technology Initiative at the Markle Foundation, is quoted as suggesting that most physicians are "not opposed to PHRs, but they anticipate challenges" (Lowes 2006). Some concerns raised by physicians may reflect less-than-full understanding of how some of the PHR offerings capture, consolidate, and coordinate information. Concern and suggestions for overcoming them include:

- Concerns about whether the average patient will faithfully and accurately maintain a "do-it-yourself" PHR, or will patients attempt to use PHRs in a fraudulent manner. It is important that any PHR a provider offers or uses be appropriately sourced, so it is clear who made each entry. Just as in a paper-based medical record or EHR, there should be access controls that do not permit deletions or alterations, but should permit amendments.

- Will physicians bother reading these PHRs? Currently, there is no reimbursement for review, although some physicians believe there are some productivity gains from patient data entry into templates that can be moved into the EHR (see figure 18.4).

- If physicians do not read the content of a PHR, it is feared that overlooking red-flag medical symptoms could increase their malpractice liability. Some attorneys are advising physicians to ask their patients to use their PHRs as important, but personal, references. They suggest that physicians be proactive in encouraging patients to maintain a record of their care for themselves and use it during an encounter as a resource to recall information, but not to supply to the physician. This is contrary to the intent of a patient-managed HIE architecture, but may also change as such an eventuality becomes more commonplace.

- Some physicians are concerned that their patients may not be able to understand the content of the record or may respond to the content by seeking potentially ill-informed help through unscrupulous Web sites. Again, education goes a long way. PHRs can be designed to hyperlink to appropriate explanatory information, and many physicians have found that a modification to their workflow to contact patients

Figure 18.4.   Patient as clinical data entry partner

One physician has created an interactive Web site that is used to make patients "clinical data-entry partners." Structured clinical interview forms help capture patient-supplied information in advance of an appointment. The clinical interview with the patient is then structured to follow the data entered by the patient, plus any remaining history questions the physician believes necessary. This physician has found that condition-specific, structured clinical interviews completed by the patient in advance of the appointment (or in the waiting room at a kiosk with or without staff assistance) has improved physician productivity significantly, reduced transcription costs, and heightened patient education and satisfaction. The notes resulting from this collaborative effort:

- Are clear, thorough, and legible, representing approximately 80 percent of the information needed for a specific visit

- Form a consistent baseline of information collected for each condition (and limit the amount of data collected to the essential)

- Create a searchable database of clinical attributes

- Aid in coding and reimbursement because physician activities and patient education are tied to the reason for the visit

Source: Blasingame 2003.

to explain results can actually save them time downstream. Highlighting for patients the need to look for (and activate) "cyberseals" of approval to validate legitimacy (Hughes 2001) on Web sites can aid patients in becoming consumer savvy.

- Physicians also are concerned about the patient's ability to share health information from one provider with another provider without the author being aware of the exchange, perhaps suggesting a competitive concern. Although this now could occur in the paper world, this is certainly a reason to promote an HIE environment where appropriate agreements concerning legal matters are addressed up front.

- Finally, physicians may have security concerns if they accept a flash drive or download from a patient. Certainly virus protection and other measures should be the norm for any provider in any information technology environment.

There are also perhaps some "deeper" challenges to the use of PHRs that have started to be raised and addressed by several individuals and organizations. Three clinics, however, have been at the forefront of PHR use and have raised some interesting issues that providers must be address. Paul Tang, MD, at the Palo Alto Medical Foundation; John Halamka, MD, at Beth Israel Deaconess; and Kenneth Mandl, MD, at Children's Hospital Boston all have different types of PHR systems, but have all posed similar questions with similar responses (Halamka et al. 2008):

- Should sensitive diagnoses be shared? All indicate yes, with appropriate security measures and where state laws do not pose legal barriers.

- Should the entire medication list be shared? All indicate yes, urging provider-based and patient-maintained lists be kept side-by-side, showing origin of documentation and updates.

- Should all lab test results be shared? Variations in workflow due to state law restrictions were noted, but in the main the expectation was to improve the timeliness of physician review so that results could be shared.

- Should all clinical notes be shared? Access should be supplied upon request.

- Should patients be authenticated to access PHR? Yes.

- Should minors have access to PHR; should patients be able to share access via proxies? Variations in practice due to state law were noted.

Finally, there are some PHR-related issues associated with health information content on the Web. Commercial, Web-based PHRs often are associated with companies that supply health information content as well a PHR. An increasing number of consumers access the Web for such information. The California HealthCare Foundation, for instance, found that 67 percent of consumers searched for condition- or disease-specific information on the Web and that online consumers are more likely to tap the Internet to search for health-related information than they are to communicate with health professionals or use a health plan, hospital, or provider Web site (CHCF 2008). Although there is an abundance of good information on the Web, there also can be risk if one does not ensure that the information is credible and up to date. Several organizations are administering e-health standards, accreditation, or

cyberseal programs, such as Health on the Net Foundation (HON), the American Accreditation HealthCare Commission (URAC), and others (Hughes 2001). Consumers and providers alike should not only look for these as they reference health information content on the Web but should also check that they are active and legitimate.

Patients and PHRs

So, despite some providers' concerns about PHRs, many are coming to understand how PHRs can be helpful both for themselves and for their patients. A number of EHR products are embedding support for PHRs in them. For example, some physician EHRs are able to provide a secure Web site where patients can view their records, add structured and context-sensitive content for their physician to view, and, in some cases, maintain a personal file as well. In other cases, the EHR is able to generate an electronic, or at least paper, summary of a visit or episode of care to provide the patient (Fahrenholz and Buck 2007).

For both providers and patients, AHIMA sponsors a Web site at www.myPHR.com that explains for consumers what a health record is, identifies consumers' health information rights, describes how to maintain a PHR, and provides additional resources on PHR products and services. It may also be useful to consider the set of questions posed in figure 18.5 as providers start to supply PHRs and patients start to use them.

Figure 18.5.   Ten Questions to Ask About PHRs

1. Will this PHR enable me to record all the health information I want?
2. Will information automatically be added to my PHR from other sources?
   - What information will be added? How will it be added? Is transfer auditable?
   - Is there opportunity to delete, correct, or add information? How? Is there an audit log?
3. Does PHR host or sponsor have any ownership rights to the information in the PHR?
4. Can the PHR host or sponsor sell the information to anyone for any reason?
   - If so, how can I ensure my privacy is protected?
   - Can I specify that my information not be sold?
5. Will my information be used for employment or insurance coverage decisions?
6. Who has access to information in my PHR?
   - Can I control who (provider, insurer, employer, caregiver, family member) has access to what information (for example, demographics/insurance, medical, behavioral) and under what circumstances (for example, specific healthcare encounter, emergency only, other)?
   - Is there an audit log of who has accessed my PHR?
7. If I no longer am employed, insured, or a patient of the host/sponsor, can I still continue to use the PHR?
8. How do I get my data if host/sponsor goes out of business? How can I transfer my PHR information to another PHR sponsor?
9. Will there be any cost for me associated with use of this PHR? Upfront, ongoing maintenance, per access, other?
10. Do you apply targeted advertisement to my PHR? If so, is there a way to use my PHR without this advertisement? How am I assured that advertisers do not get access to my health information?

Adapted from "Helping Consumers Select PHRs: Questions and Considerations for Navigating an Emerging Market," AHIMA Personal Health Record Practice Council, 2006.

Conclusion

Where EHRs are tools for clinical transformation, PHRs are becoming tools for consumer empowerment. Health 2.0 has emerged as "a new concept of healthcare wherein all the constituents (patients, physicians, providers, and payers) focus on healthcare value (outcomes/price) and use competition at the medical condition level over the full cycle of care as the catalyst for improving the safety, efficiency, and quality of healthcare." (Shreeve 2007) It has been found that informed and involved patients tend to choose less invasive (and thus less expensive) treatments, have better results, and better compliance with medical instructions (Klepper-Kahn 2007). Social networking, aided by PHR technology, is a platform that is making health consumers and clinicians peers (Sarasohn-Kahn 2008).

References and Resources

AHIMA e-HIM Personal Health Record Work Group. 2005. The role of the personal health record in the EHR. *Journal of AHIMA* 76(7):64A–D.

AHIMA Personal Health Record Practice Council. 2006. Helping consumers select PHRs: Questions and considerations for navigating an emerging market. *Journal of AHIMA* 77(10):50–56.

American Medical Association, Young physicians section. Guidelines for physician–patient electronic communications, www.ama-assn.org/ama/pub/category/2386.html.

Blasingame, J. 2003 (Mar.). Patients as clinical data entry partners. Presentation at Sixth National HIPAA Summit, Washington, DC.

California HealthCare Foundation, 2008 (March). The state of health information technology in California: Consumer perspective. www.chcf.org/topics/view.cfm?itemid=133592.

Centers for Medicare and Medicaid Services. 2008 (Feb. 20). Personal Health Records Overview. www.cms.hhs.gov/perhealthrecords.

Chesanow, N. 2006 (Feb. 17). EHRs: Where do payers fit In? *The Connected Physician,* Special Technology section, pp. TCP3–TCP6. www.memag.com/memag/article/articleDetail.jsp?id=306146.

Colwell, J. 2004 (Dec.). How two practices are taking patient visits online—and getting paid for them. *ACP Observer.* www.acponline.org/journals/news/dec04/evisit.htm.

Connecting for Health Markle Foundation. 2006 (Dec. 7). Connecting Americans to their health care: A common framework for networked personal health information. www.connectingforhealth.org.

Connecting for Health Markle Foundation. 2006 (Nov.) Survey finds Americans want electronic personal health information to improve own health care.

Conz, N., 2007 (Aug.). AHIP Looks to standardize personal health records, insurance and technology. www.insurancetech.com/showArticle.jhtml?articleID=201400212.

Fahrenholz, C. and S.L. Buck. 2007. PHRs and physician practices. *Journal of AHIMA* 78(4): 71–75.

Goldman, J. 2007 (Jan.) Issue Brief: Personal health records: Employers proceed with caution. California healthcare foundation7.

Hagland, M. 2005. Patient to partner: Will PHRs change the physician–patient relationship? *Journal of AHIMA* 76(10):38–40.

Halamka J.D., K.D. Mandl, P.C. Tang. 2008. Early experiences with personal health records, *Journal of the American Medical Informatics Association* 15(1).

HarrisInteractive. 2004 (Aug. 10). Two in five adults keep personal or family health records and almost everybody thinks this is a good idea.

HarrisInteractive. 2006 (Sept. 22). Few patients use or have access to online services for communicating with their doctors, but most would like to, *Wall Street Journal.*

HHS Office of the National Coordinator for Health Information Technology. 2007 (June 18). AHIC Consumer Empowerment: Consumer Access to Clinical Information Detailed Use Case.

HHS.gov. 2008. Value-driven health care, www.hhs.gov/valuedriven.

HITSP. 2007 (Dec 13). HITSP Consumer Empowerment and Access to Clinical Information via Networks Interoperability Specification, Healthcare Information Technology Standards Panel.

Health Industry Insights. 2006 (May). Health Industry Insights Consumer Survey.

Health Record Banking Alliance. 2006. William A. Yasnoff, MD, PhD. www.healthbanking.org.

Health Level Seven 2007 (Nov.). PHR-System Functional Model, Release 1 DSTU.

Hoover, J.N. 2006 (Dec 4). Get well soon. *Information Week*, p. 26–30.

Hughes, G. 2001. Developing "Cyberseals" of Approval. *Journal of AHIMA* 72(8):46.

Klepper B. and J. Sarasohn-Kahn, 2007 (Oct 12). A Broad Vision for Health 2.0. www.health20.org.

Krohn, R. Winter 2007. The consumer-centric personal health record—it's time. *Journal of Healthcare Information Management* 21(1).

Lowes, R. 2006 (Feb. 17). Personal health records: What's the status now? *The Connected Physician,* Special Technology Section, TCP13–TCP16.

McCallie, D. 2007 (May 23). Health record banks: A new approach to RHIOs. *HH&N Most Wired*, www.hhnmostwired.com.

Medem, 2007 (Jan.). eRisk Working Group for Healthcare's Guidelines for Online Communicatio. www.medem.com/phy/phy_eriskguidelines.cfm.

MyHealth*e*Vet 2008. www.myhealth.va.gov.

MyMedicare.gov. 2008. My Health My Medicare http://mymedicare.gov.

myPHR. 2008. Welcome to *my*PHR, AHIMA, www.myphr.com.

National Committee on Vital and Health Statistics (NCVHS), 2005 (Oct.) Personal Health Records and Personal Health Record Systems, HHS, National Center for Health Statistics, Centers for Disease Control and Prevention.

O'Donnell, A. 2006 (Dec 13). Aetna launches real-time electronic health records. *Insurance and Technology.*

Prentice S. and A, Sarner, 2003 (Jan. 3). Defining Generation V: The virtual generation, Gartner, Research ID Number: G00154114.

Rollyson C.S. and Associates Market Advisory 2007 (June 1). Consumer empowerment—A rare innovation opportunity.

Sarasohn-Kahn, J. 2008 (April). The wisdom of patients: Health care meets online social media, *ihealthreports*, California HealthCare Foundation.

SCPIE Indemnity Company, 2002. Guidelines for E-mail Communication with Patients. *Safe Practice*, 8(2).

St. Clair, D. 2005 (July). Collaborative disease management: Leveraging MCO data to improve patient outcomes. *Health Management Technology,* 28–30.

Shreeve, S. What is Health 2.0: The enabling technologies and reform initiatives for next generation health care, http://health20.org.

Terry, K. 2006 (Sept) Online "visits:" Insurers pay. *Medical Economics*, pp. 30–34.

Wolter, J. 2007 (Oct). Health record banking: An emerging PHR model. *Journal of AHIMA* 78(9):2–83.

Yasnoff, WA. Health Record Banking Alliance. www.healthbanking.org.

Zelenka, A. 2007 (Oct 6). From the Information Age to the Connected Age. http://gigaom.com/2007/10/06/from-the-information-age-to-the-connected-age.

Glossary

Acceptance testing: Final review during EHR implementation to ensure that all tests have been performed and all issues have been resolved; usually triggers the final payment for the system and when a maintenance contract becomes effective

Access control list: Provides categories of permissions to access data

Active directory: The component of the Windows operating system that manages identification of data and their relationships within a system master person index

Admissibility: Ability to introduce records into a court of law as evidence

Adoption: Utilization of a system as intended to achieve its benefits

Adverse drug event (ADE): Situation when a patient has a bad or unexpected reaction to the administration of a drug

Adverse drug reaction (ADR): Potentially anticipated but generally not preventable side effect from the administration of a drug

Aggregate data: Data extracted from individual health records and combined to form deidentified information about groups of patients that can be compared and analyzed

Algorithms: Procedures for solving mathematical problems in a finite number of steps that frequently involve repetition of an operation

Analytics: A field of study that combines use of software tools that provide a multi-dimensional view of data in relational databases to determine hidden patterns and associations, with individuals who have expertise in the underlying business who determine the potential value of the new knowledge

Ancillary department systems: Source systems in subordinate departments that support the organization's EHR infrastructure

Anecdotal benefits: Benefits expressed as a short description of an event as evidence of the usefulness of a system

Application service provider (ASP): A third-party service company that delivers, manages, and remotely hosts standardized applications software via a network through an outsourcing contract based on fixed, monthly usage or transaction-based pricing

Application specialist: Person that manages the functional changes needed in information system applications

Attributes: 1. Data elements within an entity that become the column or field names when the entity relationship diagram is implemented as a relational database. 2. Properties or characteristics of concepts

Audit controls: As relating to security services, hardware, software, and/or procedural mechanisms that record and examine activity in information systems

Authentication: 1. The process of identifying the source of health record entries by attaching a handwritten signature, the author's initials, or an electronic signature. 2. Proof of authorship that ensures, as much as possible, that log-ins and messages from a user originate from an authorized source

Balanced scorecard: Strategic planning tool that identifies performance measures related to strategic goals

Balance sheet: A report that shows the total dollar amounts in accounts, expressed in accounting equation format, at a specific point in time

Bandwidth: Capacity of a network

Bar code: Representation of information that may be read by optical scanners called barcode readers or scanned from an image by special software.

Bar code medication administration record (BC-MAR) system: Application that facilitates correct administration of medications using bar code technology (or other positive identification technology, such as radio frequency identification [RFID]) to match patient identity and medication information. *See also* Electronic Medication Administration Record (EMAR) system

Baseline: The original estimates for a project's schedule, work, and cost

Bedside terminals: Originally, terminals placed in patient rooms that connected to the hospital's mainframe computer. Many of these have been replaced with computers on wheels (COWs) for staff use, or bedside consoles, computing stations, or point-of-care computing devices often providing both access to the electronic health record for staff but entertainment, communication, information, and administrative services (for example, food ordering, survey forms, self check-out) for patients.

Benchmarking: An analysis process based on comparison

Benefits portfolio: An organization's description of value, considering both financial return on investment as well as other quality and patient safety benefits.

Benefits realization study: A study performed to determine whether anticipated benefits are realized

Best-of-breed: Information technology acquisition strategy in which an organization acquires applications from multiple vendors

Best-of-fit: Information technology acquisition strategy in which an organization acquires applications, to the extent they exist, from a single vendor

Bridge technologies: Technologies such as document imaging and/or clinical messaging that provide some, but not all, the benefits of an EHR

Case law: Unwritten law originating from court decisions where no applicable statute exists

Central processing unit (CPU):   The area of the computer where data in machine-readable form are processed, according to specific instructions (software) that also are in machine-readable form

Change control: A formal process of tracking every request for a change in a system, determining its impact on other elements of the project or the system itself, obtaining the necessary approvals or authorization for the change to be made, keeping track of the change in the event a future action is dependent on understanding what has been changed, and then carrying out the change with the necessary resources

Change management: The formal process of introducing change, getting it adopted, and diffusing it throughout the organization

Chart conversion: An EHR implementation activity in which data from the paper chart are converted into electronic form

Chief medical information officer: A physician who provides leadership in the development of the overall clinical information technology strategy, direction on the design and implementation of clinical databases and the applications that utilize them, and education and support for physicians and other users of clinical information systems regarding their purposes and functions

Client/server architecture: A computer architecture in which multiple computers (clients) are connected to other computers (servers) that store and distribute large amounts of shared data

Clinical Context Object Workgroup (CCOW):   A standard protocol developed by HL7 to allow clinical applications to share information at the point of care

Clinical data repository (CDR):   An open-structure database that is not dedicated to the software of any particular vendor or data supplier, in which data from diverse sources are stored so that an integrated, multidisciplinary view of the data can be achieved

Clinical decision support (CDS) system (CDSS):   A special subcategory of clinical information systems that is designed to help healthcare providers make knowledge-based clinical decisions

Clinical Document Architecture (CDA):   HL7 structured XML standards for clinical documents (such as discharge summaries and progress notes)

Clinical documentation system: Also called point-of-care charting, an application that guides clinicians in capturing documentation, such as nurse assessments, history and physical examination results, progress notes, not otherwise captured in other clinical applications such as bar code medication administration record systems or computerized provider order entry systems

Clinical information system (CIS):   A category of a healthcare information system that includes systems that directly support patient care

Clinical messaging: The function of electronically delivering data and automating the workflow around the management of clinical data

Clinical pathways: Tools designed to coordinate multidisciplinary care planning for specific diagnoses and treatments

Clinical pharmacy information system: An application that supports the operations of a clinical pharmacy in a hospital; advanced applications include the receipt and review of medications ordered through a computerized provider order entry (CPOE) system, support for compounding medications, and the dispensing of medications via automated dispensing devices and connectivity to a bar code medication administration record (BC-MAR) system

Clinical trials: Controlled research studies involving human subjects that are designed to evaluate prospectively the safety and effectiveness of new drugs, tests, devices, or interventions

Closed loop medication management: Comprehensive, integrated set of software applications that addresses every step in the medication use process from medication reconciliation, to ordering (computerized provider order entry [CPOE]), verification and dispensing (clinical pharmacy information system), and medication administration (bar code medication administration record [BC-MAR]) that ensures the right patient, right drug, right dose, right route, and right time

Closed system: A system that operates in a self-contained environment

Code: 1. In information systems, software instructions that direct computers to perform a specified action. **Coding** in this context refers to the writing of the instructions. 2. In healthcare, an alphanumeric representation of the terms in a clinical classification or vocabulary. **Coding** in this context refers to the process of assigning representations to data, which may be a manual process, electronically facilitated process (using an "encoder"), or fully automated process

Code set: All codes that are available in a classification or vocabulary.

Computer-based patient record (CPR):   Term originally coined by the Institute of Medicine used to describe an electronic patient record housed in a system designed to provide users with access to complete and accurate data, practitioner alerts and reminders, clinical decision support systems, and links to medical knowledge; **electronic health record** has largely replaced this term

Computerized physician order entry (CPOE):   Systems that allow physicians to enter medication or other orders and receive clinical advice about drug dosages, contraindications, or other clinical decision support; also called **computerized provider order entry**

Computer on wheels (COW):   Term used to describe a mobile cart typically outfitted with a laptop or tablet computer and battery pack, which may also include a medication drawer, utility drawer, bar code or RFID reader, ultrasound device, and other medical equipment. Also called wireless on wheels (WOW), wireless workstations, patient charting carts, and so on

Computer output to laser disk (COLD):   Systems used to capture, archive and store documents and distribute them via computer display, fax, email, Web, and print processes. Such systems currently may utilize media other than laser disk and are enhanced through indexing and workflow technology; hence, the term COLD has been superseded by the Enterprise Content Management Industry (AIIM), ANSI, and ISO with the term **enterprise report management** (ERM).

Configuration management: The process of keeping a record of changes made in an EHR system as it is being customized to the organization's specifications; also called change control

Confounding variables: Events or factors that are outside a study but occur concurrently with the study

Consensus: Collective judgment or belief, not necessarily 100 percent agreement

Consent: 1. Under the HIPAA Privacy Rule, consent for use and/or disclosure of protected health information for treatment, payment, and healthcare operations is optional, although may be required by state law or covered entity policy. 2. Consent also is the implied or expressed permission to administer care or treatment, such as one presents to a healthcare provider seeking treatment. 3. Informed consent is the ethical obligation and legal requirement (by state statute) of a provider to explain the benefits and risks and enable an informed decision by the patient before administering care and/or treatment or performing surgery and/or other medical procedures. Informed consent is required for a researcher to involve a human being as a subject in a research study covered by the Common Rule or HIPAA's Privacy Board requirements.

Consent management: Policies, processes, and technology that enable active management and enforcement of users' consent directives to control access to their electronic health information and allow care providers to meet patient privacy requirements

Consumer empowerment: In general, the investment of power or authority in those who purchase goods and services. In healthcare, consumer empowerment is embodied in providing transparency in quality and cost of healthcare, aided by personal health records (PHRs), to incentivize consumers to choose healthcare providers based on value, which in turn motivates the entire healthcare system to provide better care for less money.

Context-sensitive: An action performed by a computer program that depends on the values of the variables that are predefined to be associated with the action

Contingency plans: Documentation of the process for responding to a system emergency, including the performance of backups, the preparation of critical facilities that can be used to facilitate continuity of operations in the event of an emergency, and the process of recovering from a disaster

Continuity of Care Document (CCD):   The result of ASTM's Continuity of Care Record (CCR) standard content being represented and mapped into the HL7's Clinical Document Architecture (CDA) specifications to enable transmission of referral information between providers; also frequently adopted for personal health records

Continuity of Care Record (CCR):   A core data set of the most relevant administrative, demographic, and clinical information facts about a patient's healthcare, covering one or more healthcare encounters, developed jointly by ASTM International, the Massachusetts Medical Society, Healthcare Information and Management Systems Society (HIMSS), the American Academy of Family Physicians (AAFP), the American Academy of Pediatrics (AAP), and health informatics vendors. Initially a replacement for the Patient Care Referral Form mandated by the Massachusetts Department of Public Health, it is widely used now as a standard specification for patient health summaries and personal health records

Continuum of care: The range of healthcare services provided to patients, from routine ambulatory care to intensive acute care

Control processes: In a cybernetic system, when standards monitoring detects variation in the sensor data from the standard data

Controlled vocabulary: A predefined set of terms and their meanings that may be used in structured data entry or natural language processing to represent expressions

Conversion strategy: An organization's plan for changing from a paper-based health record to an electronic health record (EHR)

Cost–benefit analysis: A process that uses quantitative techniques to evaluate and measure the benefit of providing products or services compared to the cost of providing them

Critical path: The sequence of tasks that determine the project finish date

"C suite:" Jargon referring to the group of "chief officers" of an organization, who share nearly equal authority in their respective functional areas of responsibility, with chief executive officer (CEO), chief operating officer (COO), and chief financial officer (CFO) usually being included, and others varying by industry and organization, which in healthcare may include the chief medical officer, chief nursing officer, chief compliance officer, chief information officer, corporate development officer, and corporate human resources officer

Custodian (of records):   The individual designated responsible for maintaining a system of records, including who may have access to the records, their retention and destruction, and that they are reliable and trustworthy because they were kept in the normal course of business, and, if computer generated or computer stored, that they are authentic (that is, not altered, generated by a properly functioning computer, and the author can be identified)

Cybernetics: A theory of control systems based on communication (transfer of information) between systems and environment and within the system, and control (feedback) of the system's function in regard to the environment

Cyberseal: A mark on a Web site indicating adherence to specified policies, procedures, code of conduct, or other protections concerning privacy, security, business practices, authority, and so on

Dashboards: Reports of process measures to help leaders know what is currently going on so that they can plan strategically where they want to go next; sometimes called **scorecards**

Data administrator: Person responsible for managing the quality of data entered into a database

Data analyst: Person who processes data into information and knowledge

Data architecture: A system that consists of individual databases contributing to a central data repository from which data may be either drawn directly to supply an EHR workstation or sent to a warehouse that performs sophisticated analysis on data to supply decision support

Database administrator: Person responsible for managing the technical features of a database

Database management systems (DBMSs): Computer software that enables the user to create, modify, delete, and view the data in a database

Data comparability: The standardization of vocabulary such that the meaning of a single term is the same each time the term is used in order to produce consistency in information derived from the data

Data dictionary: A centralized repository of information about the data elements to be collected in an information system (IS) or database, such as meaning, relationships to other data, origin, usage, and format; the purpose of which is to ensure consistency of terminology

Data infrastructure: Term that refers to what data are needed to operate an enterprise and how they are structured and processed (architecture), defined (vocabulary), and quality assured

Data mart: Well-organized, user-centered, searchable database systems that usually draw information from a data warehouse to meet the specific needs of users

Data mapping: The process of creating one-way links between concepts and terms for specific purposes, such as transformation or mediation between a data source and a destination, identification of data relationships as part of data lineage analysis, discovery of hidden identifying data as part of data deidentification, or consolidation of multiple databases into a single database by identifying redundant data for consolidation or elimination

Data mining: The process of extracting information from a database and then quantifying and filtering discrete, structured data

Data-processing model: Classic model of processing data where the output of information depends on the input provided

Data set: A list of recommended data elements with uniform definitions that are relevant for a particular use

Data sharing agreement: Agreement among parties who will share data, usually within a health information exchange organization and indicating the criteria for data access, whether or not there are any conditions for certain types of use, specific (privacy, security, and other technical) standards with which the data sharing must conform, and whether the data may be deidentified

Data stewardship: The responsibilities and accountabilities associated with managing, collecting, viewing, storing, sharing, disclosing, or otherwise making use of individually identifiable health information

Data structure: The form in which data are stored, as in a file, a database, a data repository, and so on

Data use agreement: In the HIPAA Privacy Rule, an agreement required for a party to use a limited data set (that is, data that are partially but not fully deidentified) for research, public health, or healthcare operations

Data warehouses: Databases that make it possible to access data from multiple databases and combine the results into a single query and reporting interface

Decision support: A term that generally refers to information that supports decision making

Defaults: The status to which a computer application reverts in the absence of alternative instructions

Dependencies: The relationships between tasks in a project plan

Deterministic system: A system in which the parts function according to a predictable relationship

Digital signature: A form of electronic signature that binds a message to a particular individual and can be used by the receiver to authenticate the identity of the sender in a nonreputable manner

Digitized signature: A form of electronic signature that is an image of a handwritten (wet) signature

Discrete data: Data that represent separate and distinct values or observations; that is, data that contain only finite numbers and have only specified values

Dual core: IT acquisition strategy in which financial/administrative applications are largely from one vendor source and clinical applications are largely from a different vendor source

Due diligence: The actions associated with making a good decision, including investigation of legal, technical, human, and financial predictions and ramifications of proposed endeavors with another party

E-Discovery: Amendments to the Federal Rules of Civil Procedure in December 2006 (and being adopted by states) enforce the fact that electronic information, including metadata, are subject to a discovery motion

Electronic document management (EDM):   A system to capture, index, store, and manage electronic documents, largely in the form of paper documents scanned into an imaging system

Electronic health record (EHR):   "An electronic record of health-related information on an individual that conforms to nationally recognized interoperability standards and that can be created, managed, and consulted by authorized clinicians and staff across more than one healthcare organization" (The National Alliance for Health Information Technology 2008). This term has been defined by the ASTM standards development organization (E1769, 1995) and adopted by the HL7 standards development organization (2007) as "a comprehensive, structured set of clinical, demographic, environmental, social, and financial data and information in electronic form, documenting the healthcare given to a single individual." The Institute of Medicine patient record study report (1991 and 1997) defined this as "an electronic patient record that that resides in a system specifically designed to support users through availability of complete and accurate data, practitioner reminders and alerts, clinical decision support systems, links to bodies of medical knowledge, and other aids. This definition encompasses a broader view of the patient record than is current today, moving from the notion of a location or device for keeping track of patient care events to a resource with much enhanced utility in patient care (including the ability to provide an accurate longitudinal account of care), in management of the healthcare system, and in extension of knowledge."

Electronic medical record (EMR):   An electronic record of health-related information on an individual that can be created, gathered, managed, and consulted by authorized clinicians and staff within one healthcare organization (The National Alliance for Health Information Technology). In common hospital practice, a form of computer-based health record in which information is stored in whole files instead of by individual data elements; also commonly used to describe electronic records in physician offices or clinics

Electronic medication administration record (EMAR):   Application in which a schedule of medications, their dose, route, and time for administration is provided nursing staff and which is used to document such administration. May be enhanced with positive identification technology for medication five rights—*see* bar code medication administration record

Electronic prescribing (e-Rx):   When a prescription is written from the personal digital assistant and an electronic fax or when an actual electronic data interchange transaction is generated that transmits the prescription directly to the retail pharmacy's information system

Electronic signature: A form of electronic signature in which the individual utilizes a password, biometric, token, or combination thereof to provide authentication

Encryption: The process of transforming text into an unintelligible string of characters that can be transmitted via communications media with a high degree of security and then decrypted when it reaches a secure destination

Enterprisewide content management (ECM):   In general, a system to manage data collected on Web forms for customer relationship management. In healthcare, a system to manage content from a variety of digital formats, including scanned documents, electronically fed documents, e-faxes, e-mail, wave forms, sound files, and PACS

Enterprisewide content and records management (ECRM):   Convergence of electronic content management (ECM) and electronic records management (ERM) that provides functionality for managing all content across its life cycle according to legal, regulatory, and operational requirements

Enterprisewide master patient index (EMPI):   An index that provides access to multiple repositories of information from overlapping patient populations that are maintained in separate systems and databases

Enterprisewide report management (ERM):   System that manages electronic content that has been "declared" a record and must be managed throughout its life cycle according to legal, regulatory, and operational requirements

E-prescribing: In the ambulatory environment, the writing of a prescription to be filled by a retail, community, or mail-order pharmacy, instead of the ordering of a drug from a clinical pharmacy that is a department of a hospital

Ethernet: Local area network protocol for fast, wired exchange of data

Evidence-based medicine: Healthcare services based on clinical methods that have been thoroughly tested through controlled, peer-reviewed biomedical studies

E-visit: An e-mail encounter with a patient, which is reimbursable, either directly by the patient or under a benefit plan

Executive decision support: Term that refers to the use of data to help executive managers evaluate services, make decisions about major capital equipment purchases based on potential for use, and so on

Extranet: A system of connections of private Internet networks outside an organization's firewall that uses Internet technology to enable collaborative applications among enterprises

Feedback mechanisms: Processes that provide information about environmental factors that interact with the functioning of a system

Fee-for-service environment: Environment where the method of reimbursement is one where providers receive payment retrospectively based on either billed charges for services provided or annually updated fee schedules

Firewall: A computer system or a combination of systems that provides a security barrier or supports an access control policy between two networks or between a network and the Internet

Flash drive: A small, portable storage device with multigigabyte capacity that connects to a computer via a USB (universal serial bus) connection; also known by several other names, such as jump drive, thumb drive, and others

Functional needs assessment: An assessment that describes the key capabilities or application requirements for achieving the benefits of the EHR as the organization has envisioned it

Gantt chart: A graphic tool used to plot tasks in project management that shows the duration of project tasks and their dependencies. The completion of a task is a milestone

Goal: A projected state of affairs intended to be achieved

Granular: Consisting of small components or details

Graphical user interface (GUI): A style of computer interface in which typed commands are replaced by images that represent tasks (for example, small pictures [icons] that represent the tasks, functions, and programs performed by a software program)

Hacker: An individual who bypasses a computer system's access control by taking advantage of system security weaknesses and/or by appropriating the password of an authorized user

Hard skills: A skill set that includes strategic planning, portfolio management, project planning, resource leveling, issues management, and change control

Health 2.0: The use of social networking and other electronic tools to promote collaboration between patients, their caregivers, medical professionals, and other stakeholders in health

Health information exchange (HIE): The electronic movement of health-related information among organizations according to nationally recognized standards (The National Alliance for Health Information Technology)

Health information management (HIM) professionals: Individuals who have received professional training at the associate or baccalaureate degree level in the management of health data and information flow throughout healthcare delivery systems

Health information organization: An organization that oversees and governs the exchange of health-related information among organizations according to nationally recognized standards (The National Alliance for Health Information Technology); also referred to as a health information exchange (HIE) organization; and when based within a specific geographic area, regional health information organization or local health information organization

Health information service provider (HSP): As described by the U.S. HHS Office of the National Coordinator for Health Information Technology (ONC), a vendor that supplies the data integration and/or connectivity services for a health information organization

Health Plan Employer Information Data Set (HEDIS):   A set of performance measures developed by the National Commission for Quality Assurance that are designed to provide purchasers and consumers of healthcare with the information they need to compare the performance of managed care plans

Health record bank: A health information exchange (HIE) model in which an entity or entities are selected to collect, store, and appropriately disseminate all the paper and electronic health information of a consumer who opens a health records account. The consumer will have control over access to information in the account.

Hospital information system (HIS):   The comprehensive database containing all the clinical, administrative, financial, and demographic information about each patient served by a hospital

Human–computer interface: The device used by humans to access and enter data into a computer system, such as a keyboard on a PC, personal digital assistant, voice recognition system, and so on

Human systems: Systems that are organized relationships among people

Hybrid record: A health record that includes both paper and electronic elements

Icon: Type of symbol shown on a computer screen used as an indicator

Identity management: Identity management assures that a person or information system that wants to identify and locate an individual is authorized to do so and that such access is secure, tracked, and monitored

Inference engine: Software that supports decision making by maintaining a knowledge base of rules, matching the rules to the context of data being entered, and executing the rules as alerts, reminders, context-sensitive templates, and other forms of decision support that may be structured into logical constructs. *See also* rules engine

Informaticist: Individual who studies the use of technology to improve access to, and utilization of, information

Information access management: Processes that control access to personal health information

Information infrastructure: Term that refers to the full scope of functional needs, data requirements, and technical capabilities of an EHR system

Information silos: The concept that each organizational unit maintains control over information (and associated information technology [IT]) that it collects and uses, often not sharing the information seamlessly with other units or their information systems

Information technology (IT) acquisition strategy: Long-term plan for the manner in which information technology will be acquired, specifically with reference to utilizing one or many vendors

Information systems (IS) theory: Describes the technology used to process data into information that contributes value

Information theory: Describes the flow of data from its source to its ultimate destination

Infrastructure: The underlying framework and features of an information system (IS)

Input/output (I/O) devices: Peripheral devices separate from the central processing unit of the computer, many (but not all) of which perform both input and output functions

Inputs: Data entered into a hospital system (for example, the patient's knowledge of his or her condition, the admitting clerk's knowledge of the admission process, and the computer with its admitting template are all inputs for the hospital's admitting system)

Institutional review board (IRB): An administrative body that provides oversight for the research studies conducted within a healthcare institution

Integrated delivery network (IDN): Organizations that combine the financial and clinical aspects of healthcare and use different types of care delivery organizations, selected on the basis of quality and cost management criteria, to furnish comprehensive health services across the continuum of care

Integrity: The state of being whole or unimpaired

Interface: The zone between different computer systems across which users want to pass information (for example, a computer program written to exchange information between systems or the graphic display of an application program designed to make the program easier to use)

Interface engine: A software tool that manages connections among many disparate systems; sometimes called middleware

Internal rate of return (IRR): An interest rate that makes the net present value calculation equal zero

Interoperability: The ability, generally by adoption of standards, of systems to work together

Intranet: A private information network that is similar to the Internet and whose servers are located inside a firewall or security barrier so that the general public cannot gain access to information housed within the network

Issues management: The process of resolving unexpected occurrences (for example, the late delivery of needed supplies or an uncorrected system problem)

Key performance indicators: Quantifiable measurements, previously agreed on, that reflect the organization's critical success factors

Knowledge management: 1. The process by which experience (through perception, learning, communication, association, and reasoning) are added to information to provide understanding. 2. A management philosophy that promotes an integrated and collaborative approach to the process of information asset creation, capture, organization, access, and use

Knowledge sources: Various types of reference material and expert information that are compiled in a manner accessible for integration with patient care information to improve the quality and cost-effectiveness of healthcare provision

Legacy systems: Types of computer systems that use older technology but may still perform optimally

Longitudinal: A type of time frame for research studies during which data are collected from the same participants at multiple points in time

Mainframe architecture: The term used to refer to the configuration of a mainframe computer

Managed care: 1. Payment method in which the third-party payer has implemented some provisions to control the costs of healthcare while maintaining quality care. 2. Systematic merger of clinical, financial, and administrative processes to manage access, cost, and quality of healthcare

Man–machine systems: Any form of supportive operations that assist humans in the performance of their work

Manual systems: Systems that entail humans performing certain processes

Mechanical systems: Systems that are developed by humans, but that can operate without human intervention

Medical director of information systems (MDIS):   Physician responsible for supporting the design and development of clinical information systems that assist clinicians in the delivery of patient care (*see also* chief medical information officer)

Medical identity theft: Occurs when someone uses another person's identity to obtain medical services or goods

Medication reconciliation: The process of comparing a patient's medication orders to all medications the patient has been taking to avoid medication errors such as omissions, duplications, dosing errors, or drug interactions. It should be done at every transition of care in which new medications are ordered or existing orders are rewritten. Transitions in care include changes in setting, service, practitioner or level of care. (The Joint Commission, Sentinel Event Alert #35.)

Messaging standards: Standards that support the uniform format and sequence of data during transmission from one healthcare entity to another

Meta-analysis: A specialized form of systematic literature review that involves the statistical analysis of a large collection of results from individual studies for the purpose of integrating the studies' findings

Metadata: Data about data; usually including information such as meaning, relationships to other data, origin, usage, and format. *See also* data dictionary

Metrics: Measurements

Migration path: A series of steps required to move from one situation to another

Milestone: Important checkpoint or interim goal for a project; has no duration in time associated with it

Minimum necessary use standards: Guidelines or policies set in place to ensure that a patient's personal health information (PHI) is only used when absolutely needed

Modeling: A process assessment technique that describes existing processes so that conceptualization can occur and documents redesigned processes for future use (that is, implementation)

National health information infrastructure (NHII):   An infrastructure proposed by the National Committee on Vital and Health Statistics in 2002, that would be a set of technologies, standards, applications, systems, values, and laws that support all facets of provider healthcare, individual health, and public health

Nationwide health information network (NHIN):   A network of networks envisioned by the U.S. federal government that would securely connect consumers, providers, and others who have or use health-related data, using a shared architecture (standards, services, and requirements), processes, and procedures

Natural language processing: The extraction of unstructured or structured medical word data, which are then translated into diagnostic or procedural codes for clinical and administrative applications

Navigational support: With respect to a computer screen, the ability to move from one screen to another, to drill down to retrieve further detail about something, to access knowledge bases, or to request a graph or other form of display

Near miss: An unplanned event that did not result in injury, illness, or damage, but had the potential to do so. Only a fortunate break in the chain of events prevented an injury, fatality, or damage.

Net present value (NPV):   A formula used to assess the current value of a project when the monies used were invested in the organization's investment vehicles rather than expended for the project; this value is then compared to the allocation of the monies and the cash inflows of the project, both of which are adjusted to current time

Nonrepudiation: In reference to a digital signature, the means to ensure that a message is sent and received by the parties claiming to have sent and received the message. This is a way to guarantee that neither party can claim a message was not sent or received.

Objects: The basic components in an object-oriented database that include data and their relationships within a single structure

Online analytical processing (OLAP):   A data access architecture that allows the user to retrieve specific information from a large volume of data

Online transaction processing (OLTP):   The real-time processing of day-to-day business transactions from a database

Open architecture: A term that refers to the fact that elements of different information systems work together through the use of standards that are not proprietary

Open system: Process that is affected by what is going on around it and must adjust as the environment changes

Operations analysis: *See* workflow analysis.

Opt-in: A consent directive in which an action (such as a data exchange) may not occur by default unless permission is given (such as a patient supplies consent)

Opt-out: A consent directive in which an action (such as a data exchange) may occur by default unless restricted (such as by patient)

Optical character recognition (OCR):   A method of encoding text from analog paper into bit-mapped images and translating the images into a form that is computer readable

Order communication: A clerical function of transcribing orders handwritten by a physician (or other provider authorized to write orders in the hospital) into a computer system for distribution to respective ancillary department systems

ORYX: A Joint Commission initiative that supports the integration of outcomes data and other performance measurement data into the accreditation process; sometimes referred to as the ORYX initiative

Outputs: The outcomes of inputs into a system (for example, the output of the admitting process is the patient's admission to the hospital)

Outsourcing: The hiring of an individual or a company external to an organization to perform a function either on site or off site

Patient care charting: A system in which caregivers enter data into health records

Patient health summary: A list of illnesses, injuries, and other factors that affect the health of an individual patient, usually identifying the time of occurrence or identification and resolution. *See also* Continuity of Care Record.

Payback period: A financial method used to evaluate the value of a capital expenditure by calculating the time frame that must pass before inflow of cash from a project equals or exceeds outflow of cash

Pay-for-performance (P4P):   A program being sponsored by some health plans to provide incentives to healthcare organizations that can demonstrate improvement in the quality of patient care, often through the use of EHR and other health information technology. Also called pay-for-quality (P4Q)

Personal health information: As distinguished from protected health information, individually identifiable health information that is not protected under the HIPAA Privacy and Security Rules because it is not maintained or transmitted by a HIPAA-covered entity

Personal health records (PHRs):   An electronic record of health-related information on an individual that conforms to nationally recognized interoperability standards and that can be drawn from multiple sources while being managed, shared, and controlled by the individual

Pharmacy benefits management (PBM):   Companies that manage the complex rules for payers associated with benefit plans to pay for prescription drugs

Pick lists: A means of data entry in which the user selects a variable from a list in order to designate it as the desired data

Picture Archiving and Communication System (PACS):   A system that captures, stores, retrieves, and displays digital images (such as from radiologic and other medical imaging instruments)

Platforms: Combinations of hardware and operating systems on which application programs can run

Point of care (POC):   The place or location where the physician administers services to the patient

Portal: Based on Web portal technology, a point of secure access to an organization's information system applications

Practice management system (PMS):   Software designed to help medical practices run more smoothly and efficiently

Predictive modeling: Analytical process that can anticipate results from various factors

Presentation layer: The set of application programs that provides for functions such as computerized provider order entry, bar-code medication administration record, point-of-care charting, and clinical decision support

Probabilistic system: A system in which all the relationships among the parts cannot be defined in advance

Process assessment: The steps taken to understand current processes and workflows in order to identify opportunities for improvement. In EHR projects, process assessment initiates change by creating desire for improvement in capture and use of health information, identifies functional requirements of the information systems to achieve those improvements, and describes and helps educate about the nature of changes in processes and workflow to achieve improvement

Process: The manner in which work to be completed to achieve a particular result is performed

Process map: The depiction of the detailed nature of processes and workflow to enable identification of improvement opportunities

Productivity improvement: Improvement in workflow resulting in time and money savings

Pro forma cost–benefit analysis: An estimate of costs and benefits conducted before vendor selection to determine the feasibility of, and budget for, an EHR project

Program (or Project) Evaluation Review Technique (PERT) chart: A project management tool that diagrams a project's time lines and tasks as well as their interdependencies

Project management: A formal set of principles and procedures that help control the activities associated with implementing a usually large undertaking to achieve a specific goal, such as an information system project

Project management office (PMO): Sometimes referred to as a standing operational implementation team, a unit that establishes a relationship between IT and organizational business units that focuses projects on user needs

Protected health information (PHI): Under HIPAA, all individually identifiable information, whether oral or recorded in any form or medium, that is created or received by a healthcare provider or any other entity subject to HIPAA requirements

Protocols: In healthcare, detailed plans of care for specific medical conditions based on investigative studies; in medical research, rules or procedures to be followed in a clinical trial; in a computer network, protocols are used to address and ensure delivery of data

Providers: Physicians, clinics, hospitals, nursing homes, or other healthcare entities (second parties) that deliver healthcare services

Pull-down menus: The design of a data-entry screen of a computer in which categories of functions or structured data elements may be accessed through that category element

Quality improvement organizations (QIOs): Organizations that perform medical peer review of Medicare and Medicaid claims, including review of validity of hospital diagnosis and procedure coding information; completeness, adequacy, and quality of care; and appropriateness of prospective payments for outlier cases and nonemergent use of the emergency room; until 2002, called peer review organizations

Quantifiable benefits: Benefits that can be measured and achieved through cost savings, cost avoidance, revenue increases, contribution to profit, and productivity improvements

Quantitative benefits: Benefits that have a single truth (for example, by doing X, Y will surely happen)

Radio Frequency Identification (RFID): An automatic identification method, relying on storing and remotely retrieving data using devices called RFID tags, or transponders

Record locator service (RLS): Points within a health information exchange service that identifies where records for a given patient exist

Redundancy: The concept of building a backup computer system that is an exact version of the primary system and that can replace it in the event of a primary system failure

Reengineering: Fundamental rethinking and radical redesign of business processes to achieve significant performance improvements

Regional health information organization (RHIO): An organization that manages the local deployment of systems promoting and facilitating the exchange of healthcare data within a national health information network

Registry: A collection of care information related to a specific disease, condition, or procedure that makes health record information available for analysis and comparison

Remote connectivity: The ability of one computer system to exchange information with another computer system over a distance, used by providers, for example, to access lab results

Report writer: A tool used to access data in a database structure and develop meaningful tables, graphics, and other forms of reports

Request for information (RFI): A written communication often sent to a comprehensive list of vendors during the design phase of the systems development life cycle to ask for general product information

Request for proposal (RFP):   A type of business correspondence asking for very specific product and contract information that is often sent to a narrow list of vendors that have been preselected after a review of requests for information during the design phase of the systems development life cycle

Research methodology: A set of procedures or strategies used by researchers to collect, analyze, and present data

Results management: Information systems that enable not only viewing but processing of results, such as into graphics, tables, and comparisons with other data

Results retrieval: Information systems that enable viewing of results of diagnostic studies, vital signs, or other information

Retention and durability: With regard to the legality of electronic health records, the term used to refer to the fact that electronic data follow required retention schedules and can be retrieved from the electronic media on which they are stored

Return on investment (ROI):   The financial analysis of the extent of value a major purchase will provide

Risk management: A comprehensive program of activities intended to reduce the likelihood that a threat will exploit a vulnerability and result in harm, and to respond to ensuing liabilities for harm that may occur

Roll out strategy: A series of phases that identify the sequence of steps to be taken in gaining adoption of an information system, often constructed by various inpatient units, departments, physicians or other categories of users, and sites

Rules engine: A computer program that applies sophisticated mathematical models to data that generate alerts and reminders to support decision making

SCODF Personality Type Model: The identification of variations in human behavior with respect to the role (Starter, Creator, Overseer, Doer, or Finisher) an individual will play in a group

Scripting language: A type of language used by EHR vendors designed for writing programs to be executed on the Internet

Semantics: The meaning of a word or term; sometimes refers to comparable meaning, usually achieved through a standard vocabulary

Sensors: In a cybernetic system, the number of tests by category, quality control data, and resources consumed

Servers: Types of computers that make it possible to share information resources across a network of client computers

Service level agreement (SLA):   A contract between a customer and a service provider that records the common understanding about service priorities, responsibilities, guarantees, and other terms, especially related levels of availability, serviceability, performance, operation, or other attributes of the service like billing and penalties in the case of violation of the SLA.

Single sign on: A method of access control that enables a user to log in once and gain access to the resources of multiple software systems without being prompted to log in again

SMART goal: The characteristics of a goal that is Specific, Measurable, Attainable, Realistic, and Timely

Smart peripherals: The augmentation of medical devices/instruments with information processing components, such as infusion pumps with dose calculation software

Smart text: A means of documenting information in an EHR using a series of macros or codes representing the desired text

Soft skills: A skill set that includes communications, team building, change management, risk management, time management, cost management, and quality management

Source code: The software that has been written for a specific application and which is generally proprietary to the vendor and licensed for use to the customer

Source systems: Independent information system applications that contribute data to an EHR, including departmental clinical applications (for example, laboratory information system, clinical pharmacy information system) and specialty clinical applications (for example, intensive care, cardiology, labor and delivery)

Speech recognition: Situation where speech is converted to text on a screen

Standards development organization (SDO):   A private or government agency involved in the development of healthcare informatics standards at a national or international level

Standards monitoring: In a cybernetic system, an action performed by comparing the sensor data to various standards and cost/efficiency goals

Storage: Safeguarding against loss, destruction, tampering, and unauthorized use of (data) assets

Storage devices/systems: Devices or systems for storing software and data, including temporarily in the central processing unit of the computer; and in separate units or even separate networks from the main computer or computing center

Strategic plan: A broad organizationwide plan by which the facility accomplishes its strategic goals

Structured data: Binary, computer-readable data

Syntax: A term that refers to the comparable structure or format of data, usually as they are being transmitted from one system to another

System: A set of related and highly interdependent components that are operating for a particular purpose

System build: The creation of data dictionaries, tables, decision support rules, templates for data entry, screen layouts, and reports used in a system

Systems development life cycle (SDLC):   A model used to represent the ongoing process of developing (or purchasing) information systems

Systems integrators: Companies, or parts of companies, that specialize in getting disparate vendor products to work together

Task: Activity that must be completed to achieve a project goal

Team building: The process of organizing and acquainting a team, and building skills for dealing with later team processes

Templates: Patterns used in computer-based patient records to capture data in a structured manner

Terminals: A term used to describe the hardware in a mainframe computer system by which data may be entered or retrieved

Thin clients: Computers with processing capability but no persistent storage (disk memory) that rely on data and applications on the host they access to be able to process data

Token: 1. A session token is a unique identifier which is generated and sent from a server to a software client to identify an interactive session, and which the client usually stores as an HTTP cookie. 2. A security token is usually a physical device that an authorized user of computer services is given to aid in authentication

Topology: In networking terms, the physical or logical arrangement of a network

Total cost of ownership (TCO):   All costs associated with acquiring, implementing, and using an information system, not only those associated with direct licensure of the software and purchase of the hardware

Train-the-trainer: A method of training certain individuals who, in turn, will be responsible for training others on a task or skill

Transaction: A unit of work performed against a database management system that is treated in a coherent and reliable way independent of other transactions. A database transaction is atomic, consistent, isolated and durable. Examples of healthcare transaction is the entry of a medication order for a patient, the retrieval of a lab result for a patient, and the posting of temperature for a patient.

Turnkey system: A computer application that may be purchased from a vendor and installed without modification or further development by the user organization

Turnover strategy: The plan an organization will take to convert from paper to electronic system (or one electronic system to another) with respect to ensuring that the new system operates properly, including whether paper processes will cease on go-live, or whether they will be run in parallel with the electronic system for some period of time after go-live

Two-factor authentication: Use of two human factors to securely authenticate a user to a system. The most common factor for authentication is a password (something the user knows). By adding either something the user has (such as a security token, software token, ID card, or cell phone) or something the user is or does (that is, biometric) strengthens the authentication process

Unity of purpose: Characteristic of an information system that causes the collective parts of the IS to have integrity

Unstructured data: Nonbinary, human-readable data

Value-added reseller (VAR):   A vendor that adds a feature or service to an existing product and then sells it to end-users

Virtual private network: An encrypted tunnel through the Internet that enables secure transmission of data

Vocabulary: A list or collection of clinical words or phrases and their meanings

Web portal: A Web site entryway through which to access, find, and deliver information

Web services architecture (WSA):   A collection of services that are self-contained, modular applications that can be described, published, located, and invoked over a network, generally, the World Wide Web. The WSA describes three roles: service provider, service requester, and service broker; and three basic operations: publish, find and bind.

Wizard: A user interface element where the user is presented with a sequence of dialog boxes, though which the user is led through a series of steps, performing tasks in a specific sequence

Work breakdown structure: A hierarchical structure that decomposes project activities into levels of detail

Workflow: The sequence of steps and hand-offs taken within a process

Workflow management technology: Technology that allows computers to add and extract value from document content as the documents move throughout an organization

Workstation: A computer designed to accept data from multiple sources in order to assist in managing information for daily activities and to provide a convenient means of entering data as desired by the user at the point of care

Index